Brånemark/Zarb/Albrektsson, Tissue-Integrated Prostheses

Tissue-Integrated Prostheses
Osseointegration in Clinical Dentistry

Edited by

Per-Ingvar Brånemark, M.D., Ph.D.
Professor
Laboratory of Experimental Biology
Department of Anatomy, University of Göteborg
and Institute for Applied Biotechnology
Göteborg, Sweden

George A. Zarb, B.Ch.D., D.D.S., M.S. (Mich.),
M.S. (Ohio State), F.R.C.D. (C)
Professor and Chairman of Prosthodontics
Faculty of Dentistry, University of Toronto
Toronto, Canada

Tomas Albrektsson, M.D., Ph.D.
Associate Professor
Laboratory of Experimental Biology
Department of Anatomy, University of Göteborg
and Institute for Applied Biotechnology
Göteborg, Sweden

quintessence
books

Quintessence Publishing Co., Inc. 1985
Chicago, London, Berlin, São Paulo and Tokyo

Library of Congress Cataloging in Publication Data
Main entry under title:

Tissue-integrated prostheses.

  Includes bibliographies and index.
  1. Implant dentures, Endoosseous. I. Brånemark,
Per-Ingvar. II. Zarb, George A. (George Albert),
1938–   . III. Albrektsson, Tomas. [DNLM: 1. Dental
Implantation, Endoosseous. WU 640 T616]
RK667.I45T57   1985   617.6'92   85-3377
ISBN 0-86715-129-3

4th reprinting, 1990
© 1985 by Quintessence Publishing Co., Inc., Chicago, Illinois.
All rights reserved.

Lithography: Industrie- und Presseklischee, Berlin
Printing and binding: Kösel GmbH & Co., Kempten

Printed in Germany

ISBN 0-86715-129-3

Contributors

Ragnar Adell

Department of Oral Surgery
Box 330 70
S-400 33 Göteborg, Sweden

Tomas Albrektsson

Laboratory of Experimental Biology
Department of Anatomy
University of Göteborg
and Institute for Applied Biotechnology
Box 330 53
S-400 33 Göteborg, Sweden

Stig Blomberg

Department of Psychiatric Diseases
University of Göteborg
S-413 45 Göteborg, Sweden

Per-Ingvar Brånemark

Laboratory of Experimental Biology
Department of Anatomy
University of Göteborg
and Institute for Applied Biotechnology
Box 330 53
S-400 33 Göteborg, Sweden

Gunnar E. Carlsson

Department of Stomatognathic Physiology
University of Göteborg
Box 330 70
S-400 33 Göteborg, Sweden

Per-Olof Glantz

Department of Prosthetic Dentistry
Dental Clinic
Carl Gustafs Väg 34
21421 Malmö, Sweden

Torgny Haraldson

Department of Stomatognathic Physiology
University of Göteborg
Box 330 70
S-400 33 Göteborg, Sweden

Tomas Jansson — Institute for Applied Biotechnology
Box 33053
S-400 33 Göteborg, Sweden

Torsten Jemt — Department of Prosthetic Dentistry
Box 33070
S-400 33 Göteborg, Sweden

Bengt Kasemo — Department of Physics
Chalmers University of Technology
S-412 96 Göteborg, Sweden

Jukka Lausmaa — Institute for Applied Biotechnology
Box 33053
S-400 33 Göteborg, Sweden

Ulf Lekholm — Institute for Applied Biotechnology
Box 33053
S-400 33 Göteborg, Sweden

Richard Skalak — Bioengineering Institute
Department of Civil Engineering
and Engineering Mechanics
Columbia University
New York, New York 10027, U. S. A.

Karl-Gustav Strid — Institute for Applied Biotechnology
Box 33053
S-400 33 Göteborg, Sweden

A. R. Ten Cate — Dean, Faculty of Dentistry
University of Toronto
124 Edward Street
Toronto, Ontario, Canada M5G 1G6

Anders Tjellström — E.N.T. Department
Sahlgren's Hospital
S-413 45 Göteborg, Sweden

George A. Zarb — Department of Prosthodontics
Faculty of Dentistry
University of Toronto
124 Edward Street
Toronto, Ontario, Canada M5G 1G6

Table of Contents

Preface

The successful replacement of lost natural teeth by tissue-integrated tooth root analogues is a major advance in clinical dental treatment. The science behind the osseointegration method has evolved over the past three decades in both laboratory and clinical environments, and as a result of extensive multidisciplinary cooperation. This book reflects such cooperation, and we are indebted to our colleagues for making it possible.

The book is written for dental practitioners whose expertise and interests will enable them to use its principles to treat the various types of partial and complete edentulism and their consequences. Past clinical experience has underscored our previous collective inability to adequately resolve some of these patients' problems. We feel that osseointegration ushers in a new era in clinical treatment, one which is safe, predictable, and limited only by the imagination of the clinicians who use it.

Clinical texts are usually the result of joint ventures, and this book is no exception. We are grateful to the staff members at the Laboratory of Experimental Biology and the Institute for Applied Biotechnology in Göteborg, Sweden. In Toronto our assistance has come from Drs. Francis Zarb, John Cox, Claude Bergeron, Israel Tamary, Aaron Fenton, Mr. Horst Krull, and Mrs. Nancy Smith. We are indebted to these friends and colleagues who made this text possible.

Chapter 1

Introduction to Osseointegration

Per-Ingvar Brånemark

Definition of osseointegration

Osseointegration is defined as a direct structural and functional connection between ordered, living bone and the surface of a load-carrying implant. Creation and maintenance of osseointegration, therefore, depends on the understanding of the tissue's healing, repair, and remodelling capacities.

A basic prerequisite for establishing true and lasting tissue integration of a nonbiologic prosthesis with minimal risk of adverse local or general tissue reactions consists of a detailed understanding of the response behavior of highly differentiated hard and soft tissues to surgical preparation of recipient site, and installation of the prosthesis, as well as the long-term tissue adaptation to functional demands on the anchorage unit (Fig. 1-1). The time schedule, crucial for a healing process that is expected to result in restitutio ad integrum, must be determined with respect to the condition of the individual patient and tissue to be treated. Premature functional demands may result in pseudointegration accompanied by inadequate biomechanical capacities of the in-

Fig. 1-1 Diagrammatic summary of crucial problems in creating permanent tissue anchorage of prostheses penetrating skin or mucous membrane. Reliable stability must be achieved by incorporation of the anchorage element in normal bone tissue providing both adequate resistance to load and

load distribution resulting in bone remodelling. Penetration through skin or mucous membrane to allow attachment of external prosthetic devices (e.g., teeth) requires establishment of a biologic barrier between the internal and external environment in the anchorage region.

An anchorage unit consists of nonbiologic anchoring elements together with its incorporating hard or soft tissues.

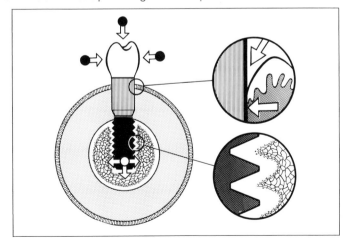

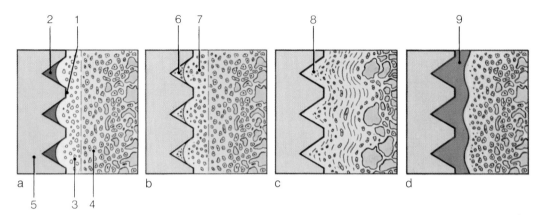

Figs. 1-2a to d   Diagrammatic representation of biology of osseointegration. (From Brånemark et al.[1])

Fig. 1-2a   The threaded bone site cannot be made perfectly congruent to the implant. Object of making a threaded socket in bone is to provide immobilization immediately after installation and during the initial healing period. The diagram is based on relative dimensions of fixture and fixture site. *1* = contact between fixture and bone (immobilization); *2* = hematoma in closed cavity, bordered by fixture and bone; *3* = bone that was damaged by unavoidable thermal and mechanical trauma; *4* = original undamaged bone; and *5* = fixture.

Fig. 1-2b   During the unloaded healing period, the hematoma becomes transformed into new bone through callus formation *(6)*. Damaged bone, which also heals, undergoes revascularization, and de-mineralization and remineralization *(7)*.

Fig. 1-2c   After the initial healing period, vital bone tissue is in close contact with fixture surface, without any other intermediate tissue. Border zone bone *(8)* remodels in response to the masticatory load applied.

Fig. 1-2d   In unsuccessful cases nonmineralized connective tissue *(9)*, constituting a kind of pseudoarthrosis, forms in the border zone at the implant. This development can be initiated by excessive preparation trauma, infection, loading too early in the healing period before adequate mineralization and organization of hard tissue has taken place, or supraliminal loading at any time, even many years after integration has been established. Once lost, osseointegration cannot be reconstituted. Connective tissue can become organized to a certain degree, but is not a proper anchoring tissue because of its inadequate mechanical and biologic capacities, resulting in creation of a locus minoris resistentiae.

terphase between the biological and technical components, whereas relative absence of functional demand on the anchorage region may not provide the necessary remodelling stimulus for the tissues encompassing the prosthesis (Figs. 1-2 a to d).

Thus, in order to provide predictable prognosis for an anchorage unit with an expected function time of several decades—perhaps 50 years—meticulous tissue handling and care is the key to clinical success. This depends on precision in *hardware* composition and design of the non-biologic implanted material, and in *software*—how to handle it, install it, and use it for anchorage of a prosthetic construction.

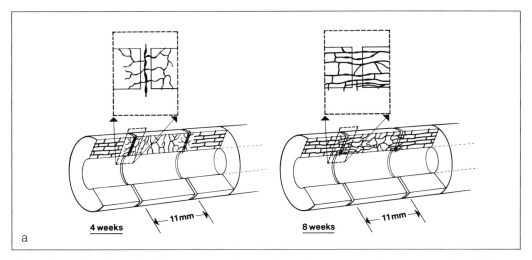

a

Figs. 1-3a and b Example of experimental study on bone tissue repair after resection of part of a long bone in the rat substituting the defect with an autologous bone graft. (From Albrektsson[2])

Fig. 1-3a Principle diagram schematically illustrates some dominating features of the vasculature in the reconstructed area four and eight weeks after transplantation. Note the preponderance of transverse vascular formations in the kerf region at the four-week stage. By eight weeks after transplantation the interfragmentary vessels are mainly longitudinally orientated. The vessels bridging the kerf at this stage are often connected with the haversian microvascular system positioned beyond the necrotic end of the head fragment. A number of wide, tortuous vessels is still noticeable in the reconstructed skeletal region.

Fig. 1-3b Schematic illustration showing some representative sequences of tissue reactions occurring in the interfragmentary region, illustrating the time schedule for bone and marrow tissue maturation.

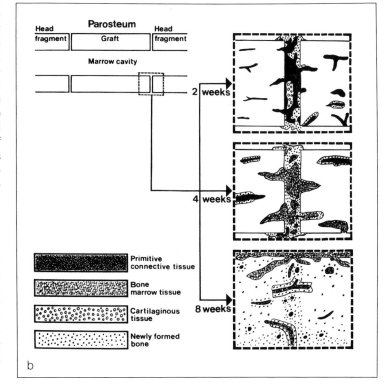

b

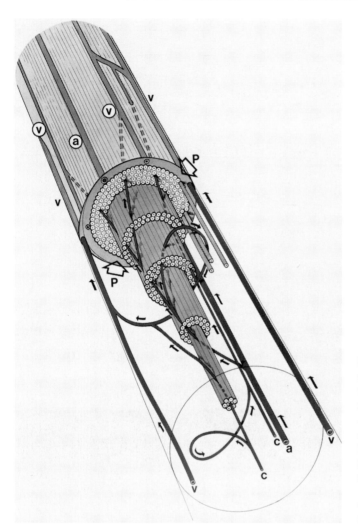

Fig. 1-4 Functional microvascular topography in peripheral nerve as analyzed by vital microscopy. P = perineurium; a = arteriol; v = venule; c = capillary. Note the capillary loops, sometimes arranged in planes perpendicular to the longitudinal axis of the nerve. Arrows denote direction of flow. (From Lundborg and Brånemark[3])

Biologic studies

Since 1952, extensive experimental and clinical studies, which have constituted the basis for permanent tissue integration of prostheses, have been performed at the Laboratory for Vital Microscopy, Department of Anatomy, University of Lund, Sweden; since 1960, at the Laboratory for Experimental Biology, University of Göteborg, Sweden; and since 1978, at The Institute for Applied Biotechnology in Göteborg, Sweden.

In a multidisciplinary, collaborative approach the authors have tried to gain a broad-spectrum knowledge on how—under controlled conditions—bone and marrow tissues can be made to repair and regenerate as such and not as low differentiated scar tissues (Figs. 1-3a and b), and how to design the nonbiologic components of the

Figs. 1-5a and b   The vascular supply to intact and healing tendons in synovial environments has been studied experimentally in rabbits.

Fig. 1-5a   Schematics of the anatomical relationship between the flexor tendon *(T)*, the pulley *(P)*, and the synovial membrane *(S)*. (1) This drawing is based on observations from the distal end of the second *P* and the proximal end of the first *P.* Note the synovial "pouch" close to the sharp edge of the *P.* (2) The synovial vascular network in the pouch region is in continuity on the non-friction side (the "outside") of the *P.* Shaded areas indicate the avascular part of the *T* and the *P* where chondrocytelike cells were observed. Thick arrows symbolize the traction and compression forces involved in active finger flexion. (From Myrhage et al.[4])

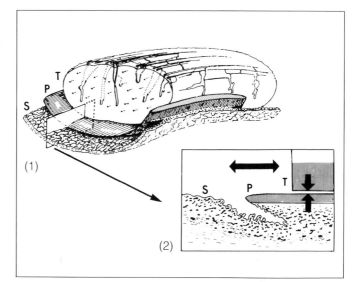

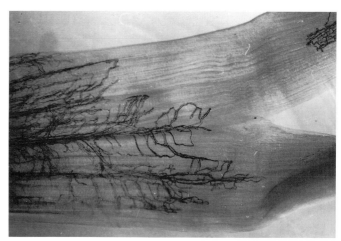

Fig. 1-5b   Avascular part of musculotendinous region.

anchorage unit to fit both tissue demands for integration at the molecular level (Å), surface anatomy of the implant to be acceptable at cellular level (μm), and also to enable surgical installation of the anchoring elements with high mechanical precision —providing initial stability—at minimal tissue injury.

Similar studies on tissue repair after experimental and clinical synovectomy supplied detailed knowledge about the revascularization phenomena, emphasizing the key role of microvascular structure and function in tissue injury and repair as well as the decisive importance of surgical trauma for tissue healing to full restitution.

The short- and long-term effects of tissue injury of mechanical, chemical, thermal, and radiation origin were evaluated in a series of studies, even in combination with controlled relative ischemia with microvascular structure and function as a common de-

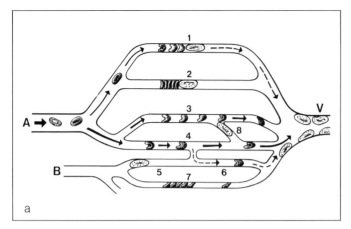
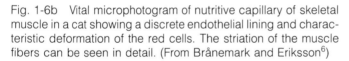

a

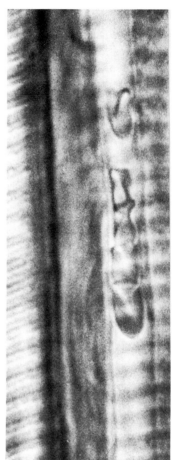

Fig. 1-6a Microvascular corpuscular rheology has been analyzed in vivo and in situ in situations of impaired flow. Semischematic drawing summarizes the different microvascular flow derangements occurring in hemorrhagic shock. Arrows indicate direction and magnitude of flow. Two terminal arterioles (A, B) lead to an interconnected capillary network, which is drained by a collecting venule (V). There is only flow in A. Readily perfused capillaries are seen at 3 and 4, and train flow is illustrated in 1. Plugging WBCs are located at 2, 5, and 8. The capillary at 6 is sparsely perfused via an intercapillary anastomosis from 4 and the capillary at 7 is arrested without any obvious plug. The venular wall is paved by WBCs. (From Amundson[5])

Fig. 1-6b Vital microphotogram of nutritive capillary of skeletal muscle in a cat showing a discrete endothelial lining and characteristic deformation of the red cells. The striation of the muscle fibers can be seen in detail. (From Brånemark and Eriksson[6])

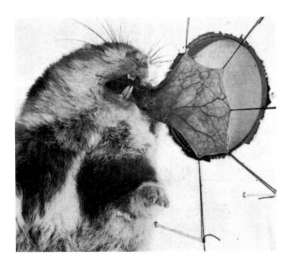

Fig. 1-7 Tissue injury and repair phenomena were studied in different standardized animal models, such as a hamster cheek pouch and a rabbit's ear and ear chamber. This figure shows a hamster cheek pouch exposed for vital microscopy in transillumination. (From Brånemark and Birch[7])

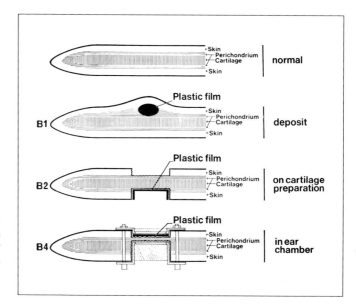

Fig. 1-8a Diagram of a normal rabbit's ear and of the various rabbit ear preparations used for vital microscopic studies on microcirculation at tissue injury. (From Brånemark and Birch[7])

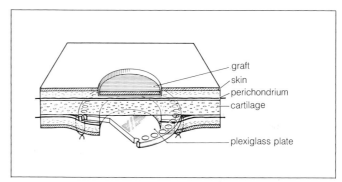

Fig. 1-8b Diagrammatic representation of a rabbit's ear chamber preparation for studies on graft recirculation. (From Birch et al.[8])

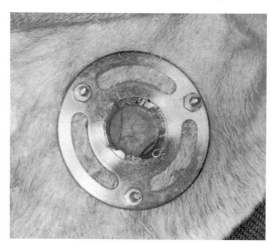

Fig. 1-8c Titanium ear chamber for long-term microvascular studies in situ in vivo. (From Brånemark and Lindström[9])

17

nominator. A variety of tissues (e.g., peripheral nerve, muscle, tendon, bone, marrow, synovial tissue, skin, and mucous membranes) were studied in various animals: mouse, rat, hamster, guinea pig, rabbit, cat, and dog (Figs. 1-4 to 1-8a to c). Even highly specialized and relatively unaccessible structures, such as the inner ear, were analyzed (Figs. 1-9a and b). In separate studies the influence of such specific factors as age, hormones, and temperature on healing tissue were investigated. A wide range of different technical procedures were used, for example, histology at light and electron microscopic resolution levels (Figs. 1-10a and b), vital microscopy including long-term studies with chamber techniques, microradiography, microangiography, and infrared thermography (Figs. 1-11a and b and 1-12a and b).

Often considerable methodological modification was required to explore and clarify the anatomy and pathophysiology of tissue injury (Figs. 1-13 and 1-14) and repair (Figs. 1-15 and 1-16) and the tissue interface toward nonbiologic prosthetic materials and constructions.

Figs. 1-9a and b Microvascular topography and function of the inner ear was studied by vital microscopy in guinea pigs.

Fig. 1-9a Diagram of the vascular areas of the cochlea showing their interrelationship. A = spiral modiolar artery; B = feeding vessels; $C1$ = vessel of the scala vestibuli; $C2$ = vessel at the vestibular membrane; D = stria vascularis; E = vessel of the spiral prominence; F = superficial short-cut vessel; $G1$ = vein of the scala tympani; $G2$ = collecting venules; H = vessel of the basilar membrane and tympanic lip; I = vessels to the limbus; J = spiral modiolar vein; K = vessels to the wall of the modiolus, acoustic nerve, and spiral ganglion; L = vertebral artery; M = basilar artery.

Fig. 1-9b Diagram shows the vascular complexity decreasing from the basal turns (left side of the diagram) to the apical turns of the cochlea. It also demonstrates the segmental type of circulation that exists in the cochlea. (From Costa and Brånemark[10])

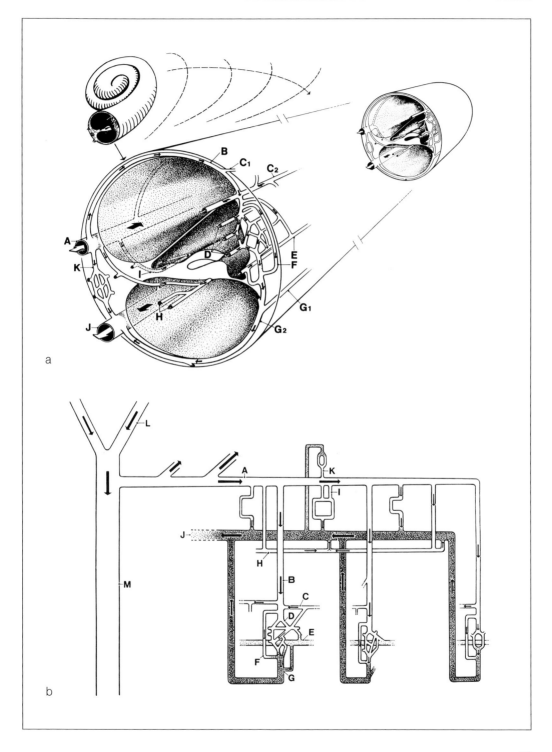

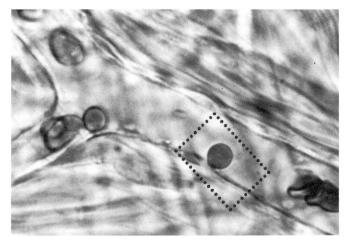

Figs. 1-10a and b Microscopic studies of blood cell behavior in situ in vivo were combined with electron microscopic evaluation of the same cells, after removing the specimen by microdissection. In this example an erythrocyte in diapedesis was examined. (From Brånemark et al.[11])

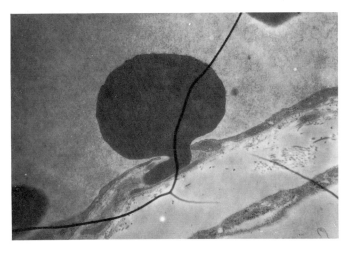

Fig. 1-10b

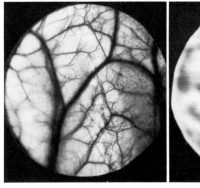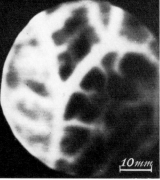

Figs. 1-11a and b Tissue response to injury was analyzed by dynamic recordings of tissue temperature by infrared thermography (in this example a rabbit's ear) (see also Fig. 1-12). (From Birch et al.[12])

Fig. 1-11a Transillumination of vascular pattern in vivo.

Fig. 1-11b Infrared thermographic emission representation of same region.

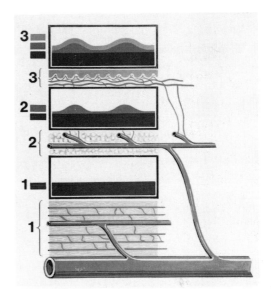

Fig. 1-12a Diagram illustrates heat transfer to skin by direct conduction via interposed tissues and by vascular connections between different tissues, forming the final emission patterns at skin surface level. *1* = muscular layer; *2* = subcutaneous tissues; *3* = cutaneous vessels and capillary bed.

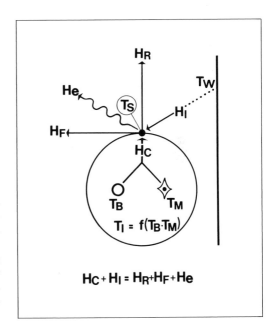

Fig. 1-12b Diagrammatic summary of factors involved in the heat flux mechanisms at the surface of a biologic body. *TS* = surface temperature heat contribution from blood *(TB)* and metabolism *(TM)*; H_I = heat contribution from incident radiant energy; H_R = heat registered by emission recording; H_F = heat loss by conduction and convection; H_e = heat loss by evaporation. (From Brånemark and Nilsson[13])

Fig. 1-13 Microvascular pathophysiology after different types, level, and duration of injury were analyzed with respect to immediate reactions and long-term consequences and recirculation or revascularization.

Diagrammatic representation of microvascular pathophysiology in tissue injury including intravascular, endothelial, and perivascular changes.

Arteriolar constriction is a common phenomenon (1). Sometimes arteriolar dilatation occurs, or even an alternation of constricted and dilated arteriolar segments. In the true capillaries the endothelial cells may swell (2), thereby reducing the capillary lumen and impairing nutritive flow of blood. This phenomenon is structurally and functionally connected with changes in the periendothelial granular cells and pericytes. Even adjacent tissue mast cells may play a role in this mechanism by disrupting and liberating the content of their granules into the ground substance, the extracellular, and the perivascular space.

Dilatation of venules and venular stasis (3) is an early and important phenomenon in tissue injury. Microvascular architecture differs in various tissues. If capillary shunts or arteriolar-venular shunts exist (4), blood may be short-circuited and thereby bypass the nutritive part of the capillary bed. Granulocytes are often rigid and may block the nutritive capillaries temporarily or even permanently (5). Wall-adhering erythrocytes (6), and granulocytes and platelets (7) are characteristic phenomena in tissue injury. Increased numbers of granulocytes which adhere to and roll along the endothelium (8) are a constant finding.

Microthrombi are formed and may consist of platelets (9), fibrin (10), a combination of fibrin and platelets (11), and may even include red cells and white cells, thereby forming a classical microthrombus (12). These wall-adhering thrombi often allow single blood cells to pass (9-12). They may, however, also completely block the lumen (13), temporarily or permanently. The erythrocytes (14) may change in shape to crenated cells, namely, acanthocytes (15), which often maintain a great deal of the plasticity of the normal red cell (16). Sometimes the red cells turn into spherocytes (17), which may disrupt, causing hemolysis. When spherocytes are compressed in a vessel, they change into characteristic hexagonal bodies (18). The white cells may exhibit different degrees of plasticity (19), but may also turn into rigid corpuscles (20). Disruption of granulocytes with liberation of their granules into the lumen has been established as an in vivo phenomenon (20), which appears to be significant in the development of tissue injury. An aggregation of red cells may, to some extent, influence nutritive flow of blood (21). Often, however, the aggregates are plastic and deformable enough to pass even narrow nutritive capillaries, and when the flow rate is increased, the cells move as solitary bodies. The noncorpuscular plasma constituents of blood may change appreciably in composition, accompanied by disturbances in microvascular rheology. Thus, significant abnormalities occur, for example, in plasma proteins, lipoproteins, and lipids.

The endothelial wall disrupts functionally with leakage of plasma, resulting in edema and the passage of single blood cells (22), or structurally, resulting in bleeding into the tissue and more or less complete breakdown of the microcirculation (23). This is then followed by derangement and necrosis of the tissue. (From Brånemark et al.[11])

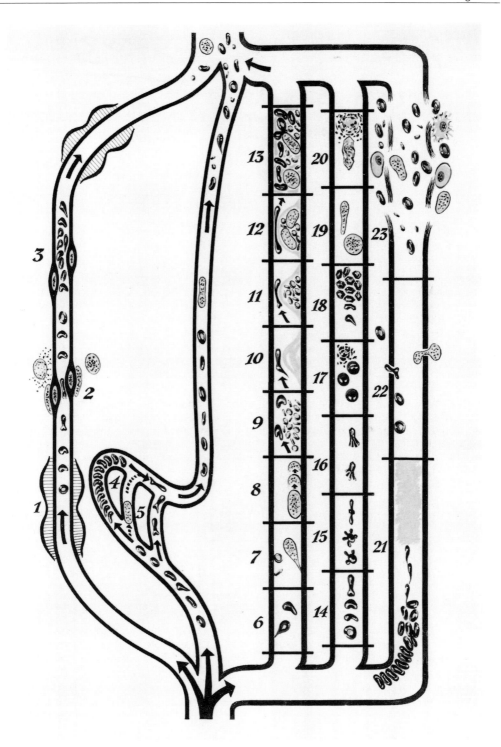

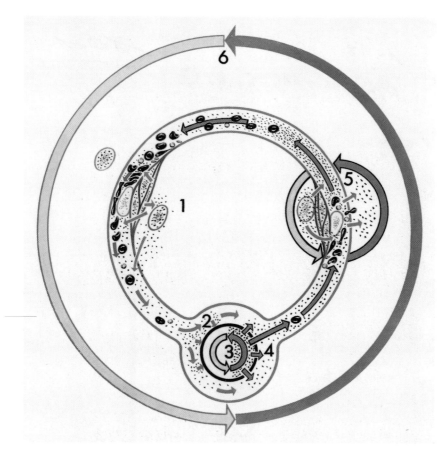

Fig. 1-14   The possible interaction between macrocirculation and microcirculation was analyzed with respect to the general communication from an injured tissue via its microcirculation to the major circulation and the possible effect of factors released locally as a consequence of the injury.

Diagram illustrating working hypothesis for the possible interaction between microvascular pathophysiology at the local site of burn *(1)*, subsequent increased permeability of capillaries in intestine *(2, 3)*, accompanied by absorption of endotoxin into the circulation *(4)*, resulting in systemic microvascular disturbances *(5)* and further injury in the burned area *(1)*. This mechanism thus establishes a vicious circle *(6)*. (From Brånemark and Urbaschek[14])

Fig. 1-15 Tissue-healing phenomena were studied by different techniques including vital microscopic chamber procedures. This figure shows diagrammatically the events in the revascularization of a tissue defect, illustrating different steps in wound healing and formation of granulation tissue with respect to the microvascular system. A tissue defect, that is, a wound (1), is first filled with a fibrin reticulum formed from plasma, leaking from damaged vessels at the edge of the wound (2). After six to 10 hours granular cells have already invaded the wound (3). These cells then extend cytoplasmatic processes, but are still moving around in the fibrin reticulum (4). Three to five days after the trauma, erythrocytes are perfusing the healing wound, thereby constituting an open circulation. In the next stage (5) granular cells stop moving and their processes connect with each other to form a cellular network which is still being perfused by red cells from vessels at the edge of the original defect. At the same time capillary sprouts are growing into the granulation tissue (6), and, finally, at five to seven days after the injury the wound is penetrated by large numbers of wide, thin-walled, newly formed capillaries (7), which are then, within three to four weeks, reduced in number to give the vascular pattern of connective tissue. (From Brånemark[15])

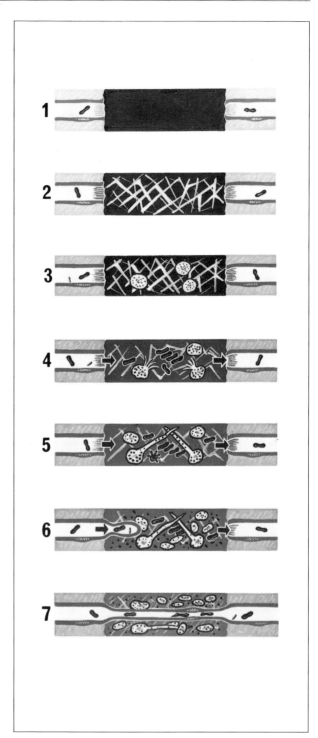

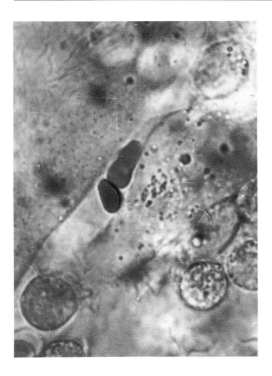

Fig. 1-16   Vital microphotograph from a rabbit's ear chamber showing a typical sprouting capillary with red cells in a newly formed tissue. (From Lindhe and Brånemark[16])

Development of the concept of osseointegration

The concept of osseointegration is based on research that began in 1952 with microscopic studies in situ of bone marrow in rabbits' fibula (Figs. 1-17a and b). This investigation was carried out with a vital microscopic technique based on extremely gentle surgical preparation, which consisted of grinding down the covering bone to a thickness of 10 μm. With the aid of specially developed microscopes unstained bone and bone marrow could be studied in vivo and in situ by transillumination at the resolution capacity of the light microscope. Blood circulation in the marrow was easily observed through the very thin bone layer. These intravital studies revealed the inti-

mate connection between marrow and bone tissue compartments (Figs. 1-18a and b). Other studies on regeneration of bone marrow emphasized the close functional connection between marrow and bone tissues during healing of bone defects. Therefore, a series of studies on bone, marrow, and joint tissues was started to determine the reaction of these tissues to different types of trauma, particularly in actual clinical situations, such as rheumatoid arthritis. Subsequently, efforts were directed at diminishing the negative effects of various traumatic agents on repair processes in these tissues. With the aim of complete restitutio ad integrum at reconstructive surgical procedures traumatic factors detrimental to the healing process were further identified in differentiated tissue such as relative ischemia, local

Figs. 1-17a and b Preparation of bone window 10 to 30 μm over marrow cavity in a rabbit's fibula with maintained microcirculation and undisturbed intravascular rheology in bone and marrow vessels.

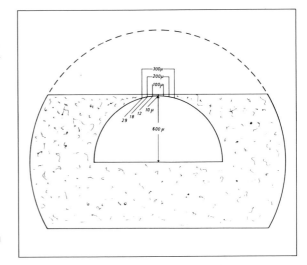

Fig. 1-17a Transverse sectional diagram of prepared fibula.

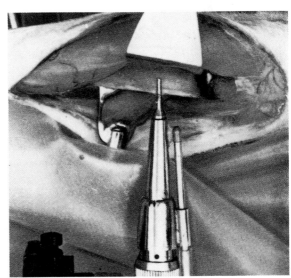

Fig. 1-17b Removal of covering bone tissue by grinding using specially developed cutting tools. (From Brånemark[17])

tissue temperature, and use of topically applied drugs (e.g., sodium fluorides, steroids, ENT drugs, and wound disinfectants). The effects of anti-inflammatory drugs and roentgen contrast media were also analyzed. Furthermore, to follow bone and marrow over a longer period of time, in vivo microscopy of these tissues was carried out, using an implanted titanium chamber containing an optical system for transillumination of a thin layer of original or newly formed tissue. Pure titanium was chosen instead of tantalum, which had been used previously for vital microscopic chambers. Titanium seemed to have better mechanical and surface characteristics for implantation in a biologic environment (Figs. 1-19a to d). These studies, in the early 1960s, indicated

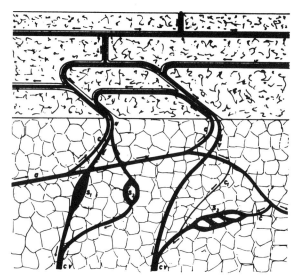

Fig. 1-18a Vascular anatomy and flow patterns in bone and marrow in a rabbit's fibula according to vital microscopic observations.

The bone marrow arteriole (a) divides dichotomously into capillaries (c). These capillaries run to sinusoids, which are sometimes hexagonal (s_2) and sometimes spindle-shaped (s_1). Sinusoids unite to form sinusoidal systems (s_3). The sinusoids are drained by venules into collecting venules (cv). The sinusoids vary rhythmically in degree of dilation with accompanying variation in the velocity of flow within them. Some blood cells bypass a sinusoid by flowing from a capillary via a shunting capillary (c_1) directly into a venule. Capillaries stemming from marrow arterioles enter the haversian canals to supply endosteal parts of the diaphyseal bone. The capillaries then swing back into the marrow to empty via venules (v) into sinusoids or directly into collecting venules. Sometimes two streams flowing in opposite directions are seen in one and the same haversian canal. The blood flow in the bone capillaries is fairly steady and the velocity is higher than in the marrow capillaries. (From Brånemark[17])

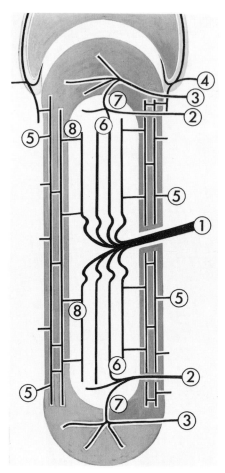

Fig. 1-18b Schematic review of the main sources of vascular supply to bone, marrow, and joint tissues. The interrelations between the different vascular areas are indicated. 1 = vasa nutritia which anastomose with metaphyseal (2) and epiphyseal (3) vessels. 6 and 7 = vascular connections between epiphyseal, metaphyseal, and nutrient marrow vessels. Even the joint vasculature (4) has direct connections (via bone vessels) with the marrow cavity. The vascular system in compact and trabecular bone (5) is in close anatomical and functional contact (8) with the medullary vessels. (From Brånemark[18])

Figs. 1-19a to d   Titanium chamber for long-term vital microscopy of bone and marrow tissues in situ.

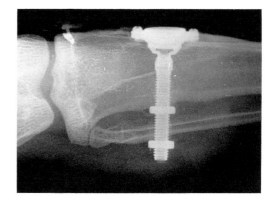

Fig. 1-19a   Chamber in situ.

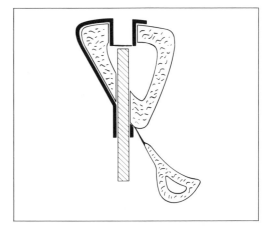

Fig. 1-19b   Diagrammatical transverse section of a rabbit's tibiofibula showing positioning of chamber device. (From Brånemark et al.[19])

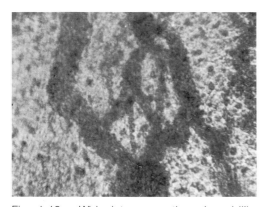

Fig. 1-19c   Wide interconnecting sinusoidlike vessels with thin endothelial lining. Three weeks postoperative. (From Brånemark et al.[19])

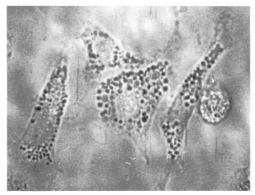

Fig. 1-19d   Typical granular cells in regenerating marrow. Three weeks postoperative in rabbit. Vital microscopy 1,000x. (From Brånemark et al.[19])

Figs. 1-20 a and b   Formation of bone and marrow in isolated segment of rib periosteum in rabbits and dogs was analyzed in studies on the osteogenetic potential of periosteal tissues. (From Brånemark and Breine[20])

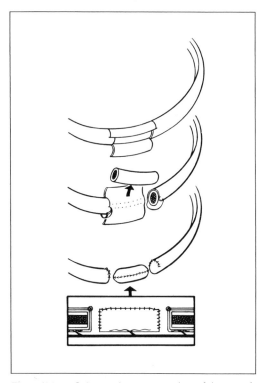

Fig. 1-20a   Schematic presentation of the surgical procedure for isolating rib periosteum with preservation of vascular supply.

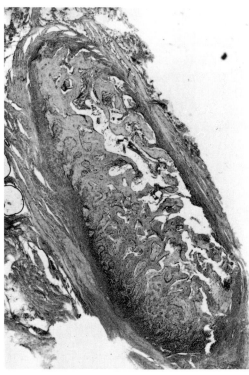

Fig. 1-20b   Typical example of regenerated tissue in periosteal tube in dog after 35 days showing trabecular bony tissue surrounded by connective tissue layer. Light microscopy 20x.

the possibility of establishing true osseointegration in bone tissue, because the optical chambers used could not be removed from the surrounding bone once they had healed. The titanium framework had become completely incorporated in the bone, and the mineralized tissue completely congruent with the microirregularities of the titanium surface.

Interdisciplinary, clinical research, together with plastic and ENT surgeons, brought about the study of repair of mandibular defects and replacement of middle ear ossicles by means of autologous bone grafts. Because of the unpredictable outcome of immediate grafts consisting of cortical bone, marrow, and spongious bone as repair material for defects in hard tissue, attempts were made to develop a grafting technique with a more predictable outcome. A procedure was designed to *preform autologous bone transplants* in rabbits and dogs (Figs. 1-20a and b to 1-22a to c). With this experimental experience various clinical

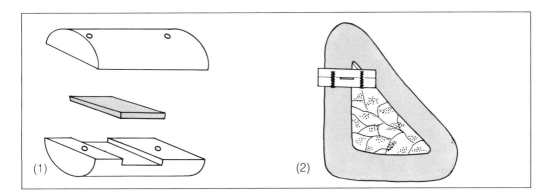

Figs. 1-21a to d   The procedure of preforming autologous bone grafts with specific topographical anatomy was developed in a series of experimental studies in rabbits and dogs.

Fig. 1-21a   *(1)* Sketch showing the principles of the titanium mold used when preforming a bone transplant of lamellar form. *(2)* Cross section of the proximal tibial metaphysis with the titanium mold in position. (From Hallén et al.[21])

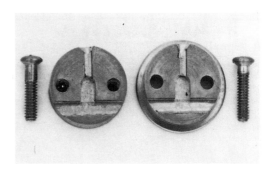

Fig. 1-21b   Titanium mold for the creation of a facsimile ossicle which was used in experiments on dogs, installed into the proximal tibial metaphysis.

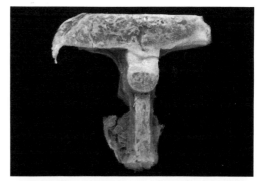

Fig. 1-21c   The preformed transplant removed. (From Hallén et al.[21])

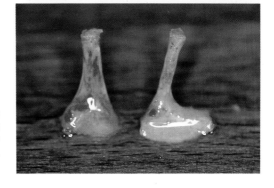

Fig. 1-21d   Two preformed autologous ossicles from the upper tibial metaphysis of a patient who received one of the grafts for middle ear repair with uncomplicated good function still after seven years follow-up.

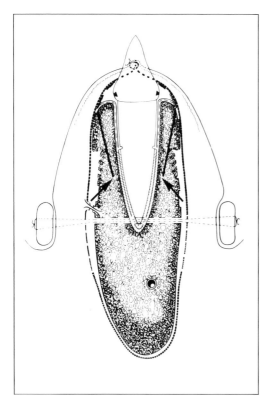

Figs. 1-22a to c   Preformed autologous bone graft from the rib of a dog used for reconstruction of the differentiated periodontal tissues and adjacent jawbone in experimental horizontal defects. (From Adell[22])

Fig. 1-22a   Diagrammatic representation of an experimental area immediately after transfer of the graft has been carried out. Close approximation of the apical spongious surface of the preformate to the multiple perforated marginal cortical plate of the alveolar process via titanium pins. There is a plate of the preformate facing the root and a periosteal layer between this cortical plate and the root surface.

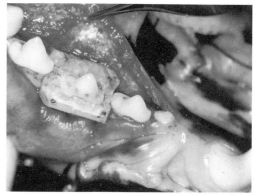

Fig. 1-22b   Application of preformates against the root surface and the multiple perforated alveolar process. The two preformates have been stabilized by titanium pins providing tight fitting of the preformates.

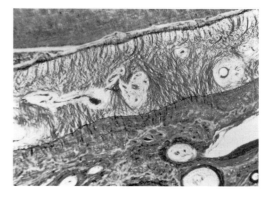

Fig. 1-22c   Histologic section of reconstructed periodontium with adjacent jawbone in an experimental horizontal defect.

Figs. 1-23a and b   Major skeletal defects were produced in a dog's mandible and tibial diaphysis. Reconstruction was performed using integrated titanium fixtures as anchorage for titanium splints providing fragment stability in the defect space. All periosteum was removed in the defect which was filled with autologous bone and marrow graft. (From Brånemark[23])

Fig. 1-23a   Schematic representation of experimental defects in mandible and tibia in a dog that were reconstructed by means of autologous marrow and spongious bone grafts stabilized by titanium splints secured to osseointegrated fixtures in remaining bone distal and proximal to the defect.

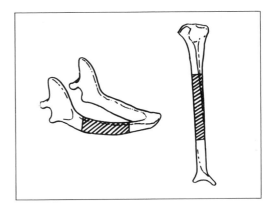

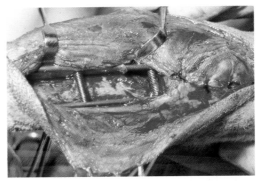

Fig. 1-23b   Topography of lower leg in a dog at the time of resection of the tibia. Two lateral titanium stabilizers were used. Periosteum was completely removed in the area of defect.

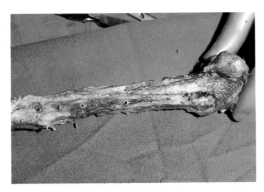

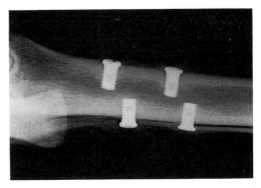

Fig. 1-23c   Reconstructed tibia three years later with stabilizers removed.

Fig. 1-23d   Radiograph illustrates anatomy of integrated fixtures prior to resection. (From Brånemark[23])

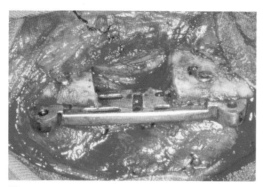

Fig. 1-24a   Experimental defect in a dog's mandible reconstructed with stabilizing buccal and lingual titanium splint connected to previously integrated fixtures on both sides of the defect, which was filled with a graft composed of autologous marrow and spongious bone.

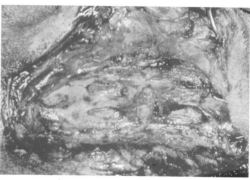

Fig. 1-24b   Reconstructed area six months later. (From Brånemark[23])

applications were made possible in situations where special demands are put on the structure and function of skeletal reconstructions requiring grafting of tissues.

Development of procedure for rehabilitation of edentulism

One animal series comprised the study of repair of large mandibular and tibial defects in dogs where different reconstruction possibilities were evaluated. The best results were obtained when titanium fixtures were allowed to become incorporated in positions proximal and distal to the defect prior to creation of the bone defect. This two-stage procedure enabled titanium splints to be connected to the integrated fixtures at

the time of creating the skeletal defect, and allowed for immediate functional loading of the reconstructed bone (Figs. 1-23a to d and 1-24a and b).

As a consequence of successful experimental and clinical repair of major defects in the jaw skeleton, resulting in skeletal continuity but without replacement for teeth, a demand was created for a jawbone-anchored substitute for teeth. Accordingly, studies on healing and mechanical stability of jawbone-anchored prosthetic elements were carried out, using anchoring elements of pure titanium of different sizes and designs. It was found that an implant, inserted in the marrow space and allowed to heal immobilized, without initial loading, became surrounded by a layer of compact bone (Figs. 1-25a to c). No sign of soft tissue was

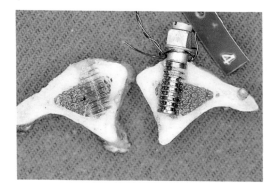

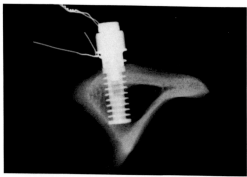

Figs. 1-25a to c   Different designs of titanium fixtures were tested in long bones and in jawbones of dogs. A constant phenomenon found was condensation of bone tissue toward the titanium surface in the marrow cavity in addition to integration in cortical bone. (From Brånemark[23])

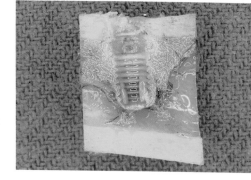

detected between bone and implant surface. There was a positive correlation between the microtopography of the titanium surface, absence of contamination, gentle surgical preparation of implant site, and the condition of bone and marrow at roentgenological and histological analyses of these tissues at the interphase. Osseointegration could be established in different parts of the skeleton (e.g., cranium, jawbone, long bones, and also tail vertebrae of dogs) in experimental animals—rats, rabbits, and dogs—even when transcutaneous abutments were connected (Fig. 1-26).

Based on these observations on tissue repair and integration of titanium fixtures, further experimental work was conducted aiming at development of clinical procedures for the rehabilitation of edentulism using fixed-bridge constructions, particularly in cases with severe resorption of the alveolar jawbone. A combination of osseointegrated fixtures and autologous bone transplants were thought to be useful in these cases.

In these studies, dogs were made partially edentulous; the anterior teeth, canines included, were maintained; premolars and the first molars were extracted. After bone healing of the extraction sockets the dogs were provided with prosthetic constructions similar to dental bridges attached to osseointegrated screw-shaped titanium fixtures—4 mm in diameter and 10 mm long with a particular microarchitecture of the surface—that were allowed to heal into the jawbone during a period of three to four months under unloaded conditions (Figs. 1-27a to d and 1-28a to e). Radiological and

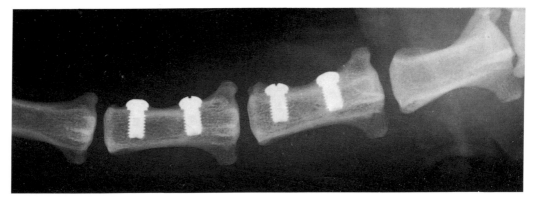

Fig. 1-26   Osseointegrated titanium fixtures installed in dorsoventral direction in the vertebrae of a dog's tail.

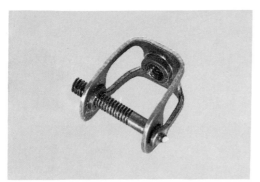

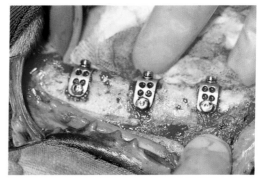

Figs. 1-27a and b   After reconstruction of the experimental defects in a dog's mandible (see Figs. 1-23 and 1-24) attempts were made to compensate for lost teeth using a combination of subperiosteal and transosseous titanium implants. (Fig. 1-27a from Brånemark et al.[24]; Fig. 1-27b from Brånemark[23])

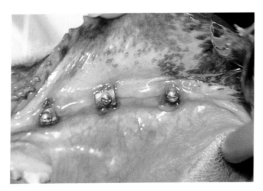

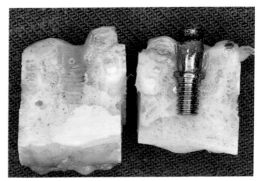

Fig. 1-27c   This was found to provide anchorage but also unpredictable soft-tissue reactions.

Fig. 1-27d   Separate screw-shaped titanium fixtures were developed, which were finally designed after experimental evaluation of about 50 different configurations and dimensions of implants. (From Brånemark[23])

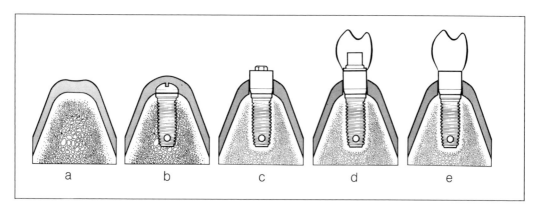

Figs. 1-28a to e   In the experimental studies in dogs a two-stage procedure was developed for integration of screw-shaped titanium fixtures at the initial procedure.

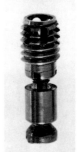

Figs. 1-28a and b   The fixture was installed in the jawbone after reflecting the mucoperiosteum. A very gentle technique for bone preparation was used with profuse saline irrigation to reduce heat injury.

Figs. 1-28c to e   The mucoperiosteal flap was then closed. After a healing period of two to three months the mucoperiosteum was removed over the fixture and a mucosa piercing abutment cylinder was connected to the fixture providing attachment for a prosthetic device substituting teeth. (From Brånemark[23])

histologic analyses indicated that integration and bridge stability could be maintained for 10 years in dogs without significant adverse reactions in hard or soft tissues despite the fact that oral hygiene procedures were applied only once or twice a year in these dogs. The load-bearing capacity of single implants was 100 kg for the lower jaw and 30 to 50 kg for the upper jaw. At the time the animal was killed it was observed that the titanium fixture could not be removed without causing fractures in the surrounding bone, whereas the interface between bone and titanium remained intact. This was also true for implants inserted in the near vicinity of the nasal cavity or the mucoperiosteum of the maxillary sinus (Figs. 1-29a to e through 1-32a to c).

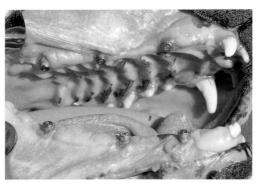

Fig. 1-29a Partially edentulous upper and lower jaw in a dog with three fixtures integrated in each jaw and with connected mucosa penetrating abutments. (From Brånemark[23])

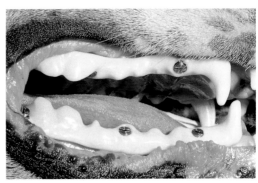

Fig. 1-29b Acrylic resin prosthesis. (From Brånemark[23])

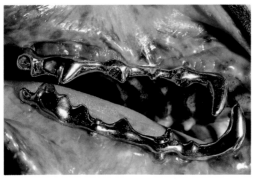

Fig. 1-29c Chrome-cobalt superstructure. (From Brånemark[23])

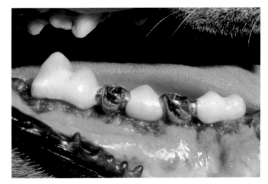

Fig. 1-29d Two fixtures support a prosthesis made of porcelain baked to metal with molar tooth as cantilevered abutment. (From Brånemark[23])

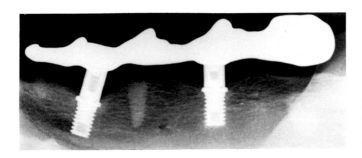

Fig. 1-29e Radiogram of anchoring bone four years after connection of bridge. (From Brånemark et al.[24])

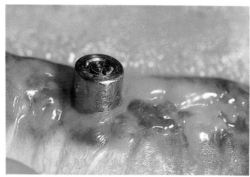

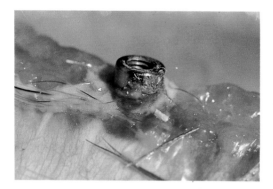

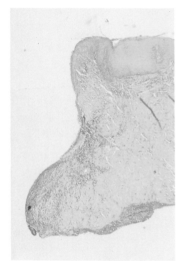

Figs. 1-30a to e   The dogs in long-term experiments were only subjected to gingival hygiene control once or twice a year at time of radiographic examination. Typical example of mucoperiosteal situation before and after local cleaning of abutment region with a superficial inflammatory reaction responding to local tissue hygiene procedures. (From Brånemark et al.[24])

Fig. 1-30a *(top left)*   Shows characteristic debris, hair, etc., and gingival reaction before oral hygiene began. Fifty-three months, 3x.

Fig. 1-30b *(top right)*   After two weeks' oral hygiene. Fifty-three and a half months, 3x.

Fig. 1-30c *(left)*   Biopsy corresponding to Fig. 1-30b illustrates the situation in the tissue. Only scattered round cells in the adjacent epithelium and connective tissue. Fifty-three and a half months, 30x.

Fig. 1-30d *(bottom left)*   Shows that the inflammatory process is concentrated to the superficial soft tissues leaving the anchoring bone unaffected.

Fig. 1-30e *(bottom right)*   The typical encapsulation in compact bone follows exactly the anatomy of the fixture even at its apical part.

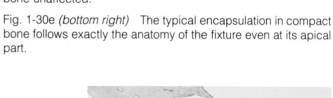

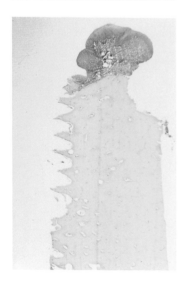

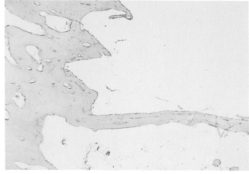

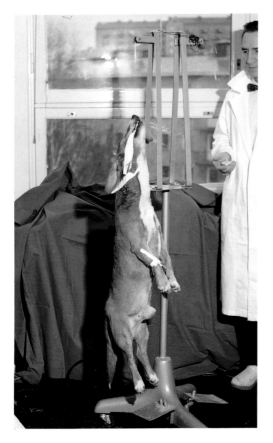

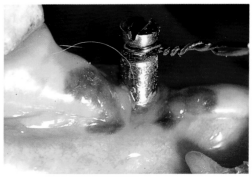

Figs. 1-31a and b The anchorage capacity of integrated fixtures was illustrated by suspending the dog via wires connected to separate fixtures.

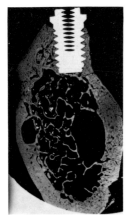

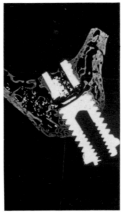

Figs. 1-31c and d Microradiograms of ground sections show the pattern of remodelling and density of the mineralized tissue around the fixtures.

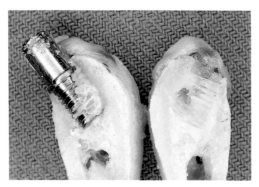
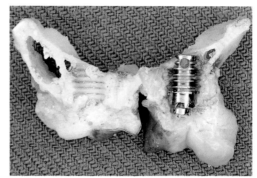

Figs. 1-32a and b   Fixtures in situ in upper and lower jaws after exposing the fixture by cutting the bone in two segments. The fixture is still incorporated in bone tissue, which cannot be removed from the titanium surface. (From Brånemark et al.[24])

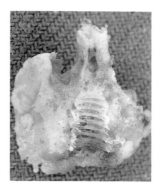

Fig. 1-32c   Fixture in upper jaw removed from bone to illustrate remodelling of bone with formation of dense capsule in the trabecular bone; 32 months.

Combination of osseointegration and bone grafting

In order to reconstruct severely resorbed edentulous jaws, a special transplantation technique was developed that procured a *preformed* graft from the donor site that corresponded to the desired anatomy (Figs. 1-33a to c). A titanium mold was used to control the remodelling of the preformed graft, and fixtures were integrated simultaneously in the graft-to-be. The tibia and rib bone of the dog and rabbit were used as donor sites. Long-term experimental studies indicated the possibility of achieving bone anchorage for titanium fixtures that could accept unlimited functional load from prosthetic substitutes for teeth, similar to tooth-borne bridges. This anchorage function was established both for fixtures installed in the original experimentally edentulous jawbone and for fixtures incorporated in transplanted bone tissue.

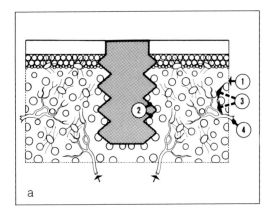

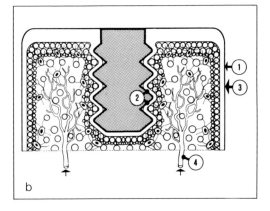

Figs. 1-33a and b   Diagrammatic comparison between immediate (Fig. 1-33a) and preformed autologous bone grafts (Fig. 1-33b). Basically, the immediate graft is cut to the desired anatomical shape at the time of grafting and accordingly damaged and devitalized, whereas the preformed graft is biologically molded and remodelled to an adequate anatomy by controlled bone healing. The trauma inflicted to the graft, and especially its superficial parts, at procurement and transfer is thus drastically reduced. The operation time required is also minimized, but instead two operations are required, one for preparation and the other for transfer of the graft. Some important differences between preformed and immediate bone grafts containing endoprosthetic components are shown schematically: *1* = surface tissue of graft not damaged by preparation to adjust shape as in immediate grafting; *2* = implant devices incorporated in remodelled, vital bone means greater strength of anchorage; *3* = graft protected against invading granulation tissue by remodelled cortical bone layer with vital cells; and *4* = microvascular architecture adapted to the topography at the site of reconstruction. At the donor site there is a stepwise adaptation to the removal of the graft, which is to a large extent relieved of the load taken by this part of the skeleton. Therefore, there is a minor trauma to the donor area at the actual transfer of the graft. The strength of the host skeleton is less reduced than at immediate grafting. As a consequence of preformation the graft is more fit to become incorporated at the recipient site with less risk for disturbances in the course of healing and with minimal loss of the transplant due to resorption. (From Breine and Brånemark[25])

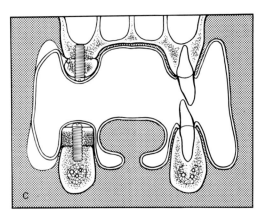

Fig. 1-33c   Topography of reconstructed jawbone using preformed autologous bone and marrow graft in comparison with the original anatomy.

Vital microscopic studies on microcirculation

Soft-tissue penetration of titanium abutments caused no side effects in the reconstructed edentulous jaw. Similar results were obtained at skin penetration of titanium chambers employed in vital microscopy of bone and marrow tissues in situ in rabbit and dog tibiae.

In extensive long-term studies on human microcirculation aimed at understanding the intravascular corpuscular behavior of blood as a mobile tissue, titanium chambers containing optical systems were used to enable continuous observation in situ in vivo of intravascular rheology of blood in microvascular units. These titanium chambers were inserted in a twin-pedicled skin tube on the inside of the left upper arm of healthy volunteers and a group of patients suffering from diabetes (Figs. 1-34a to f).

In addition to these fundamental studies on the intravascular anatomy of human blood, special investigations were performed on microvascular reactions to complete or relative ischemia in humans (Figs. 1-35a and b through 1-38). The observations indicated a remarkable capacity of microvascular repair and reconstitution of microcirculation even after several hours of controlled ischemia. Integrity of the interface between skin and subcutaneous tissues and titanium was maintained, providing strong support for plans to use osseointegration of titanium prosthesis in situations of human tissue defects even when the integumentum—skin or mucous membrane—has to be penetrated.

The chamber tissue reactions were evaluated by studying intravascular rheological phenomena. There were no long-standing inflammatory processes in the chamber tissue or in the regions of skin penetration.

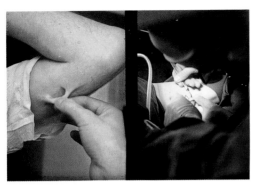

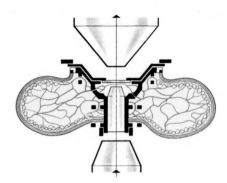

Fig. 1-34a Microcirculation in humans was studied by vital microscopy in implanted titanium optical chambers in twin-pedicled skin tubes on the inside of the upper arm. (From Brånemark[26])

Fig. 1-34b Transverse section of chamber, skin tube, and microscope elements, as positioned during observation.

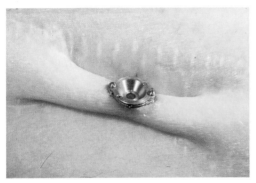

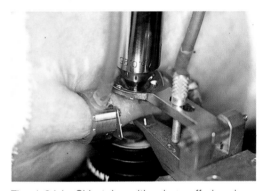

Fig. 1-34c Skin tube with chamber. (From Brånemark[26])

Fig. 1-34d Skin tube with microcuffs in microscope for controlled ischemia experiment.

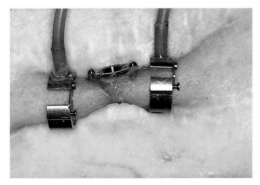

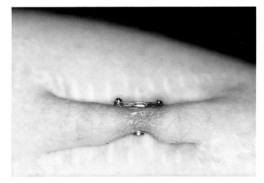

Fig. 1-34e Inflammatory response after release of cuff occlusion during six hours.

Fig. 1-34f Same specimen as in Fig. 1-34d, 24 hours later showing recovery of the compressed tissue and maintained integration of the chamber in the skin tube.

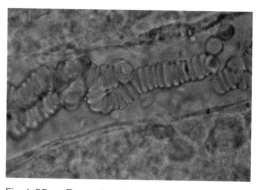 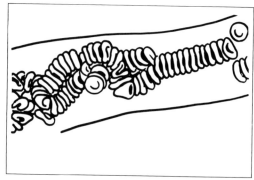

Fig.1-35a Example of red blood cell behavior in a low flow situation forming rouleaux in a skin tube chamber in humans.

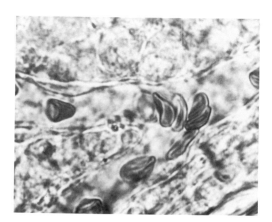 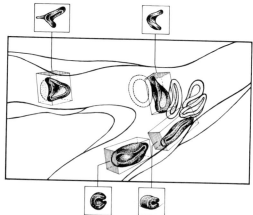

Fig. 1-35b The biconcave red cells often give the impression of having a peripheral rim, tending to maintain their original three-dimensional form. (From Brånemark[26])

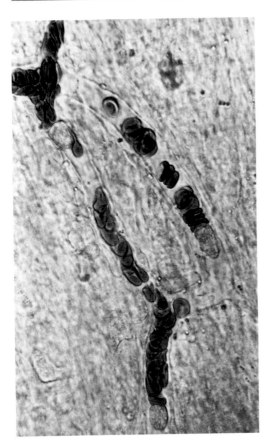

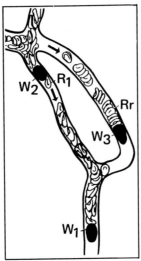

Fig. 1-36 Typical microvascular segment in human skin tube chamber. There are three granulocytes seen: one moving ahead of the red cell column, only slightly reducing flow (W_1), another granulocyte (W_2) almost completely blocks the vascular lumen but occasional red cells (R_1) are still capable of passing between the white cell and the endothelium. Erythrocytes (R_r) are piling up behind the flow-obstructing third white cell (W_3). (From Brånemark[26])

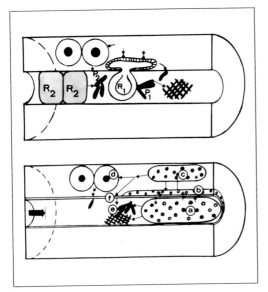

Fig. 1-37 The intravascular behavior of blood cells was studied in a series of investigations concentrating on the interaction between the different corpuscular elements of blood and their relation to the vascular endothelium. Examples of these studies are erythrocyte diapedesis (R_1) and the blocking effect of granulocytes due to their relative rigidity as compared to the easily deformable red cell. Possible tissue injury mechanisms are represented by a platelet aggregate (P_1). R_2 indicates the effect of blockage of red cells with the possible release of substances initiating platelet aggregation (P_2). a = intravascular granulocyte; b = periendothelial granular cell; c = mast cell; d = tissue cell; e = platelets; f = endothelium. (From Brånemark et al.[27])

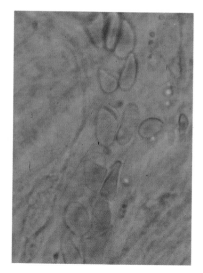 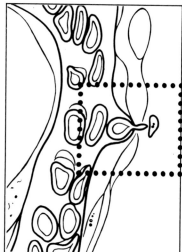

Fig. 1-38 Attempted diapedesis of erythrocytes in human skin venule as observed in vivo. (From Brånemark[26])

Clinical application of osseointegration

On the basis of these successful long-term experimental studies on bone anchorage of, and soft-tissue behavior at, titanium devices, and the additional favorable information on interface integrity in the human skin tube chamber, the first edentulous patient was treated in 1965, according to the osseointegration principle, using a two-stage technique.

A modified reconstruction procedure was applied in those edentulous jaws where the remaining bone was insufficient to allow for fixture anchorage. A *preformed graft* was created in the proximal tibial metaphysis, and fixtures were allowed to become integrated in the graft-to-be during the primary remodelling period (Fig. 1-39). The combination of preformed transplants and integrated fixtures have resulted in favorable long-term clinical results with more than 15 years follow-up. This procedure has the advantage of a high degree of prognostic predictability, but the disadvantage of requiring two surgical procedures.

Therefore, an alternative one-stage reconstruction program using autologous bone and marrow grafts, immediately transferred and anchored to the recipient site via titanium fixtures, later to be used also as bridge support, was tried. The long-term clinical results, with a follow-up of more than 10 years, indicate that it is possible to achieve good results even with immediate autologous bone and marrow grafts, provided a gentle surgical technique is used (Fig. 1-40). Evaluated radiographically, the directly transferred bone graft behaves and develops as the original jawbone, and the mucoperiosteum creates a well-functioning barrier toward the oral cavity.

In patients where there is a discontinuity of the mandible, sometimes including the joint region requiring a new capitulum mandibulae to be created, a preformed autologous graft from the ilium has been used and given good, predictable, long-term results with minimal graft resorption even in cases subjected to therapeutic radiation prior to reconstruction (Fig. 1-41).

The same basic principles as for preformed

47

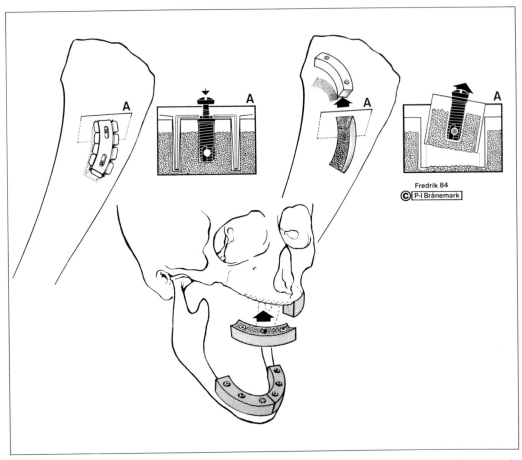

Fig. 1-39 Diagrammatic summary of two-stage clinical reconstruction technique for severely resorbed edentulous jawbone, using preformed autologous bone and marrow graft with integrated titanium fixtures from the proximal tibial metaphyses on both sides.

alveolar bone grafts were applied (see Fig. 1-39). The graft-to-be, encased in os ilium, was partially surrounded by titanium molds. The fixtures were inserted in two directions, horizontally and vertically, in order to allow both a splint to connect the transplant to the remaining part of the mandible, into which horizontal fixtures were installed at the primary procedure, and a bridge to be at-tached to the vertical fixtures. Clinical long-term results indicate that the graft keeps its original shape even when the caput man-dibulae has been replaced and that bridge stability has the same favorable prognosis as in the original jawbone.

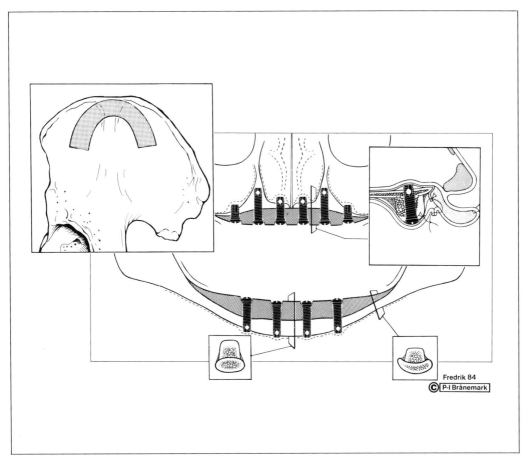

Fig. 1-40   Schematic representation of procedure for one-stage reconstruction treatment of edentulous jawbone with advanced resorption, using immediate grafting of autologous bone and marrow from donor site in the iliac bone.

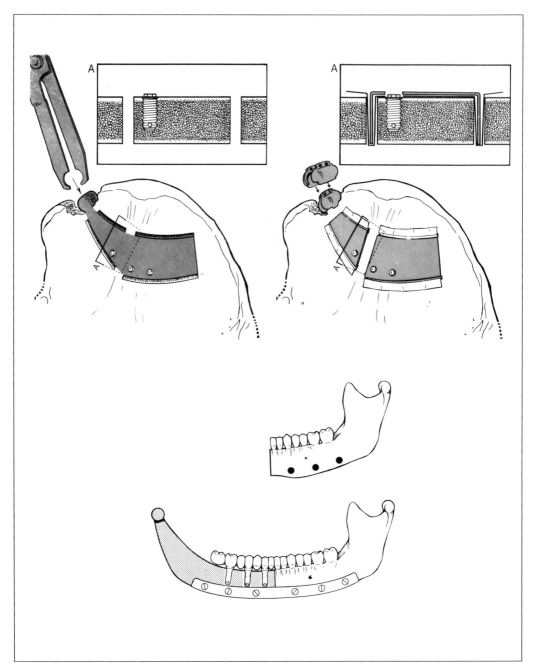

Fig. 1-41 Diagrammatic summary of reconstruction of the defective mandible using a preformed autologous bone and marrow graft from os ileum in combination with osseointegrated fixtures for attaching a stabilizing splint and anchoring a bridge device. A special mold is used for shaping a new capitulum.

Osseointegration in clinical dentistry

The edentulous jaw is a typical example of a tissue defect that causes different degrees of functional impairment. A well-fitting removable prosthesis appears to be an acceptable alternative to natural teeth, provided the anatomy of the remaining hard and soft tissues allow good retention for the denture and the patient can function orally and totally with this prosthetic device. Progressive loss of alveolar bone presumably related to, for instance, inadequate load remodelling stimulus to the jawbone via the denture (Figs. 1-42a to e) often results in instability of the prosthesis, causing more or less serious functional and psychosocial problems.

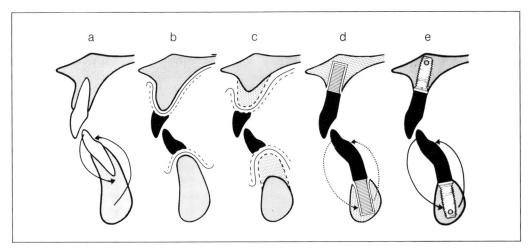

Figs. 1-42a to e   Diagrammatic representation of jawbone anatomy in a sagittal section of the frontal jaw region illustrates the biomechanical situation for implants in relation to various degrees of resorption of the alveolar process. In extreme resorption there is very unfavorable leverage. This is due to the increasing distance between the jawbone and the occlusal plane, and the sometimes accompanying unfavorable topography of implants because of resorption anatomy, particularly in the horizontal plane. Figures 1-42c and d show the lack of direct connection between the tooth substitute and the jawbone resulting in inadequate stability of the prosthetic device and inadequate remodelling stimulus for bone remodelling.

Fig. 1-42a   Arrows show mechanical interrelation between teeth and jawbone illustrating how the jawbone anchors teeth or prostheses, thus providing adequate bone remodelling stimulus for the jawbone by maintaining bone volume and density.

Fig. 1-42b   Denture-compensated edentulism.

Fig. 1-42c   The jawbone has been augmented by biologic or nonbiologic material using onlay procedures.

Fig. 1-42d   Prosthetic device anchored in soft tissue provides inadequate mechanical stability and insufficient load-remodelling stimulus.

Fig. 1-42e   Osseointegrated prosthetic device provides both stability and bone-remodelling stimulus.

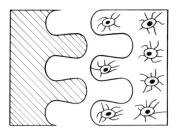 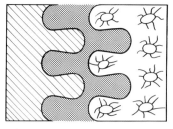

Figs. 1-43a to f Schematic representations of different kinds of interface zones.

Figs. 1-43a and b Use of so-called bone cement to fill anatomical discrepancies between implant and bone. As a consequence of surgical trauma and the impact of the cement the bone tissue is more or less severely damaged. (From Albrektsson et al.[28])

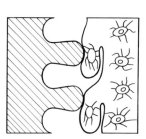 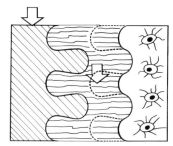

Figs. 1-43c and d Noncemented prosthetic installation where the preparatory damage to the bone results in bone resorption and a connective tissue interface with low mechanical capacity and also low resistance to inflammatory processes. (Fig. 1-43c from Albrektsson et al.[28])

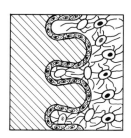 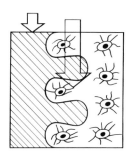

Fig. 1-43e Noncemented anchorage but with thin cellular layer of connective tissue between more or less normal bone and implant. Even in this situation there is a locus minoris resistentiae and a less predictable long-term result.

Fig. 1-43f Direct connection between implant and living bone. Experimentally and clinically this type of implant anchorage has proven to be superior to the others and the only one in which the long-term outcome in the individual case is predictable. (From Albrektsson et al.[28])

Various attempts have been made to anchor dental prostheses in soft or hard tissues. Judging from available long-term clinical follow-up studies, these methods have not resulted in good long-term function, particularly in those cases most in need of a stable device, namely, patients with extreme resorption of the alveolar bone in the maxilla and mandible. Unfortunately, the result often has been local tissue derangement, leaving the edentulous patient in a much worse situation for retention of a conventional denture than before the implants were inserted, and sometimes with long-standing inflammatory processes, osteitis, nerve lesions, pain condition, etc. Attempts to insert an implant to be anchored by regenerated tissue, believed to simulate the periodontal ligament, have not been successful. According to the literature, a loaded implant inserted directly into living bone does not function over longer periods of time because (1) rejection mechanisms inevitably lead to formation of low differentiated connective tissue, which separates the implant from bone tissue, and (2) local inflammatory reactions, despite antibiotic treatment, which inevitably not only cause loss of stable anchorage but also, via long-standing osteitis, lead to severe loss of jawbone.

Thus, the prevailing opinion is that attempts to make biologic and nonbiologic materials exist and work together inevitably lead to failure. Contrary to this view, our long-term experience of jawbone-anchored prostheses in partially or completely edentulous jaws according to the principle of osseointegration strongly suggests that the hard and soft tissue prognosis is good and predictable. Therefore, osseointegration seems to provide a realistic treatment alternative for rehabilitation of edentulism.

Orthopedic reconstruction (e.g., endoprostheses for joint repair, using nonbiological prosthetic material) is commonly based on anchorage in bone by means of a space-filling bone cement, such as methylmethacrylate. This procedure causes inevitable osteocyte death at the site of insertion because of mechanical, thermal, and chemical injury. After an initial period of implant retention bone resorption takes place, accelerated by functional loading, and the implant will eventually become surrounded by a layer of low differentiated soft tissue. Subsequently, the implant becomes separated from healthy bone by a layer of non-mineralized tissue, resulting in inadequate retention. Furthermore, the surrounding bone is not given sufficient loading stimulus to promote bone remodelling (Figs. 1-43a to f).

This series of events will occur even if the implant originally is stably anchored to bone without any nonbiologic space-filler, but where the interphase consists of a tissue which, at insertion of the prosthesis, has been damaged to such an extent that it will not heal into organized bone and marrow tissues. Surgical and loading trauma will bring about the development of a thin layer of low differentiated scar tissue between implant and bone. In the long run, such an interface will become mechanically insufficient, allowing uncontrolled movements between implant and bone. If the implant is connected with an abutment penetrating skin or mucous membranes, these relative movements at functional loading add a risk for inflammatory reactions and bacterial invasion from the external environment to the site of anchorage. This transport of noxious agents can eventually be propagated by the pumping micromovements that occur when the soft tissue is being deformed because of displacement of the implant in its topographic relation to the surrounding bone. In the long-term prognostic perspective this situation should be compared with the osseointegrated fixtures that are directly united to living, remodelling bone without an intermediate soft-tissue layer and therefore with the implant moving with, and as a mechanical part of, the incorporating hard tissue; thus, load is transferred directly to the anchoring bone. The crucial point is that *bone and marrow must be made to heal as highly differentiated tissues and not allowed to develop into low differentiated scar tissue.*

In order to create osseointegration it is necessary to prepare the bone with a minimum of tissue injury. In the treatment of edentulous jaws it is imperative to respect certain important principles that are true for all implant procedures. A minimal volume of remaining bone should be removed and the original jawbone topography must as far as possible be left intact. As a consequence, the removal of fixtures in case of nonosseointegration is not detrimental to the original jaw anatomy: substitutional new bone will grow into the previous implant site and restore bone topography to its preoperative state. If osseointegration cannot be achieved and the implant has to be removed, or if the patient wants to return to the use of a conventional prosthesis, it is important that the retention anatomy is the same as it was before installing the fixtures.

Logically, only one basic shape of implant is required. After 30 years of experimental and 20 years of clinical development work, the authors have chosen a fixture design of a screwlike implant of pure titanium, which has an outer diameter of 3.7 mm and lengths varying from 7 to 18 mm (Figs. 1-44a to c). This anchoring element can be used in any edentulous jaw irrespective of volume and quality of the remaining bone tissue provided it is installed, allowed to become incorporated, and loaded via a bridge according to the requirements of the procedure.

Both prostheses and abutments are connected to the fixtures with screws, allowing removal for technical adjustment. The abutments can also be removed and the fixtures again covered with mucoperiosteum for a short period or even indefinitely (Fig. 1-45). This system of a fixed bridge construction attached to a set of anchoring units provides a high degree of mechanical flexibility and also a wide choice of bridge designs and materials.

Figs. 1-44a to d Reconstructive procedures to be used in defect situations that are not life threatening must be designed so that if the procedure fails, the patient is not in a worse situation than before the treatment was applied. In rehabilitation of edentulism this means that the patient should be able to return to a denture, with basically the same retention anatomy as before installation of the fixtures.

To minimize negative effects in the long-term perspective the nonbiologic components in the anchorage unit should be of minimal volume and surface area, the microarchitecture of the titanium surface should fit the requirements of the ground substance and cells of the hard and soft tissues, and the surface must be completely clean and noncontaminated minimizing the risk for creating a local tissue rejection reaction.

Small separate anchorage elements give optimal flexibility in the clinical reconstruction situation and require removal of minimal volume of remaining bone tissue to provide a site for the anchorage element. Also, if one element fails, the remaining integrated fixtures because of excessive anchorage capacity will provide stable anchorage for the bridge, allowing the patient continued good oral function with a stable bridge, while additional fixtures, if required, are being integrated.

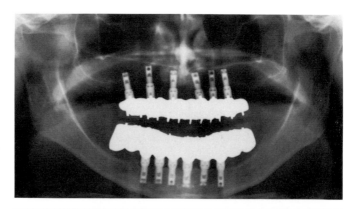

Fig. 1-44a Typical topography of fixtures in reconstructed maxilla and mandible. (From Brånemark[23])

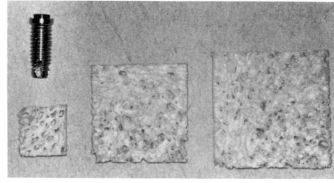

Fig. 1-44b Shows the relative dimensions between the fixtures, overall length of 10 mm and diameter of 3.75 mm, and the anchoring surface for one, four, and six fixtures, respectively.

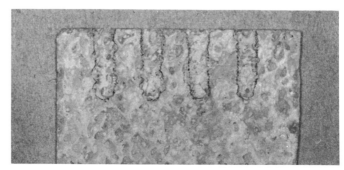

Fig. 1-44c Shows a complete failure situation with loss of all anchoring fixtures. The retention anatomy for a conventional denture is the same as before fixture installation.

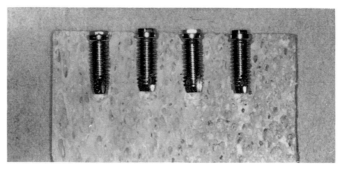

Fig. 1-44d After healing under the covering mucoperiosteum new fixtures can be installed in the previous sites which meanwhile have been filled by new bone formation. Additional fixtures could also be installed after a short intermediate period in the bone tissue between the original fixture sites.

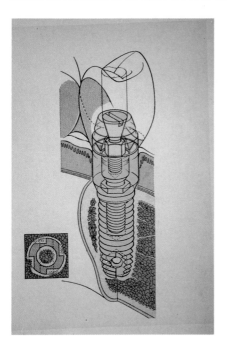

Fig. 1-45 Schematic representation of anchorage unit based on principle of screw-connected components: fixture, abutment, and center screw for prosthesis attachment. The apical part of the titanium fixture is designed to cut and thread the bottom of the bone site. (From Adell et al.[29])

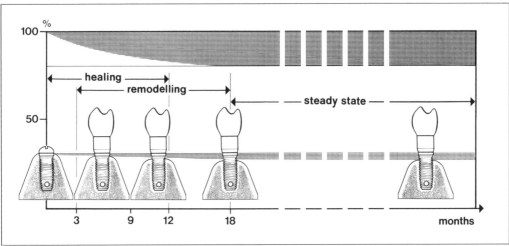

Fig. 1-46 The dynamic relation between the fixture and the jawbone can be distinguished in time into three—partly overlapping—periods. During the *healing* phase new bone is formed close to the immobile, resting implant. When the implant is exposed to masticatory forces, the newly formed bone *remodels* according to the magnitude, direction, and frequency of the applied load. After about 18 months a *steady state* is achieved, which means that there is a balance between the forces acting on the implant and the remodelling capacities of the anchoring bone. The hatched area at the top of the diagram illustrates the reduction in height of anchoring bone, expressed in percent of the original level of embedding jawbone, which occurs during the healing and remodelling phase. (From Brånemark et al.[1])

Handling of hard and soft tissues

The healing time of bone tissue after fixture insertion in the jaw has been empirically estimated, in large clinical series, at three to six months, with the fixtures unloaded except for the normal functional load of that particular edentulous bone region (Fig. 1-46). When the prosthesis has been connected to the abutments the jawbone around the anchoring element will continue to remodel during several years until a "steady state" has been reached (Fig. 1-47). Due to the surgical trauma at fixture insertion and the gradual adaptation to the load, some marginal bone is lost during the remodelling phase, whereas once the steady state has been reached, negligible bone resorption takes place as evaluated at yearly radiographic examinations using computerized periodic identical radiography.

Even if great care is taken at the time of surgery, one cannot avoid some bone damage and, thus, the long healing period of three to six months (see Figs. 1-2a to d). When controlled functional loads are applied, the bone will remodel to a shape and density that relates to the direction and size of the load. If the surgical trauma has been too large, or if excessive loads are applied, the process of osseointegration will be disturbed and soft-tissue formation may take place. The demineralization phase, which occurs as an important part of the bone-healing process when osseointegration is established, is particularly sensitive to dynamic load transfer and subsequent deformation and displacement between the fixture surface and the young osteoid tissue. Even then implant retention may be adequate, but will not last in the long run. It appears that with time the soft-tissue layer increases in width; it is advisable to remove a nonosseointegrated fixture.

When designing the surgical procedure it is important to minimize risks of damaging sensitive tissues such as nerves and vessels in the upper and lower jaw. Because of

Fig. 1-47   The dynamic load stimulus conveyed to the bone tissue via the osseointegrated fixtures provides adequate remodelling stimulus for the bone tissue between the fixtures to remain in height and volume and eventually to increase in density (see Fig. 1-51). According to 10-year follow-up studies the load also seems to preserve the bone tissue distal to the foramina in the lower jaw, apparently markedly reducing the "physiological" resorption of the edentulous jaw.

In the edentulous mandible, fixture sites were located between the mental foramina and not distal to them for two major reasons.

First of all, in a situation where the load, even of a full bridge construction, could be taken of fixtures located mesial to the foramina, the risk of nerve and vessel lesion was avoided.

Secondly, in a completely edentulous mandible fixtures placed distal to the foramina and joined by a rigid construction to fixtures in mesial position might interfere with normal load deformation of the mandible, thereby possibly exerting a negative influence on flow and remodelling of bone in the lower jaw.

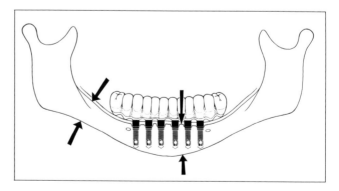

Figs. 1-48a to g   Radiographs of main types of resorption anatomy in patients comprising our clinical material.

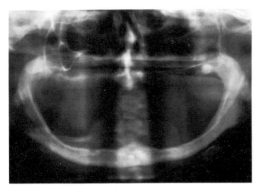

Fig. 1-48a   Orthopantomogram showing advanced resorption.

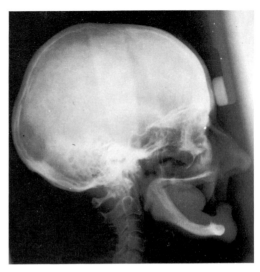

Fig. 1-48b   Profile radiogram showing extreme resorption.

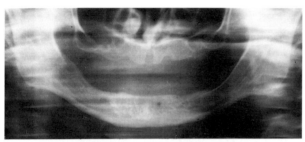

Figs. 1-48c to e   Typical progressive bone loss in edentulous jaw at five-year intervals.

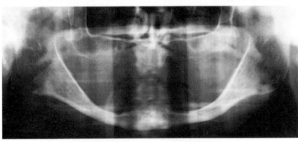

Fig. 1-48d

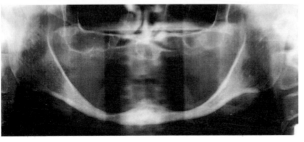

Fig. 1-48e

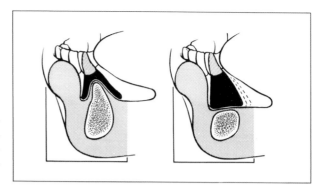

Fig. 1-48f Diagrammatic representation of lower jaw morphology corresponding to jawbone topography represented in Figs. 1-48c and e, respectively.

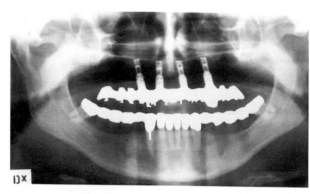

Fig. 1-48g Reconstruction using four fixtures in an extremely resorbed maxilla.

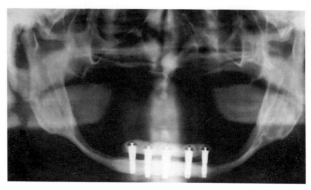

Fig. 1-48h Extreme resorption of edentulous mandible with fixtures, which at installation penetrated the lower border of the lower jaw (see Fig. 1-54).

the anchorage capacity of osseointegrated fixtures, loaded under controlled conditions, fixture placement can be restricted to the area between the mental foramina in the lower jaw and between the anterior recesses of the sinuses in the upper jaw (Figs. 1-48a to h and 1-49a to e). Cantilevered extensions can be used so that an adequate fixed replacement dentition can be provided. A minimum of four fixtures, well inte-

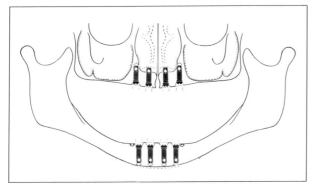

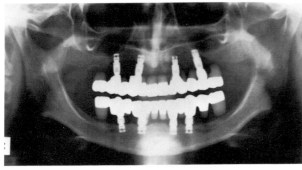

Fig. 1-49a Diagrammatic representation of a case with four osseointegrated fixtures supporting upper and lower full arch prostheses. (From Adell et al.[29])

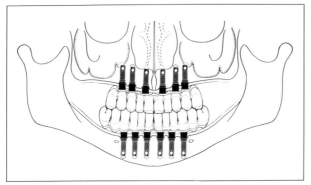

Fig. 1-49b Orthopantomographic representation. (From Brånemark et al.[1])

Figs. 1-49c and d If adequate space is available between maxillary sinuses or mandibular foramina, six fixtures are installed as support. (Fig. 1-49c from Adell et al.[29])

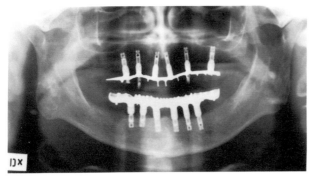

Fig. 1-49d

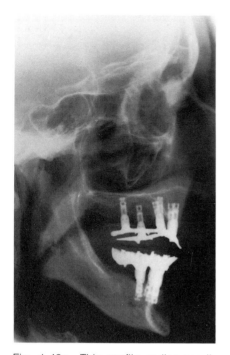

Fig. 1-49e This profile radiogram illustrates how the bridge can be extended to provide an adequate dentition even in the premolar region.

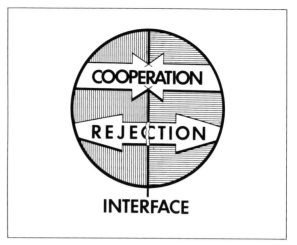

Fig. 1-50 Prognostic predictability is provided by extreme precision at surgical installation of noncontaminated titanium components with correct surface microarchitecture in combination with occlusal adjustments of the fitting bridge superstructure distributing the load to the fixtures. Cooperation at the interface level between molecular, cellular, and tissue components creates a strong dynamic connection between biologic and nonbiologic material. Once established after careful control of healing and initial loading, rejection can be prevented by careful control of the condition of the soft and hard tissues. (From Brånemark[23])

grated in bone of good quality, is sufficient for a functionally adequate prosthetic replacement in an edentulous jaw. Nevertheless, if topographically possible, six fixtures are recommended as a safety measure, should integration not be achieved or later fail for one of the anchorage elements, or should mechanical failure occur.

While a gentle surgical technique is essential to establish osseointegration, careful prosthetic procedures and control of the healthy state of the mucoperiosteum is vital for the maintenance of osseointegration (Fig. 1-50). Frequent checkups and adjustments of occlusion are of great importance. In order to provide a mechanical substitute for the resilience of the periodontium, the artificial teeth are made of a plastic material which will function as a shock absorber. Most patients treated with the os-

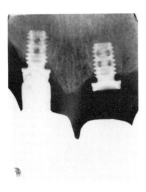

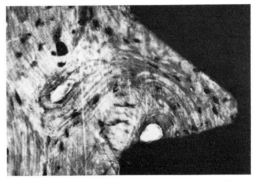

Bone ——→|←— Fixture ——→|←— Bone

Fig. 1-51a An upper jaw fixture with surrounding bone removed because of failure of mechanical components after six years of function with persisting integration. (From Brånemark[23])

Fig. 1-51b Densitometric analysis of radiograph in Fig. 1-51a, taken immediately before removing the fixture, shows osseointegration without any intermediate soft tissue, and increased density of bone close to the fixture.

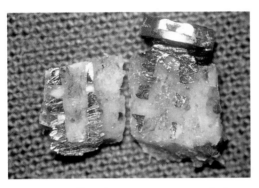

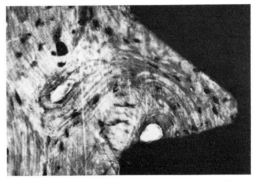

Fig. 1-51c Specimen was removed by a trephine and cut longitudinally into two halves with a diamond disk, but with bone tissue still firmly—and inseparably—adhering to the titanium surface.

Fig. 1-51d Ground section of bone and fixture showing integration (40x). (From Brånemark[23])

Figs. 51d and f produced in collaboration with T. Albrektsson, Dept. of Anatomy, University of Gothenburg, Sweden.

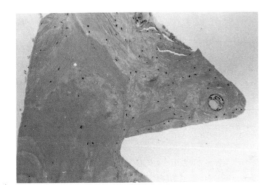

Fig. 1-51e In light microscopy, bone threads of the fixture site are clearly defined. (From Brånemark[23])

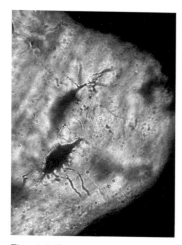

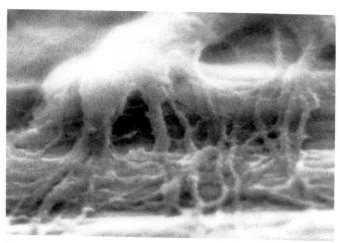

Fig. 1-51f At higher resolution of the ground section in Fig. 1-51d two osteocytes in their lacunae, with interconnecting system of canaliculi, indicate normal microstructure of bone close to the titanium surface.

Fig. 1-51g High resolution scanning electron micrograph of an osteoblast with its cellular processes adapted to surface of fixture shown in Fig. 1-51c.

seointegration method show an extreme loss of alveolar bone preoperatively. The vertical size of this tissue defect must be substituted for by the prosthesis and requires particular designing skill in order to assure adequate load distribution at mastication and to meet phonetic and cosmetic requirements.

Objective evidence of permanent osseointegration of loaded fixtures was obtained through the analysis of osseointegrated implants removed from patients because of mechanical rather than biological failure (Figs. 1-51a to g). Typical for these fixtures is that they cannot be removed from the implant site without causing fracture in the bone rather than cleavage at the actual interface between bone and titanium. Cellular processes of osteoblasts spreading onto the titanium surface indicate acceptance of the implanted material at the cell membrane level. Biopsies from the mucoperiosteum surrounding the transepithelial abutment show soft-tissue cells, collagen, and ground substance which appear to create a seal toward the oral cavity, similar to crevicular epithelium and subgingival tissues at teeth (Figs. 1-52a to g and 1-53).

Biophysical and chemical analyses of clinical fixtures after long-term function indicate that there is in fact an ongoing active interchange between the surface oxides on implanted titanium fixtures and the hard and soft tissues (Figs. 1-54a to e).

Criteria for clinical success or failure

The basic aims of applying osseointegration in clinical dentistry to provide reconstruction in cases of partial or total edentulism is to bring the patient back to a state similar to a dentate condition, irrespective of the re-

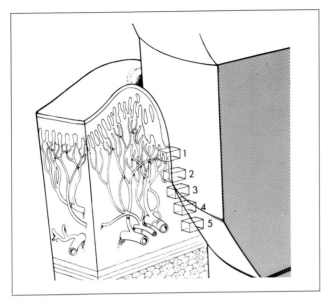

Fig. 1-52a A three-dimensional schematic of the relationship between the gingiva and a titanium abutment. The numbers indicate the localization of the electron microscopic sections (see below). The light and electron micrographs in Figs. 1-52a to g were processed and analyzed by Dr. L. E. Ericson and Dr. P. Thomsen, Dept. of Anatomy, University of Göteborg, Sweden.

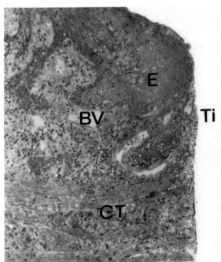

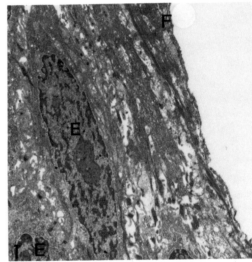

Fig. 1-52b Light micrograph of the tissue adjacent to an oral titanium abutment connected to an osseointegrated fixture after six years of uneventful function. The junction between the (removed) titanium implant (Ti) and the epithelium (E) and subepithelial connective tissue (CT) is shown. Blood vessels (BV) are present beneath the epithelium surrounded by perivascular infiltrates of macrophages and lymphocytes. No inflammatory cells are present in the connective tissue close to the implant (original magnification 150x).

Fig. 1-52c (1) Electron micrograph of the surface of the gingival epithelium not in contact with the titanium implant. Filamentous material (F) is present on the surface. E = epithelial cells (original magnification 5000x).

Fig. 1-52d *(2)* Electron micrograph of the junction between the gingival epithelial cells and the subepithelial connective tissue adjacent to the (removed) titanium abutment *(Ti)*. The epithelial cells are furnished with desmosomes *(arrows)* and hemidesmosomes *(arrowheads)*. The epithelial basal lamina *(open arrows)* separates the epithelial cells from the connective tissue containing collagen *(Co)*. The interface between tissue and implant consists of filamentous material probably originating from disintegrated epithelial cells (*) (original magnification 7000x).

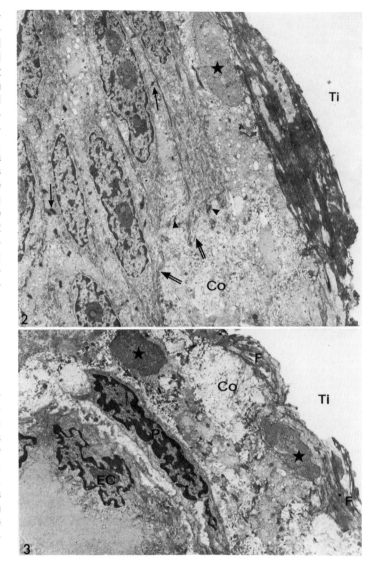

Fig. 1-52e *(3)* Electron micrograph of a capillary located close to the titanium abutment *(Ti)*. A pericyte is located in close proximity to an endothelial cell *(EC)*. Filamentous material *(F)*, disintegrating epithelial cells (*), and collagen *(Co)* form the interface between tissue and implant (original magnification 9000x).

sorption anatomy of the edentulous jaw and bone quality (Figs. 1-55a and b). This means stable, safe, and reliable anchorage of a prosthetic substitute for teeth, functioning as a fixed bridge on natural teeth with a predictable duration—without significant complications—for the patient's lifetime.

This presupposes that the functional anatomy of the remaining edentulous jawbone can be maintained by subjecting it to controlled, adequate load stimuli, resulting in remodelling and activation of the bone tissue. The long-term healthy state of the anchoring bone and the covering mucosa

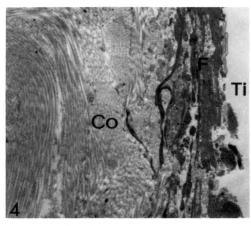

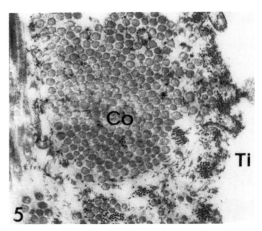

Fig. 1-52f *(4)* Subepithelial connective tissue close to the (removed) titanium abutment *(Ti)*. Filamentous material *(F)* separates the surface of the abutment from collagen fibers *(Co)* (original magnification 8000x).

Fig. 1-52g *(5)* Deep part of the subepithelial connective tissue close to the titanium abutment *(Ti)*. Collagen *(Co)* and filamentous material are in close contact with the surface of the abutment. In the dense connective tissue, composed by orderly arranged collagen bundles and fibrils close to the titanium surface, there are no signs of inflammation (original magnification 33,000x).

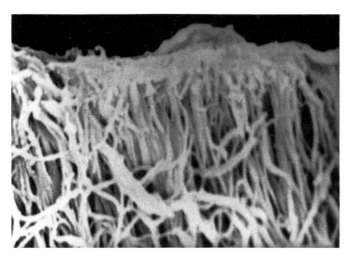

Fig. 1-53 Topographical arrangement of collagen fiber bundles in the mucosa close to a titanium abutment from a clinical case as visualized by SEM.
The three-dimensional interwoven pattern of collagen results in the formation of a mechanical cuff, which participates in creating a structural and functional seal between the oral cavity and the anchorage region.

must be preserved both by precise control of masticatory load distribution via a perfectly fitting prosthetic construction and by maintaining the mucoperiosteal functional barrier toward the oral cavity at the piercing abutments without persisting deep inflammatory processes. With these precautions

osseointegration has been successfully used in jaws of varying degrees of resorption anatomy and bone quality in patients of ages ranging from 20 to 79 years at fixture installation. Good long-term results have been obtained even in cases of supposedly low healing capacity of hard and soft tis-

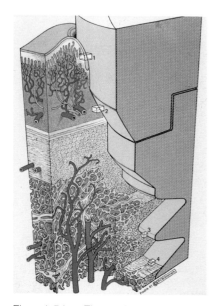

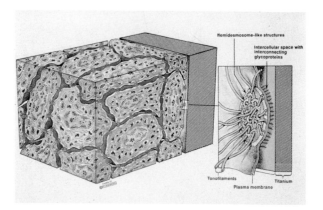

Fig. 1-54b Enlarged schematic of gingiva-titanium oxide contact zone. Inset demonstrates a hemidesmosomelike structure anchoring the epithelial cells to the implant surface.

Fig. 1-54a Three-dimensional diagram of tissue-titanium interrelationship showing an overall view of the intact interface zone around osseointegrated implants. The numbers 1 to 4 indicate the localization of the detailed interface descriptions visualized in Figs. 1-54b to e.

Fig. 1-54c High resolution drawing of subgingival connective tissue at the boundary zone. Fibroblast processes are seen in immediate contact with the titanium oxide surface, in reality though separated from it by a thin layer of proteoglycanes. A network of collagen and blood vessels approaches the titanium surface and surrounds a normal blood vessel.

Fig. 1-54d Interface between cortical bone and titanium. An osteocyte with numerous processes in canaliculi approaches the titanium oxide surface. The calcified ground substance around the osteocyte is removed to show details. A meshwork of collagen surrounds the bone cell. There is an intimate contact between the ground substance of the haversian bone and the titanium oxide.

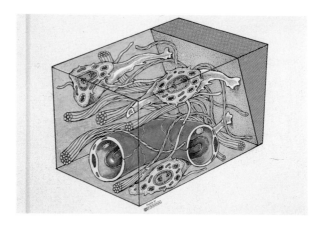

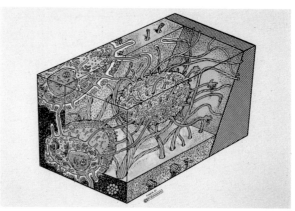

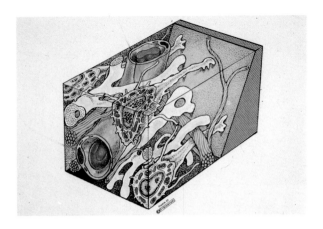

Fig. 1-54e Contact layer between cancellous bone and implant. Note fibroblast and osteoblast processes approaching the titanium surface. The bone trabeculae are seen in close relationship to the implant surface and to a blood vessel. (From Albrektsson et al.[30])

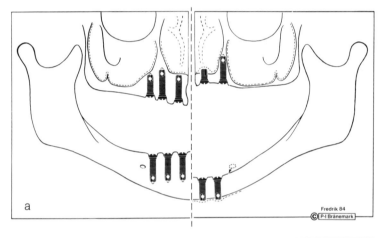

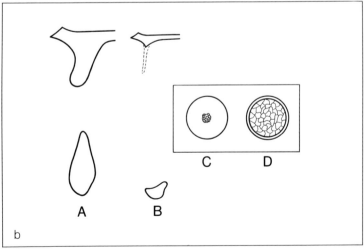

Figs. 1-55a and b Diagrammatic representation of range of jawbone defect anatomy and varying qualities of bone where the osseointegration procedure has been successfully applied. (A) Minimal resorption. (B) Maximal resorption. (C) Maximal bone density. (D) Minimal bone density.

sues, such as long-standing diabetes and after therapeutic doses of radiation.

Criteria for clinical success or failure when using implanted nonbiologic prostheses in human hard or soft tissues must be defined both with respect to the patient's need for permanent structural and functional reconstruction, and the reactions of the anchoring hard and soft tissues being ultimately responsible for the long-term survival and function of the reconstruction.

The patients must be well informed about the perspectives of the procedure. Its basic aim is stable anchorage of a prosthetic device. It is important to *exclude* those patients with psychiatric problems (dysmorphoparanoia, neuroses, drug abuse, etc.) where even a perfectly reconstructed oral tissue situation is not accompanied by psychosocial rehabilitation. It is, however, equally important to *include* for treatment those patients whose edentulism is a causal factor behind their psychiatric or social problems. Because of the importance of correct patient selection, a psychiatrist has been included, since 1968, in the treatment team in Göteborg, collaborating both preoperatively and postoperatively during the development period for all cases and thereafter for patients with a special psychiatric history.

The patients' appraisal of the prosthesis, its stability and likeness to their natural teeth, their unawareness of the previous edentulism, the lack of local tissue problems, etc., are important for identifying a successful clinical rehabilitation effect. However, such a patient might have a hard- and soft-tissue condition that is far from acceptable from the biologic and prognostic point of view.

Therefore, it is imperative that ordinary clinical criteria are used to establish objective definitions of the state of the tissues. Stability of bridge and separate anchorage units can be evaluated manually with the superstructure removed, and modifications of routine procedures for examinations of gingival conditions can be used. The state and remodelling of the anchoring jawbone can be objectively evaluated by controlled radiography, and numerically interpreted and followed with the aid of computerized image analyses based on the fact that the fixtures are anatomically identical and of symmetric geometry (see Figs. 1-51a to g).

Combining information on the patient's oral and total function and local soft- and hard-tissue condition, it is possible to prognosticate fairly accurately the long-term oral function for a specific patient. This requires that individual estimates are related to and based on numerical information from consecutive long-term clinical materials of representative resorption anatomy and bone character. That means that, to provide reliable reference statistics, every patient treated, and every fixture installed, must be followed up for at least 10 years with regular clinical controls. In addition, the preoperative resorption anatomy of this clinical material must represent the entire range of jawbone anatomy and quality. It goes without saying that the procedure, in order to be really useful in oral rehabilitation for patients most in need of a tissue-integrated prosthesis, must be equally applicable to the edentulous mandible and maxilla in their different stages of resorption anatomy and with varying bone quality (see Figs. 1-55a and b).

The present state of long-term clinical prognosis can be illustrated by results obtained in a consecutive series of edentulous patients, who were treated with bridges on osseointegrated fixtures during 1965 to 1974. In this material, with a follow-up period of 10 to 19 years, and with every patient controlled at least once a year, there were 161 jaws – 85 upper and 76 lower. Bridge stability was found to be 99% in lower jaws and 89% in upper jaws. Radiographic examination including computerized image

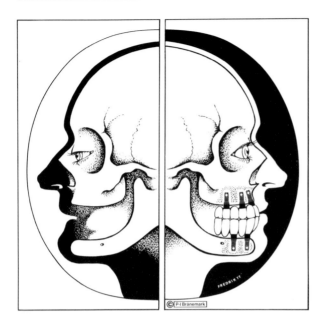

Fig. 1-56 Reconstruction with tissue-integrated prostheses in partial or complete edentulism provides a structural and functional restitution to a state similar to the dentate situation also preventing further bone resorption. In addition to the local oral rehabilitation effects there are also positive consequences for the entire psychosocial condition of the previous oral invalid. (From Brånemark et al.[1])

analysis of bone remodelling at the interface showed that the anchoring bone had reached a steady state for marginal height with a yearly loss of less than 0.1 mm and with increasing density. The mucosa at the abutment penetrations was, as a rule, clinically healthy.

Stomatognatho-physiological investigations on patients with jawbone-anchored bridges using electromyographic recordings, measurement of maximal masticatory forces and force as when chewing, foil discrimination tests and chewing time determination, as well as analysis of the three-dimensional movement of the rehabilitated mandible towards the maxilla and circumoral muscle behavioral patterns revealed that bridges on osseointegrated fixtures bring the edentulous patient back to an oral function similar to that of a dentate situation with the same extension of the dentition. Furthermore, long-term follow-up analysis with 10 years interval indicates that after installation of a jawbone-anchored bridge, the maximal bite force increases about 30% and the bite force as when chewing increases 100% over the same time period indicating a positive dynamic interaction between the tissue-anchored prosthetic device and the neuromuscular system of the edentulous patient.

On the basis of the long-term clinical results obtained with osseointegration in oral rehabilitation it seems justified to conclude that complete and partial edentulism can be safely treated with jawbone-anchored prostheses, and without risks of untoward tissue reactions, provided proper handling of the host tissues and load distributions is followed (Fig. 1-56).

Acknowledgements

The late Viktor Kuikka provided invaluable assistance in the development of titanium components and surgical instruments for experimental and clinical application of the osseointegration procedure.

Illustrations were made by Fredrik Johansson.

References

1. *Brånemark, P.-I., et al.*
Osseointegrated implants in the treatment of the edentulous jaw. Experience from a 10-year period. Scand. J. Plast. Reconstr. Surg. 16 (Suppl.), 1977.

2. *Albrektsson, B.*
Repair of diaphyseal defects. Thesis, University of Göteborg, Sweden, 1971.

3. *Lundborg, G., and Brånemark, P.-I.*
Microvascular structure and function of peripheral nerves. Adv. Microcirc. 1:66-68, 1968.

4. *Myrhage, R., et al.*
Nutrition and healing of flexor tendons in synovial environment. Adv. Biomater. Vol. 4, 1982.

5. *Amundson, B.*
Skeletal muscle microcirculation and metabolism in hemorrhagic shock. Thesis, University of Göteborg, Sweden, 1979.

6. *Brånemark, P.-I., and Eriksson, E.*
Method for studying qualitative and quantitative changes of blood flow in skeletal muscle. Acta Physiol. Scand. 84:284-288, 1972.

7. *Brånemark, P.-I., and Birch, J.*
Microvascular damage produced by a plastic film wound dressing. Scand. J. Plast. Reconstr. Surg. 2:71-76, 1968.

8. *Birch, J., Brånemark, P.-I., and Lundskog, J.*
The vascularization of a free full thickness skin graft. II. A microangiographic study. Scand. J. Plast. Reconstr. Surg. 3:11-17, 18-22, 1969.

9. *Brånemark, P.-I., and Lindström, J.*
A modified rabbit's ear chamber. High-power, high-resolution studies in regenerated and preformed tissues. Anat. Rec. 145:533-540, 1963.

10. *Costa, O., and Brånemark, P.-I.*
Vital microscopic evaluation of the microvessels of the cochlea. Adv. Microcirc. 3:96-107, 1970.

11. *Brånemark, P.-I., et al.*
Microvascular pathophysiology of burned tissue. Ann. NY Acad. Sci. 150:474-494, 1968.

12. *Birch, J., et al.*
Vascular reactions in an experimental burn studied with infrared thermography and microangiography. Scand. J. Plast. Reconstr. Surg. 2:97-103, 1968.

13. *Brånemark, P.-I., and Nilsson, K.*
Thermographic and microvascular studies of the peripheral circulation. Proc. of a Boerhaave Course for Postgrad. Med. Education, Leiden, The Netherlands, 1968. Bibl. Radiol. 5:130-142, 1969.

14. *Brånemark, P.-I., and Urbaschek, G.*
Endotoxins in tissue injury. Angiology 18:667-671, 1967.

15. *Brånemark, P.-I.*
Capillary form and function. The microcirculation of granulation tissue. Bibl. Anat. 7:9-28, 1965.

16. *Lindhe, J., and Brånemark, P.-I.*
Observations on vascular proliferation in a granulation tissue. J. Periodont. Res. 5:276-292, 1970.

17. *Brånemark, P.-I.*
Vital microscopy of bone marrow in rabbit. Thesis, University of Lund, Sweden. Scand. J. Lab. Invest. 11 (Suppl. 38):1-82, 1959.

18. *Brånemark, P.-I.*
Bone marrow microvascular structure and function. Adv. Microcirc. 1:1-65, 1968.

19. *Brånemark, P.-I., et al.*
Regeneration of bone marrow. A clinical and experimental study following removal of bone marrow by curettage. Acta Anat. 59:1-46, 1964.

20. *Brånemark, P.-I., and Breine, U.*
Formation of bone marrow in isolated segment of rib periosteum in rabbit and dog. Blut 10:236-252, 1964.

21. *Hallén, O., et al.*
Preformed autologous ossicles. Experimental studies. Acta Otolaryngol. 82:394-401, 1976.

22. *Adell, R.*
Regeneration of the periodontium. Diss., Göteborg, Sweden. Scand. J. Plast. Reconstr. Surg. 11 (Suppl.), 1974.

23. *Brånemark, P.-I.*
Osseointegration and its experimental background. J. Prosthet. Dent. 50:399-410, 1983.

24. *Brånemark, P.-I., et al.*
Intra-osseous anchorage of dental prostheses. I. Experimental studies. Scand. J. Plast. Reconstr. Surg. 3:81-100, 1969.

25. *Breine, U., and Brånemark, P.-I.*
Reconstruction of alveolar jawbone. An experimental and clinical study of immediate and preformed autologous bone grafts in combination with osseointegrated implants. Scand. J. Plast. Reconstr. Surg. 14:23-48, 1980.

26. *Brånemark, P.-I.*
Intravascular anatomy of blood cells in man. Monograph. Basel: S. Karger, 1971, pp. 1-80.

27. *Brånemark, P.-I., Haljamäe, H., and Lundborg, G.*
Pathophysiology of microvascular and interstitial compartments in low flow states. pp. 321-343 *In* Les Solutés de Substitution Rééquilibration Métabolique. Paris: Librairie Arnette, 1971.

28. *Albrektsson, T., et al.*
Osseointegrated titanium implants. Requirements for ensuring a long-lasting, direct bone anchorage in man. Acta Orthop. Scand. 52:155-170, 1981.

29. *Adell, R., et al.*
A 15-year study of osseointegrated implants in the treatment of the edentulous jaw. Int. J. Oral Surg. 10:387-416, 1981.

30. *Albrektsson, T., et al.*
The interface zone of inorganic implants in vivo: Titanium implants in bone. Ann. Biomed. Eng. 11:1-27, 1983.

Further Reading

Adell, R., et al. Intra-osseous anchorage of dental prostheses. II. Review of clinical approaches. Scand. J. Plast. Reconstr. Surg. 4:19-34, 1970.

Adell, R., Skalak, R., and Brånemark, P.-I. A preliminary study of rheology of granulocytes. Blut 21:91-105, 1970.

Albrektsson, T., et al. The preformed autologous bone graft. An experimental study in rabbits. Scand. J. Plast. Reconstr. Surg. 12:215-223, 1978.

Albrektsson, T., et al. Ultrastructural analysis of the interface zone of titanium and gold implants. pp. 137-138 *In* Proc. 2nd Europ. Conf. on Biomaterials, Göteborg, Sweden, 27-29 Aug. 1981. Adv. Biomater. 4:167-177, 1982.

Albrektsson, B., and Brånemark, P.-I. Early microvascular reactions to slow and rapid thawing of frozen tissue. Adv. Microcirc. 2:37-68, 1969.

Albrektsson, T., Brånemark, P.-I., and Lindström, J. Osseointegrerade benimplantat, undersökning av interfacezonen. Abstract. Hygiea 89:386, 1980.

Albrektsson, T., Brånemark, P.-I., and Lindström, J. Transcutaneous titanium implants in clinical practice. Adv. Biomater. 4:157-166, 1982.

Asano, M., and Brånemark, P.-I. Cardiovascular and microvascular responses to smoking in man. Adv. Microcirc. 3:125-158, 1970.

Asano, M., and Brånemark, P.-I. Microcirculation studied by microphotoelectric plethysmography in man. pp. 81-85 *In* Proc. 6th Europ. Conf. on Microcirculation, Aalborg, Denmark. Basel: S. Karger, 1971.

Asano, M., and Brånemark, P.-I. Cutaneous microcirculatory responses to venous and arterial occlusion in man. Bull. Inst. Publ. Health 23:1-8, 1974.

Asano, M., Brånemark, P.-I., and Castenholz, A. A comparative study of continuous qualitative and quantitative analysis of microcirculation in man. Microkymography and microphotoelectric plethysmography applied to microvascular investigation. Adv. Microcirc. 5:1-31, 1973.

Asano, M., Brånemark, P.-I., and Myrhage, R. Microcirculatory responses to venous and arterial occlusions in man. Microvasc. Res. 3:444, 1971.

Bagge, U., et al. Three-dimensional observations of red blood cell deformation in capillaries. Blood Cells 6:231-239, 1981.

Bagge, U., and Brånemark, P.-I. White blood cell rheology. An intravital study in man. Adv. Microcirc. 7:1-17, 1977.

Bagge, U., and Brånemark, P.-I. Red cell shapes in capillaries. Abstract, Int. Symp. on Filterability and Red Blood Cell Deformability, Göteborg, Sweden, Sept. 1980.

Bagge, U., and Brånemark, P.-I. Red cell shapes in capillaries. Scand. J. Clin. Lab. Invest. 41 (Suppl.):156, 1981.

Bagge, U., Brånemark, P.-I., and Skalak, R. Measurement and influence of white cell deformability. *In* A. Lowe et al. (eds.) Clinical Aspects of Blood Viscosity and Cell Deformability. Berlin: Springer Verlag, 1981.

Birch, J., and Brånemark, P.-I. The vascularization of a free full thickness skin graft. I. A vital microscopic study. Scand. J. Plast. Reconstr. Surg. 3:1-10, 1969.

Birch, J., Brånemark, P.-I., and Lundskog, J. The influence of a vasodilator on the revascularization of a skin graft. Scand. J. Plast. Reconstr. Surg. 2:77-82, 1968.

Birch, J., Brånemark, P.-I., and Nilsson, K. The vascularization of a free full thickness skin graft. III. An infrared thermographic study. Scand. J. Plast. Reconstr. Surg. 3:18-22, 1969.

Brånemark, P.-I. Considerations on new fields and new methods of vital microscopy. Bibl. Anat. 1:38-45, 1961.

Brånemark, P.-I. Effect of nicotinic acid and histamine on capillary circulation of bone marrow in rabbit. Acta Haematol. 25:71-79, 1961.

Brånemark, P.-I. Experimental investigation of microcirculation in bone marrow. Angiology 12:293-305, 1961.

Brånemark, P.-I. The sinusoid. Bibl. Anat. 1:239-244, 1961.

Brånemark, P.-I. Vitalmikroskopie. Eine Methode für gleichzeitiges mikroskopisches Studium von Struktur und Funktion. Leitz Mitt. Wiss. u. Techn. 11:73-76, 1962.

Brånemark, P.-I. Capillary function in connective tissue. Acta Rheum. Scand. 9:3-9, 1963.

Brånemark, P.-I. Intracapillary rheological phenomena. pp. 459-473 *In* Paper presented at 4th Int. Congr. of Rheology, Providence, R. I., Aug. 1963. Symposium on Biorheology, 1963.

Brånemark, P.-I. Experimental biomicroscopy. Bibl. Anat. 5:51-55, 1964.

Brånemark, P.-I. Intracapillary behaviour of the blood. Proc. 2nd Europ. Conf. on Microcirculation, Pavia, Italy, 1962. Bibl. Anat. 4:491-495, 1964.

Brånemark, P.-I. Studies in the effect of ionizing radiation on capillary structure and capillary function. Swed. Cancer Soc. Yearbook 4:345-346, 1964.

Brånemark, P.-I. Infrarödtermografi. Medicinsk användning av värmebildsteknik. Spectrum International 2, Utg. Pfizer AB, 26-40, 1965.

Brånemark, P.-I. Infraröd-termografi. Registrering av vävnadstemperatur. Paper presented at Kärlsymposium Diabetesangiopati, Bofors, 1965.

Brånemark, P.-I. Die Infrarotthermographie in der Klinik. Dtsch. Med. Wochenschr. 20:961-962, 1966.

Brånemark, P.-I. Intravitial microscopy: Its present status and its potentialities. Med. Biol. 16:100-108, 1966.

Brånemark, P.-I. Local tissue effects of sodium fluoride. Odontol. Rev. 18:273-294, 1967.

Brånemark, P.-I. Rheological aspects of low flow states. pp. 161–180 *In* Microcirculation as Related to Shock. New York: Academic Press Inc., 1968.

Brånemark, P.-I. Pathophysiologie der Mikrozirkulation im Schock und ihre Beziehung zu metabolischen Veränderungen. pp. 33-43 *In* W. E. Zimmerman and I. Staib (eds.) Schock, Stoffwechselveraenderungen und Therapie, Proc. Symp. on Shock, Freiburg, West Germany, 1969. Stuttgart: F. K. Schattauer, 1970.

Brånemark, P.-I. Blood circulation in joints in rheumatoid arthritis and its pathogenetic importance. pp. 221-237 *In* W. Müller (ed.) Rheumatoid Arthritis. London: H. G. Harwerth & K. Fehr. Acad. Press, 1971.

Brånemark, P.-I. Rehabilitering med käkbensförankrad bettersättning. Läkartidningen 69:4813-4824, 1972.

Brånemark, P.-I. The light microscope in microvascular research, problems and measurements. Proc. 7th Europ. Conf. on Microcirculation, Aberdeen, Scotland, 1972, Part I. Bibl. Anat. 11, 219-227, 1973.

Brånemark, P.-I. Microvascular function at reduced flow rates. pp. 1-12 *In* Proc. Strathclyde Bioengineering Seminars, Glasgow, Scotland, Aug. 1975.

Brånemark, P.-I. Osseointegrering: Temanummer. Läkartidningen 74:3749-3757, 1977.

Brånemark, P.-I., et al. Capillary structure and function in rheumatoid arthritis. Acta Rheum. Scand. 9:284-292, 1963.

Brånemark, P.-I., et al. The contributions and limitations of refined classical methods. J. Royal Micr. Soc. 83:29-35, 1964.

Brånemark, P.-I., et al. Biological and clinical evaluation of infrared thermography. J. Radiol. 48:1-2, 69-76, 1967.

Brånemark, P.-I., et al. Diabetesangiopati studerad med infraröd termografi. Nord. Med. 78:959, 1967.

Brånemark, P.-I., et al. Infrared thermography in diabetes mellitus. A preliminary study. Diabetologia 3:529–532, 1967.

Brånemark, P.-I., et al. Mandibelrekonstruktion med titanskelett. Nord. Med. 77:640-641, 1967.

Brånemark, P.-I., et al. Synovectomy in rheumatoid arthritis. Experimental biological and clinical aspects. Acta Rheum. Scand. 13:161-189, 1967.

Brånemark, P.-I., et al. Thermographic evaluation of diabetic angiopathy. A preliminary study. Excerpta Med. Int. Congress Series No. 140, Sixth Congress of the Internat. Diabetes Federation, Stockholm, Sweden (se Svensk Nord. Med.), 1967.

Brånemark, P.-I., et al. Tissue injury caused by wound disinfectants. J. Bone Joint Surg. 49A:48-62, 1967.

Brånemark, P.-I., et al. Mikrozirkulatorische Reaktionen bei Gewebeschädigung und Entzündung. Verhandlungen der Gesellschaft für exp. Medizin der Deutschen Demokratischen Republik. Vol. 13:103, Dresden: Verlag Theodor Steinkopff, 1968, pp. 103-115.

Brånemark, P.-I., et al. Thermographic evaluation of patch-test and tuberculin reactions. Acta Derm. Venereol. 48:385-390, 1968.

Brånemark, P.-I., et al. Experimentella studier av intraosseal förankring av dentala proteser. Göteborgs Tandläkare-Sällskaps Årsbok 359:2-25, 1969.

Brånemark, P.-I., et al. The influence of some anti-inflammatory drugs on original and regenerating synovial tissue. Acta Orthop. Scand. 40:279-299, 1969.

Brånemark, P.-I., et al. Tissue response to chymopapain in different concentrations. Clin. Orthop. 67:52-67, 1969.

Brånemark, P.-I., et al. Repair of defects in mandible. Scand. J. Plast. Reconstr. Surg. 4:100-108, 1970.

Brånemark, P.-I., et al. Käkrekonstruktion och benförankrad bettersättning. Läkartidningen 68:3105-3116, 1971.

Brånemark, P.-I., et al. Studies in rheology of human diabetes mellitus. Diabetologia 7:107-112, 1971.

Brånemark, P.-I., et al. Microvascular behaviour of platelets in man. pp. 183-195 *In* K. M. Brinkhous et al. (eds.) Thrombosis. Risk Factors and Diagnostic Approaches. Stuttgart: F. K. Schattauer Verlag, 1972.

Brånemark, P.-I., et al. Local tissue effects of surface-applied ENT drugs. Acta Otolaryngol. 80:128-136, 1975.

Brånemark, P.-I., et al. Reconstruction of the defective mandible. Scand. J. Plast. Reconstr. Surg. 9:116-128, 1975.

Brånemark, P.-I., et al. Osseointegrated Implants in the Treatment of the Edentulous Jaw. Experience from a 10-year Period. Stockholm: Almqvist & Wiksell, 1977.

Brånemark, P.-I., et al. Osseointegrated titanium implants in the rehabilitation of the edentulous patient. Adv. Biomater. 4:133-141, 1982.

Brånemark, P.-I., et al. An experimental and clinical study of osseointegrated implants penetrating the nasal cavity and maxillary sinus. J. Oral Maxillofac. Surg. 42:497, 1984.

Brånemark, P.-I., and Albrektsson, T. Microcirculation and healing of artificial implants in bone. Proc. 2nd World Congress for Microcirculation, 2:59-60, 1979.

Brånemark, P.-I., and Albrektsson, T. Titanium implants permanently penetrating human skin. Scand. J. Plast. Reconstr. Surg. 16:17-21, 1982.

Brånemark, P.-I., Albrektsson, T., and Bagge, U. Microvascular phenomena in grafted bone. pp. 379-390 In Proc. 2nd Conf. on Osseous Circulation, University of Toulouse, France, 1977.

Brånemark, P.-I., and Asano, M. Mikrovaskulära effekter av tobaksrökning. Läkartidningen 67:54-59, 1970.

Brånemark, P.-I., Aspegren, K., and Breine, U. Microcirculatory studies in man by high resolution vital microscopy. Angiology 15:329-332, 1964.

Brånemark, P.-I., and Bagge, U. Intravascular rheology of erythrocytes in man. Blood Cells 3:11-24, 1977.

Brånemark, P.-I., and Bagge, U. Erythrocytes, leukocytes and platelets in the human microcirculation. In J. F. Stolz (ed.) Proc. Europ. Symp. on Hemorheology and Diseases, Nancy, France, Oct. 1979, 1981.

Brånemark, P.-I., and Ekholm, R. Pictorial recording of the microcirculation. pp. 13-40 In W. L. Winters and A. N. Brest (eds.) The Microcirculation, Proc. Conf. Heart Assoc. Southeastern Pennsylvania, Philadelphia, Pa. Springfield, Ill.: Charles C. Thomas, Publ., 1966.

Brånemark, P.-I., and Ekholm, R. Adherence of blood cells to vascular endothelium. Blut 16:274-288, 1968.

Brånemark, P.-I., Ekholm, R., and Goldie, I. To the question of angiopathy in rheumatoid arthritis. An electron microscopic study. Acta Orthop. Scand. 40:153-175, 1969.

Brånemark, P.-I., Ekholm, R., and Lindhe, J. Colloidal carbon used for identification of vascular permeability. Med. Exp. 18:139-150, 1968.

Brånemark, P.-I., and Goldie, I. Observations on the action of prednisolone tertiary butyl acetate (Codelcortone TBA) and methylprednisolone acetate (Depomedrone) on normal soft tissues. Acta Rheum. Scand. 13:241-256, 1967.

Brånemark, P.-I., and Goldie, I. Physiologic aspects on the timing of synovectomy in rheumatoid arthritis. In W. Hijmans et al. (eds.) Proc. Symp. Early Synovectomy in Rheumatoid Arthritis, Amsterdam, 1967, Excerpta Medica, 11-22, 1969.

Brånemark, P.-I., Goldie, I., and Hirsch, C. Den frusna axeln. Klinik och patomorfologi. Läkartidningen 65:549-554, 1968.

Brånemark, P.-I., Goldie, I., and Lindström, J. Observations on the action of intraarticularly administered prednisolon tertiary butyl acetate (Codelcortone TBA) and methylprednisolon acetate (Depomedrone) in the normal rabbit knee joint. A vital microscopic and histologic study. Acta Orthop. Scand. 38:247-258, 1967.

Brånemark, P.-I., and Harders, H. Intravital analysis of microvascular form and function in man. Lancet 7:1197-1199, 1963.

Brånemark, P.-I., Helander, E., and Lindström, J. Effect of ultrasound in therapeutic doses on tissue circulation. Europa Medicophysica 2:213-216, 1966.

Brånemark, P.-I., Helander, E., and Lindström, J. Experimental investigation of the effect of pulsotherapy. Europa Medicophysica 2:209-212, 1966.

Brånemark, P.-I., Jacobsson, B., and Sörensen, S. E. Microvascular effects of topically applied contrast media. Acta Radiol. Scand. 8:547-559, 1969.

Brånemark, P.-I., and Johansson, B. W. Thermography as an aid in hibernation research. Acta Physiol. Scand. 73:300-304, 1968.

Brånemark, P.-I., and Jonsson, I. Determination of the velocity of corpuscles in blood capillaries. A flying spot device. Biorheology 1:143-146, 1963.

Brånemark, P.-I., and Jonsson, I. Photomicrographic and cinematomicrographic equipment for use with flash illumination. J. Royal Micr. Soc. 82: 245-249, 1963.

Brånemark, P.-I., and Jonsson, I. A diathermy unit for microsurgical preparations. Scand. J. Clin. Lab. Invest. 16:119-122, 1964.

Brånemark, P.-I., Laine, V., and Vainio, K. Vascular reactivity in rheumatoid arthritis. A pilot study in synovectomized and nonsynovectomized knee joints. Acta Rheum. Scand. 12:35-46, 1966.

Brånemark, P.-I., and Lindström, J. Studies in the function of nutritive capillaries in the connective tissue in rabbit's ear chamber. J. Anat. 97:323-332, 1963.

Brånemark, P.-I., and Lindström, J. Microcirculatory effects of emulsified fat infusions. Circ. Res. 15:124-130, 1964.

Brånemark, P.-I., and Lundskog, J. Biological aspects on the bio-implant interface. *In* Symp. on Biomaterials, 3rd Int. Conf. Medical Physics and Medical Engineering, Chalmers University of Technology, Göteborg, Sweden, 1972.

Brånemark, P.-I., Lundskog, J., and Albrektsson, B. Studies in flow of blood and heat in bone. pp. 133-142 *In* Proc. 1st Conf. on Osseous Circulation, University of Toulouse, France, 1973.

Broman, T., et al. Intravital and postmortem studies on air embolism damage of the blood-brain barrier tested with trypan blue. Acta Neurol. Scand. 42:146-152, 1966.

Costa, O., and Brånemark, P.-I. Microvascular physiology of the cochlea. Adv. Microcirc. 3:108-114, 1970.

Haljamäe, H., et al. Pathophysiology of shock. Pathol. Res. Pract. 165:200, 1979.

Hansson, B. O., Lindhe, J., and Brånemark, P.-I. Microvascular topography and function in clinically healthy and chronically inflamed dento-gingival tissues—a vital microscopic study in dogs. Periodontics 6:264-271, 1968.

Hirsch, C., Goldie, I., and Brånemark, P.-I. Frozen shoulder. Clinical and pathomorphological aspects. Egypt. Orthopaedic J. 7:70-79, 1972.

Hjortsjö, C. H., et al. A tomographic study of the rotation movements in the temporomandibular joint during lowering and forward movement of the mandible. Odontol. Rev. 5:81-110, 1954.

Hjortsjö, C. H., Brånemark, P.-I., and Sonesson, B. Studies on the shape of the articular eminence with its relation to the mechanism in the temporomandibular joint. Odontol. Rev. 4:187-202, 1953.

Holm-Pedersen, P., Nilsson, K., and Brånemark, P.-I. Vascular proliferation during wound healing in young and old rats. J. Periodont. Res. 4 (Suppl.):27-28, 1969.

Holm-Pedersen, P., Nilsson, K., and Brånemark, P.-I. The microvascular system of healing wounds in young and old rats. Adv. Microcirc. 5:80-106, 1973.

Hugoson, A., Lindhe, J., and Brånemark, P.-I. Revascularization of regenerating gingiva in female dogs treated with progesterone. Odontol. Rev. 1-12, 1971.

Lindblad, G., Brånemark, P.-I., and Lindström, J. Capillary form and function in dogs with experimental hepatitis contagiosa canis. An intravital microvascular study. Acta Vet. Scand. 5:1-10, 1964.

Linder, L., et al. Electron microscopic analysis of bone-titanium interface. Acta Orthop. Scand. 54:45-52, 1983.

Lindhe, J., Birch, J., and Brånemark, P.-I. Vascular proliferation in pseudo-pregnant rabbits. J. Periodont. Res. 3:12-20, 1968.

Lindhe, J., Birch, J., and Brånemark, P.-I. Wound healing in estrogen treated female rabbits. J. Periodont. Res. 3:21-23, 1968.

Lindhe, J., and Brånemark, P.-I. Changes in microcirculation after local application of sex hormones. J. Periodont. Res. 2:185-193, 1967.

Lindhe, J., and Brånemark, P.-I. Changes in vascular permeability after local application of sex hormones. J. Periodont. Res. 2:239-265, 1967.

Lindhe, J., and Brånemark, P.-I. The effects of sex hormones on vascularization of granulation tissues. J. Periodont. Res. 3:6-11, 1968.

Lindhe, J., and Brånemark, P.-I. Experimental studies on the etiology of pregnancy gingivitis. J. West. Soc. Periodontol. 16:50-51, 1968.

Lindhe, J., Brånemark, P.-I., and Birch, J. Microvascular changes in cheek-pouch wounds of oophorectomized hamsters following intramuscular injections of female sex hormones. J. Periodont. Res. 3:180-186, 1968.

Lindhe, J., Brånemark, P.-I., and Lundskog, J. Changes in vascular proliferation after local application of sex hormones. J. Periodont. Res. 2:266-272, 1967.

Lindhe, J., Hansson, B. O., and Brånemark, P.-I. The effect of topical application of fluorides on the gingival tissues. J. Periodont. Res. 6:211-217, 1971.

Lindström, J., and Brånemark, P.-I. Capillary circulation in the joint capsule of the rabbit's knee—A vital microscopic study. Arthritis Rheum. 5:226-236, 1962.

Lindström, J., Brånemark, P.-I., and Albrektsson, T. Mandibular reconstruction using the preformed autologous bone graft. Scand. J. Plast. Reconstr. Surg. 15:29-38, 1981.

Lundskog, J., and Brånemark, P.-I. Microvascular proliferation produced by autologous grafts of nucleus pulposus. Adv. Microcirc. 3:115-124, 1970.

Lundskog, J., Brånemark, P.-I., and Lindström, J. Biomicroscopic evaluation of microangiographic methods. Adv. Microcirc. 1:152-160, 1968.

McQueen, D., et al. Auger electron spectroscopic studies of titanium implants. Adv. Biomater. 4:179-185, 1982.

Olofsson, J., Bagge, U., and Brånemark, P.-I. Influence of white blood cells on the distribution of blood in microvascular compartments. Proc. 7th Europ. Conf. on Microcirculation, Aberdeen, Scotland, 1972, Part I. Bibl. Anat. 11, 405-410, 1973.

Romanus, M., et al. Intravital microscopy of the microcirculation in man during and after experimentally controlled ischemia. Scand. J. Plast. Reconstr. Surg. 12:181, 1978.

Rydevik, B., et al. Effects of chymopapain on nerve tissue. An experimental study on the structure and function of peripheral nerve tissue in rabbits after local application of chymopapain. Spine 1:137-148, 1976.

Rydevik, B., et al. Letter to the editor (Tissue effects of chymopapain) Spine 3:282-283, 1978.

Rydevik, B., et al. Microvascular response to locally injected collagenase. Scand. J. Plast. Reconstr. Surg. 1985 (in press).

Schatzker, J., and Brånemark, P.-I. Intravital observations on the microvascular anatomy and microcirculation of the tendon. Acta Orthop. Scand. 126 (Suppl.): 1-23, 1969.

Skalak, R., and Brånemark, P.-I. Deformation of red blood cells in capillaries. Science 164: 717-719, 1969.

Skalak, R., Brånemark, P.-I., and Ekholm, R. Erythrocyte adherence and diapedesis. Angiology 21:224-239, 1970.

Tjellström, A., et al. A clinical pilot study on preformed, autologous ossicles. I. Acta Otolaryngol. 85:33-39, 1978.

Tjellström, A., et al. A clinical pilot study on preformed, autologous ossicles. II. Acta Otolaryngol. 85:232-242, 1978.

Tjellström, A., et al. Analysis of the mechanical impedance of bone anchored hearing aids. Acta Otolaryngol. 89:85-92, 1980.

Tjellström, A., et al. The bone-anchored auricular epithesis. Laryngoscope 91:811-815, 1981.

Tjellström, A., et al. Osseointegrated titanium implants in the temporal bone. A clinical study on bone-anchored hearing aids. Am. J. Otol. 2:304-310, 1981.

Urbaschek, B., Brånemark, P.-I., and Nowotny, A. Lack of endotoxin effect on the microcirculation after pretreatment with detoxified endotoxin (Endotoxoid). Experientia 24:170, 1968.

Chapter 2

Nature and Significance of the Edentulous State*

George A. Zarb

Tooth loss and its consequences have plagued mankind for many centuries. The clinical disciplines of prosthodontics and oral surgery can claim an ancient, if not always distinguished, heritage. The Phoenicians and Egyptians left evidence of fixed prostheses, which consisted of carved ivory teeth attached with gold wire to adjacent natural teeth. Few dentists appreciate what the first complete dentures actually looked like and what kept them in place. Still fewer know that Queen Elizabeth I used rolls of cloth to pad out her lips or that the American presidential world cruise was ruined for President Grant when his teeth were lost overboard. A little more than a century ago, artificial teeth were so insecure that they were commonly removed during eating, and many denture-wearing ladies did much of their eating in the privacy of their bedroom. For most patients, the loss of even a few teeth is mutilating, and provides a strong incentive to seek dental care to preserve and restore normal speech, masticatory function, and a socially acceptable appearance. To most dentists the loss of teeth poses an even greater mutilation: the destruction of part of the facial skeleton and the distortion of the morphology and function of soft tissues (Figs. 2-1 and 2-3c and d).

The morphologic changes associated with the edentulous state, particularly when combined with aging changes, tend to manifest themselves as an appearance of compromised facial support. The individual compo-
nents that contribute to such undermined cosmetic changes include narrowing of the lips, deepening of the nasolabial groove, loss of labiomental angle, increase in the columella-philtral angle, and decrease in the horizontal labial angle (Fig. 2-2). A brief review of the salient features that profoundly affect the edentulous state will include some of the implications of support for prostheses, the effects of aging, and the adaptive responses to wearing prostheses.

Support for prostheses

The masticatory apparatus is involved in the process of acquisition and trituration of food,[1] with direct responsibility for these tasks falling on the teeth and their supporting tissues. The attachment of teeth in sockets is one of the many important modifications that took place during mammalian evolution.

Teeth function properly only if adequately supported. This support is provided by the periodontium, an organ composed of soft and hard connective tissues. In the edentulous patient, the entire mechanism of functional and parafunctional load transmission is modified dramatically because of a loss of periodontal support. Watt[2] computed the

* This chapter is based in part on the paper "The Edentulous Milieu," *Journal of Prosthetic Dentistry* 49:825-831, 1983. Figures 2-1, 2-3, and 2-4 are reproduced courtesy of The C. V. Mosby Co., St. Louis, Mo.

Figs. 2-1a and b   The edentulous state almost invariably leads to varying degrees of bone reduction in the denture-bearing areas. This undermining of the integrity of the facial skeleton leads to distortion of the overlying soft tissues.

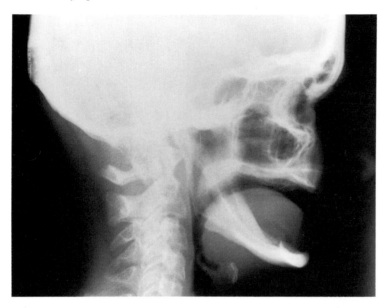

Fig. 2-1a   Lateral view.

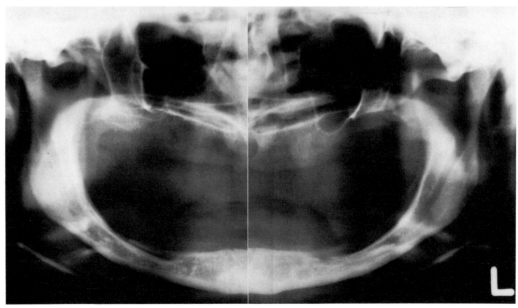

Fig. 2-1b   Orthopantogram.

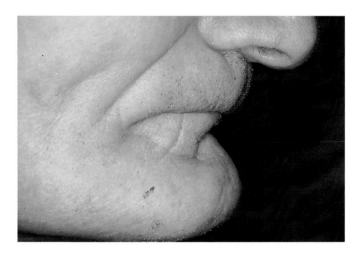

Fig. 2-2 The edentulous predicament is frequently associated with distinct and adverse cosmetic changes in a patient's appearance. These changes result from morphological alterations, which tend to be emphasized by the aging process.

mean area of periodontium in each arch to be 45 cm², with this area becoming variably depleted as teeth are lost. It eventually shrinks to 23 cm² in the edentulous maxilla, and 12 cm² in the edentulous mandible. The size of the available residual ridge can be compromised even further as a result of congenital anomalies or surgical interventions (Figs. 2-3a and b).The prosthodontist is therefore confronted with both a quantitative and qualitative compromise in the edentulous arches' load-bearing potential. The mucosa demonstrates little tolerance or adaptability to denture wearing, a tolerance that can be reduced still further by the presence of systemic diseases such as anemia, hypertension, diabetes, and nutritional deficiencies. In fact, it is tempting to suggest that any disturbances of the normal metabolic process may lower the upper limit of mucosal tolerance and initiate inflammation.[1]

Several longitudinal studies indicate that residual alveolar bone appears to be vulnerable to denture wearing and responds by an ongoing and insidious reduction that is irreversible and probably inevitable (Fig. 2-3c). An atrophic mandible is a common

consequence and is frequently associated with superficial muscle attachments that tend to preclude retentive prostheses. Furthermore, the clinical problem is frequently complicated by the possible adverse effects of aging and/or the presence of poor neuromuscular control.

The prosthesis support problem is therefore a serious one, not only because of both qualitative (loss of periodontal ligaments) and quantitative (reduction in size of stress-bearing areas) compromises, but also because different resorptive patterns can result in several localized or related morphological changes which singly or together pose clinical problems. These changes include (1) sharp, spiny residual ridges; (2) uneven residual ridges; (3) prominent mylohyoid and internal oblique ridges; (4) prominent genial tubercles; (5) prominent mentalis eminence; (6) absent or minimal attached mucosa usually with unfavorable frenal attachments; (7) vulnerably placed neurovascular structures; (8) hypermobile ridge tissue; (9) enlarged tongue; and (10) atrophic mucosa.

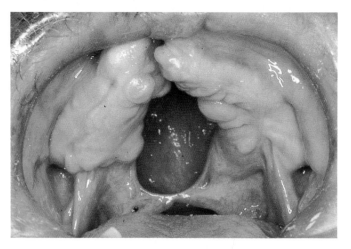

Figs. 2-3a to h The potential denture-bearing area can be dramatically compromised.

Fig. 2-3a Cleft palate patient.

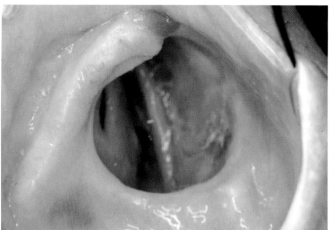

Fig. 2-3b Patient who has undergone hemimaxillectomy.

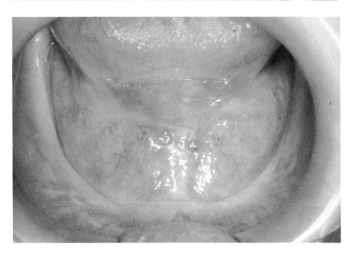

Fig. 2-3c The type of advanced resorption in this edentulous mandible frequently precludes fabrication of a retentive and stable denture.

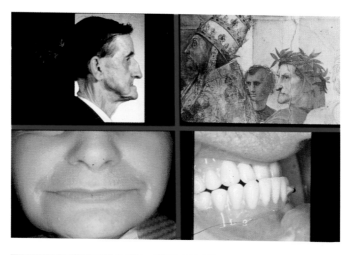

Fig. 2-3d Spatial mandibular changes that accompany unmonitored dental aspects of aging can modify functional demands on both ridges and temporomandibular joints. While adaptive changes are frequently observed, a progression to degenerative arthritis may also occur.

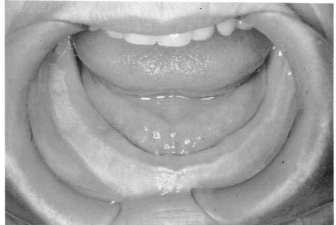

Fig. 2-3e Surgical need to achieve wide, deep sulcus is prescribed by the prosthodontist, and an interpremolar vestibuloplasty also reduces adverse mentalis muscle activity.

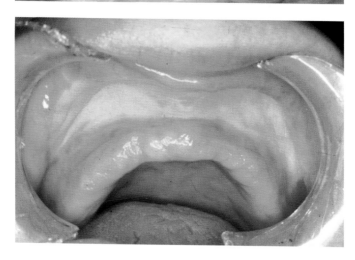

Fig. 2-3f A broad vestibuloplasty is needed in the maxilla because several dislodging muscles are involved, as opposed to the dominant mentalis muscle in the mandible.

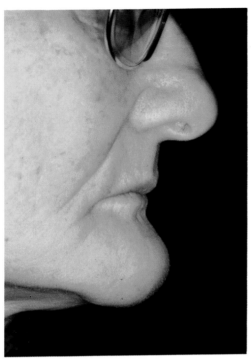

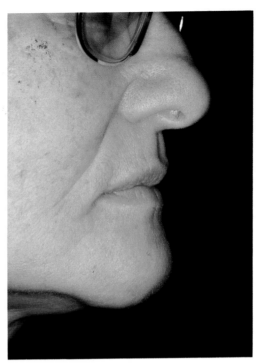

Fig. 2-3g Preprosthetic surgical view of a patient whose advanced residual ridge resorption led to distortion of her circumoral soft tissue support. Powerful mentalis muscle activity led to a cosmetic and functional compromise.

Fig. 2-3h Patient was treated with a vestibuloplasty; posttreatment result was excellent.

Effects of aging

The incidence of documented edentulism in Western countries is staggering, with surveys in various parts of the world showing a high percentage of edentulous patients among the elderly. The oral aspects of aging currently receiving increasing attention in the curricula of dental schools and in the edentulous patient include the mucosa; residual bone, maxillomandibular relations; the tongue and taste; and salivary, nutritional, and psychologic changes. Regardless of what happens in preventive and restorative dentistry, many of today's middle-aged patients (who will be the geriatric patients of

tomorrow) have already lost their teeth. Furthermore, our life expectancy is longer and the world population is growing. Patients who start wearing complete dentures in their 30s and 40s will probably pose very difficult prosthodontic problems, because time and long-term denture wearing will continue to exact a biologic price from their oral supporting tissues.

It should be emphasized that the association of depleted dentitions with adverse biomechanical joint loading frequently precedes the edentulous state (Fig. 2-3d), and that this can combine with consequences of aging to play a role in degeneration of the temporomandibular joints. The hypothesis has been proposed that degenerative arthritis is a process rather than a disease entity,[3] somewhat analogous to heart failure, and that joint changes occur as part of a continuum of adverse loading that may be related to dental morphologic features. These changes reflect the balance in adaptation and degeneration that result from alterations in functional demands on or in functional capacity of the joints. This hypothesis can be reconciled with current thinking on the pathogenesis of degenerative arthritis and may be a useful teaching clinical model for analyzing the edentulous milieu in a broader context.

Adaptive responses

Many patients who wear complete dentures experience considerable difficulty adapting to their prostheses.[4] They may present no obvious signs of injury or disease in the denture-bearing area, and their symptoms are difficult to pin down both verbally and geographically. Most of these patients fail to respond to treatment, which is usually of a technical nature, and they are frequently dismissed as having difficult mouths or experiencing difficulty in adapting to the dentures.

The presence of inanimate foreign objects (prostheses) in an edentulous mouth is bound to elicit different stimuli in the sensory-motor system, which in turn influences oral motor behavior. Both exteroceptors and proprioceptors are probably affected by the size, shape, position, and pressure from, and mobility of, the prostheses. However, the role of mucosal and other stimuli in the control of jaw movement and other motor behaviors needs clarification. The findings of several authors[1,2,4] strengthen the assumption that denture wearing is a matter of skilled performance. Once this skill is acquired, the patient relies much less on pure-

ly physical factors such as adhesion and cohesion for denture control.

The acceptance of any prosthesis is accompanied by a process of habituation, or a gradual diminution of responses to continued or repeated stimuli.[5] The tactile stimuli that arise from the contact of complete prostheses with the richly innervated oral cavity are probably ignored after a short period of time. Because each stage of the decrease in response is related to the memory patterns of the previous application of the stimulus, storage of information from the immediate past is an integral part of habituation. Difficulty in the storage of information of this type tends to accompany old age, which accounts for the problems of some older patients in getting used to all types of removable prostheses such as distal-extension partial dentures, complete dentures, and maxillofacial prostheses. Age may also play an important role in determining the facility with which a patient adapts to prosthetic therapy. The facility for learning and coordination appears to diminish with age, probably as a result of progressive atrophy of elements of the cerebral cortex. Clinical experience suggests that stimuli must be specific and identical to achieve habituation, and that when a stimulus does not elicit a strong response from an organism, repetition will result in a decreased response. If the stimulus response is strong, sensitization will result.[6] Habituation appears to involve more than a passive process in that experience, attention, and interest may modify the fineness of sensory discrimination. It is still undetermined whether the lowered sensory threshold in the difficult denture patient is primarily a motor problem or whether such factors as individual variation in experience, attention, and interest are involved to any significant degree.

Psychologic inventories have been used to assess the personality characteristics of the difficult denture patient,[1] and studies have shown that a large proportion of such patients score high on indexes of neuroticism. Both learning and skilled performance show optimal relationships with anxiety, while levels of anxiety that are too high or too low appear to be incapacitating. While this suggests that only the most anxious patients should experience difficulty with their denture, clinical experience suggests that such a conclusion may be a narrow and restrictive one.

The overall impression is that denture wearing is a matter of skilled performance and that once this skill is acquired, there is less reliance on purely physical factors.

Clinical treatment

Prosthodontists have been remarkably successful in treating difficult edentulous patients with complete dentures. However, clinical experience confirms the existence of a large number of patients with "varying degrees" of prosthetic success, and a smaller number with no success at all. It appears that most of these patients' problems are related to depleted residual ridge support, with the ridge often covered by thin, nonresilient mucosa, and accompanied by unfavorable patterns of neuromuscular control. Furthermore, the increase in life span, accompanied by the biologic effects of aging, elicits changes in the masticatory system that tend to militate against successful long-term prosthodontic treatment.

In a clinical therapeutic context, the edentulous elderly patient with advanced residual ridge reduction presents one of the greatest challenges facing the dental profession today. While the literature offers many techniques to cope with such a challenge, the problem has often been approached mechanically, with too little attention paid to the biologic reactions of the oral tissues. Two exciting and innovative techniques, enlargement of the denture-bearing area and use of dental implants, have offered considerable scope for coping with this challenge.

Enlargement of denture-bearing areas

Vestibuloplasty (Fig. 2-4)

With a vestibuloplasty the oral surgeon detaches the origin of muscles on either the labial or lingual side, or both sides, of the edentulous residual ridges, enabling the prosthodontist to increase the vertical extensions of the denture flanges. When horizontal shelving is present in the mentalis muscle region, the surgical procedure is less successful, and its relative efficacy is due to the modification of the powerful mentalis muscle's activity.

In recent years, close cooperation between the two involved disciplines has resulted in a clearer understanding of what the surgical intervention should achieve. A wide and deep sulcus has not appeared to be essential for success (Fig. 2-3e), and the vestibuloplasty can be restricted to the inter-premolar region since the buccinator muscles are not the major cause of the problem of denture instability.[1, 7] Displacement of the mentalis muscle and adjacent muscle slips allows for the production of a looser lower lip, along with a wound margin down low in the sulcus. This leads to an increase in both stability and depth of the labial flange (see Fig. 2-4). The situation varies in the maxillae, where the surrounding musculature lacks the mentalis muscle's unstabilizing potential. A broader vestibuloplasty is indicated here (Fig. 2-3f). In Figs. 2-3g and h the excellence of the therapeutic result is quite evident.

While lingual vestibuloplasties can provide for an increase in the denture's lingual flange, the procedure is a traumatic one,

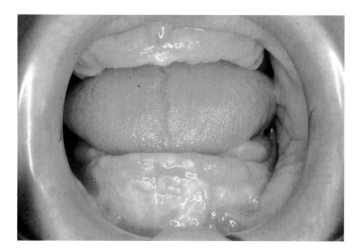

Fig. 2-4a Mucosal graft vestibuloplasty fulfills the objective of an increased vertical extension for labial flange.

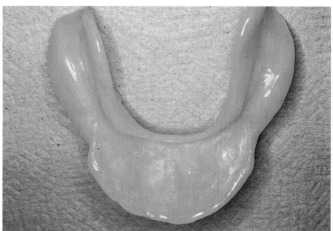

Figs. 2-4b and c Relative "migration" of mentalis muscle insertion that accompanies advanced ridge resorption is reversed following vestibuloplasty, and room for a new deeper labial flange is now possible.

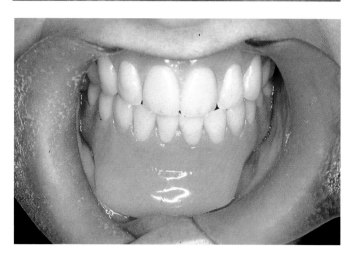

Fig. 2-4c

Table 2-1   Comparison of skin, mucosal, and collagen grafts

(Biological covers for surgically denuded areas protect the area by resisting bacterial growth on the tissue surface and minimizing wound contracture.)

Split-skin grafts	Well tolerated.
	Some postoperative shrinkage.
	Graft does not show metaplastic change.
	Difference in color and consistency of grafted site. Occasional hair growth.
	Some degree of morbidity associated with donor site healing. In elderly patients skin is often inelastic and atrophic.
Mucosal grafts	Theoretically a more satisfactory graft.
	Limited quantity of mucosa is available.
	Uniformly thin graft removed with a mucotome is costly and difficult.
	A degree of morbidity associated with a palatal donor site.
Heterologous collagen graft	Readily available for immediate use.
	No morbidity apparent.

particularly in frail and elderly patients, and therefore not frequently recommended. The long-standing clinical impression that free skin grafts lose resiliency and develop nuisance crinkling was confirmed by Moller and Jolst.[8]

Skin grafts tend to develop a marked increase in parakeratosis with subsequent clinical sogginess. Furthermore, they seem to exhibit poor denture cohesion and adhesion when compared with mucosa. Whenever possible, mucosal grafts are preferred.

Recent reports[9] underscore the efficacy of employing biological dressings for areas of denuded mucous membrane. Collagen xenografts appear to offer the advantage of immediate use without the disadvantages inherent in the use of split skin or mucosa for grafting. Table 2-1 attempts a comparison of the relative merits of skin, mucosal, and collagen grafts.

Ridge augmentation

Surgeons have attempted to restore mandibular bulk by placing onlay bone grafts from the iliac or ribs sources above or below the mandible. Follow-up reports of this approach suggest that the end result generally leaves much to be desired with respect to long-term maintenance of ridge height, after the ridge is exposed to functional and parafunctional stress. Other methods of dimensional increase of the mandible by means of a "visor" and "sandwich" osteotomy have also been proposed. The report by de Koomen et al.[10] suggests optimism for the procedure, although a cautious approach is recommended because it can be a formidable undertaking for some patients.

Use of dental implants

The notion of successfully implanting artificial tooth roots is an exciting one. However, the literature on oral implantology has tended to be dominated by anecdotal reports that could mislead dentists into thinking that implantology is a predictably successful clinical treatment method that can be readily incorporated into routine practices.

It seems that insufficient data are available to enable the clinician to predict the number of years of success of any alloplastic oral implant.[11] Premature dissemination of alloplastic implant materials, methods, and techniques has tended to precede prior scientific animal and clinical research.[11, 12] In fact, it is tempting to suggest that there has been far too much testing of dental implants in humans and far too little evaluation of dental implant design and materials in laboratory animals.[13]

At no time in the history of surgical implants has there been such an unrealistic reporting of results as in the dental implant field. Yet, dentists persist in their endeavors to restore missing teeth with implants, frequently ignoring simpler, safer, and more predictable solutions for the prosthodontic problems confronting them.[1] Implant placement on this basis is often tantamount to the creation of an instant, advanced periodontal disease-like predicament.

It appears that most of the conventionally used implants behave unpredictably and will eventually fail, with some types of implants failing more slowly than others. Most clinical educators believe that the use of such clinical experimental techniques should be limited to those few situations in which the patient is aware of the experimental nature of the procedure and its short-lived potential. In 1959 Obwegeser[14] concluded that implants should be advocated only as long as they are intended for use for a limited time. Johns[15] observed that until the development of a pseudocementum that could evoke the formation of tissues analogous to Sharpey's fibers, neither a satisfactory pseudojunctional epithelium nor a well-contoured bone support around an abutment may be possible.

Regrettably, most reported implant techniques do not survive scientific scrutiny. Thus it is understandable why most prosthodontic and oral surgical departments limit their teaching on dental implants to a mere presentation of scientific facts coupled with a strong reluctance to prescribe the technique clinically.

A recent conference sponsored by the Na-tional Institutes of Health (NIH) attempted to establish guidelines for the use of various types of implants *already* in clinical use.[16] A group of dentists involved with dental implants looked at retrospective clinical data provided by several clinicians. These recommendations, while clearly limited by the retrospective nature of the study and the diversity of opinion offered by the conference participants, acknowledged the lack of well-controlled scientific documentation. A list of minimal clinical guidelines was, however, drawn up. While this author's observations reflect a dissatisfaction with the biomechanical implications of current implant techniques, this is not meant to indict the possible use of dental implants. Several health disciplines are committed to a constant search for better tissue and organ replacements, and clinical dentistry is no exception. However, a conscientious and tenacious commitment to research in the field of tooth and supporting alveolar bone replacement demands scientific methodology that has been lacking. In this context a quote from the Draft Statement re National Guidelines for Health Planning, USA, 1978, is quite relevant: "The effectiveness and safety of clinical procedures should be determined *before* they are incorporated into common practice, and monitored on a continuing basis; when found effective and safe, they should be introduced in ways that enhance economy, equity, and quality."

It is only the work of Brånemark et al.[17] and Adell et al.[18] that suggests the possibility of a scientific breakthrough in this field, because their clinical implant studies are the only ones that survive longitudinal scientific scrutiny.

References

1. *Hickey, J. C., and Zarb, G. A.*
   Boucher's Prosthodontic Treatment for Edentulous Patients. 8th ed. St. Louis: The C. V. Mosby Co., 1980.

2. *Watt, D. M.*
   Morphological changes in the denture-bearing area following the extraction of teeth. Thesis, University of Edinburgh, Scotland, 1961.

3. *Editorial*
   Pathogenesis of osteoarthrosis. Lancet 2:1131, 1973.

4. *Zarb, G. A.*
   Oral motor patterns and their relation to oral prostheses. J. Prosthet. Dent. 47:472, 1982.

5. *Glaser, E. M.*
   The Physiological Basis of Habituation. London: Oxford University Press, 1966.

6. *Thompson, R. F., et al.*
   A dual-process theory of habituation: Theory and behavior. *In* V. S. Pecke and M. J. Herz (eds.) Habituation. Vol. 1. New York: Academic Press, 1973.

7. *Qualyle, A. A.*
   The atrophic mandible: Aspects of technique in lower labial sulcoplasty. Br. J. Oral Surg. 16:169, 1978-1979.

8. *Moller, J. F., and Jolst, O.*
   A histologic follow-up study of free autogenous skin grafts to the alveolar ridge in humans. Int. J. Oral Surg. 1:283, 1972.

9. *Mitchell, R.*
   A new biological dressing for areas denuded of mucous membrane. Br. Dent. J. 155:346, 1983.

10. *de Koomen, H. A., et al.*
    Interposed bone-graft augmentation of the atrophic mandible. J. Maxillofac. Surg. 7:129, 1979.

11. *Boucher, L. J.*
    Alloplastic tooth implants. J. Prosthet. Dent. 36:567, 1976.

12. *Shulman, L. B.*
    Moderator summary, section on implants. Symposium Proceedings, Dental Biomaterials-Research Priorities. HEW Publ. no. 74-548, 134-137, 1974.

13. *Hubert, S. F.*
    Discussion on "biomaterials." J. Dent. Res. 54 (Special issue B):174, 1975.

14. *Obwegeser, H. L.*
    Experiences with subperiosteal implants. Oral Surg. 12:777, 1959.

15. *Johns, R. B.*
    Experimental studies on dental implants. Proc. R. Soc. Med. 69:1, 1976.

16. *U. S. Department of Health and Human Services.*
    Dental implants: Benefit and risk. National Institutes of Health—Harvard Consensus Development Conference. Dec., 1980.

17. *Brånemark, P.-I., et al.*
    Osseointegrated implants in the treatment of the edentulous jaw—Experience from a ten-year period. Monograph. Stockholm: Almqvist and Wiksell, 1977.

18. *Adell, R., et al.*
    A 15-year-old study of osseointegrated implants in the treatment of the edentulous jaw. Int. J. Oral Surg. 6:387, 1981.

Chapter 3

Nature of Implant Attachments

George A. Zarb and Tomas Albrektsson

The masticatory apparatus is involved in the process of trituration of food. Direct responsibility for this task falls on the teeth and their supporting tissues. The attachment of teeth in sockets, in the jawbones, is one of the many modifications that took place during the period when the earliest mammals were evolving from their reptilian predecessors. The success of this modification is indicated by its rapid adaptation throughout the many different groups of emerging Mammalia. Teeth tend to function properly only if adequately supported. This support is provided by the periodontium, which is an organ composed of hard connective tissues (cementum and bone) and soft connective tissues (the periodontal ligament and the lamina propria of the gingiva). The periodontium is regarded as a functional unit, and is attached to the dentin by cementum, and to the jawbone by the alveolar process. Continuity between these two hard tissue components is maintained by the periodontal ligament and the lamina propria.

Periodontal ligament

In the natural dentition, the periodontal ligament comprises a well-innervated, highly vascular, and cellular fibrous connective tissue which is also metabolically very active. It is called a ligament because it consists of dense regular bundles of collagen fibers that are inserted into both tooth and bone (Sharpey's fibers), and are oriented in groups, in a manner that resists both vertical and horizontal forces applied to the tooth. This resilient suspensory apparatus demonstrates four roles: (1) shock absorption, (2) sensory function, (3) regulation of osteogenesis, and (4) as an accomodator of tooth movements.

Shock absorption

The periodontal ligament is very well suited to cope with the stresses of functional and parafunctional occlusal contacts. The alignment of the principal fibers of the ligament follows a wavy course at rest, but the fibers are stretched taut as a result of occlusal force application. The ligament's vascularity also provides a hydraulic dampening effect to counter occlusal forces. Furthermore, the presence of glycosaminoglycans in the extracellular component of the ligament enables these macromolecules to bind large amounts of water from the tissue fluid. This bound water contributes to the hydraulic dampening effect and gives the ligament viscoelastic properties. The sudden loading of a tooth leads to fluid displacement through foramina in the inner cortical plate or lamina dura, and to nonloaded regions of the ligament. The net effect of the fluid shift along with fiber tension displacement tends to dissipate the applied stress. It has been

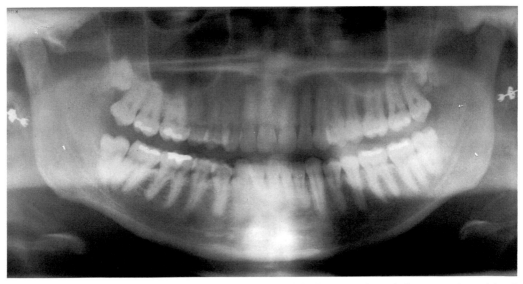

Fig. 3-1a   Orthopantomogram of a dentulous young adult illustrates the relative area of combined periodontal ligaments available for fulfilling the resilient suspensory apparatus's four roles.

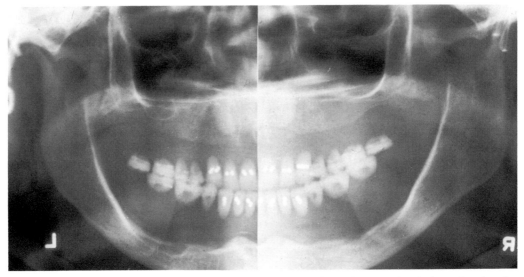

Fig. 3-1b   In this middle-aged edentulous patient, the periodontal ligament's role is undertaken by the denture-bearing areas of mucoperiosteum. This clearly represents a qualitative and quantitative role compromise.

estimated that the ligament covers a combined area of 45 cm^2 in each dental arch, and that it is from 0.15 to 0.38 mm wide. Although this width tends to decrease with age, the ligament's functions are not necessarily compromised (Fig. 3-1).

Sensory function

The periodontal ligament is a sensory organ. It contains numerous nerve endings that are thought to be pain receptors, along with other nerve endings that are associated with blood vessels, and may represent autonomic nerve fibers with a vasomotor function. These nerve endings are branches of the fifth cranial nerve and also include specialized nerve endings believed to be mechanoreceptors. The nerve endings have the protective function of preventing the development of potentially excessive forces, and they are also involved in stereognosis and in the control of mandibular movements.

Regulation of osteogenesis

It has been observed that teeth with a normal periodontal ligament do not usually undergo ankylosis. This suggests that the ligament possesses control mechanisms to prevent its obliteration by osteogenesis or cementogenesis. On the other hand, teeth that have been avulsed and replanted without significant amounts of viable periodontal ligament on their root surfaces will become ankylosed and suffer extensive root resorption.

Adaptive tooth movements

The ligament is a very active tissue, which demonstrates a high rate of turnover and remodelling. It therefore plays an important role in occlusion by permitting adaptive tooth movements. As soon as teeth erupt into the oral cavity and occlusal contact is established, the nonfunctional orientation of the periodontal fibers changes into a functional arrangement. This fiber arrangement gives maximal stabilization to the tooth in the alveolar socket and, at the same time, allows a physiologic range of tooth mobility in all directions. Gradual changes in force patterns occur during growth and eruption of the teeth. Abrupt alterations are produced as a result of loss or removal of an opposing or an adjacent tooth, or the placement of a fixed or removable prosthesis. The position normally occupied by a tooth in the dental arch depends on the balance of all the forces acting on that tooth over an extended period of time. Sustained alterations in the magnitude or duration of the forces may cause the position of the tooth to change. This change is produced in the structural elements of the periodontium as a result of the position gradually assumed by the tooth in the alveolus. It appears that changes in force patterns acting on the teeth over extended periods of time elicit adjustments in the supporting tissues. Consequently the application of consistently greater loads during mastication tends to cause an increase in the width of the periodontal ligament and in both the number and density of principal fibers. Very little change of tooth position occurs, however. More sustained, but smaller, forces cause a change in tooth position so that an equilibrium position is reestablished. The specific thresholds of force and time that are required for these changes to occur are unknown, and they probably vary in different people.

Forces acting on the dentition

The greatest forces acting on the teeth are normally produced during mastication and deglutition, and they are essentially vertical in direction. Each thrust is of short duration, and for most people, at least, chewing is restricted to short periods of time. Deglutition, on the other hand, occurs about 500 times a day,[1] and tooth contacts during swallowing are usually of longer duration than those occurring during chewing.[2] Loads of a lower order, but of a longer duration, are produced throughout the day by the tongue and perioral/circumoral musculature. These forces are predominantly horizontal. Estimates of peak forces from the tongue, cheeks, and lips have been made, and tongue force appears to exceed labiolingual force during activity. During rest or inactive periods, the total forces may be similar in magnitude.

During mastication, biting forces are transmitted through the bolus to the opposing teeth whether the teeth make contact or not. These forces increase steadily (depending on the nature of the food fragment), reach a peak, and abruptly return to zero. The magnitude, rise time, and interval between thrusts differ among individuals, and depend on the consistency of the food and the point in time in a specific chewing sequence. The direction of the forces is principally perpendicular to the occlusal plane in normal function, but the forward angulation of most natural teeth leads to the introduction of a horizontal component that tends to tilt the teeth mesially, as well as buccally or lingually. Upper incisors may be displaced labially with each biting thrust; these tooth movements quite probably cause proximal wear facets to develop.

In healthy dentitions, teeth are not in occlusion except during the functional movements of chewing and deglutition, and during the movements of parafunction. Graf calculated that the total time during which the teeth are subjected to functional forces of mastication and deglutition during an entire day amounts to approximately 17.5 minutes.[3] More than half of this time is due to jaw-closing forces applied during deglutition. Graf concluded that this total time and the range of forces seem to be well within the tolerance level of healthy periodontal tissues.

Masticatory loads are much smaller than those that are produced by conscious effort (approximately 45 kg), and are approximately 20 kg for the natural dentition. The loads generated during parafunctional jaw movements—grinding or bruxing, and clenching—are greater than the masticatory loads, and tend to be prolonged as well as occurring diurnally and nocturnally.

The ligament does not function independently from the other tissues of the periodontium. It must be remembered that the entire functional unit also includes the gingiva and the alveolar bone. In fact, deformation of this bone contributes to the absorption of occlusal forces. Regrettably, little is known about the sensory innervation of bone, but it appears reasonable to suggest that receptors may be present that contribute to the control of occlusal function.

This brief review underscores the fact that the periodontal ligament is well suited for its diverse roles of support and protection of the natural dentition. The remit to the researcher in the field of dental implants has been one of developing a predictable method of implant attachment, one which preferably would be analogous with most of the roles the periodontal ligament serves. Any effort to simulate its functional attachment role is bound to be a complex one, since it must reconcile several basic and clinical science disciplines. Research directed towards the development of a peri-implant ligament that could simulate some, if

I	II	III
Interfacial adhesive/fixative	Fibrous encapsulation	Osseointegration
e.g., Acrylic resin, cement	e.g., endosseous blade vent	e.g., Brånemark's T.I.P.
— Low tissue differentiation		— Interfacial osteogenesis
— Development of nonadherent capsule		— Predictable longevity
— Unpredicatable clinical performance		

Fig. 3-2 Implant attachment objective is a simulated periodontal ligament. Reported alternatives to this objective suggest these three systems of interfacial response. Methods I and II seem to represent a halfway biotechnology, and a palliative one at best.

not all, of a periodontal ligament's functions would be very worthwhile. Such an induced structure would then create an analogous interfacial stress situation to that encountered in the natural dentition, with the structure having to attach to both bone and implant.

The diverse efforts to anchor implants in bone can be classified in the context of the elicited host bone response. Such an "interfacial" classification suggests at least four mechanisms: (1) attachment via highly differentiated fibrous tissue, (2) attachment via low differentiated fibrous tissue, (3) anchorage via use of artificial fixatives (such as acrylic resin cement), and (4) direct anchorage in vital bone. Figure 3-2 is a speculative analysis of the bone response to different implant attachment methods.

Attachment via highly differentiated fibrous tissue

tooth is anchored to the bone by the highly differentiated periodontal ligament which represents the ideal form of anchorage of a tooth substitute. Unfortunately, restoration and maintenance of a proper periodontal ligament around a dental implant has not yet been reported. The most promising experimental approach was reported by Pilliar et al., who described orthopedic implants anchored by a particular type of highly differentiated fibrous tissue with fibers arranged in a manner similar to those of a periodontal ligament.[4] However, this research was very short term, and it remains uncertain whether a highly differentiated periodontal ligament-like anchorage around clinically functioning implants is possible.

Attachment via low differentiated fibrous tissue

An analysis of bone response to the majority of implants in current clinical use by dentists suggests that one of two events tends to occur. The first event would reflect a tissue rejection with an acute or chronic inflammatory response and early loss of the implant. The second event, which has frequently been construed as a successful response, is one in which a nonadherent fibrous encapsulation of varying thickness around the implant takes place. In these situations, evidence is lacking to suggest that such an encapsulation constitutes a "pseudoperiodontium" or a "periodontiumlike" structure.

Clinical observation of the second type of response suggests that a time dependent shift to an acute rejection can occur. In fact, such a situation can be considered analogous to what happens when teeth with chronic advanced periodontal disease develop periodontal abscesses. The premise here is that both clinical situations are characterized by a compromised and therefore vulnerable attachment mechanism whose behavior in the context of function, long-term maintenance, and oral systemic health relationships is unpredictable.

Some authors have persisted in regarding the development of such a low differentiated fibrous tissue response to metallic implants as a mandatory one,[5-9] indicating that such implants were most secure immediately after their insertion and would become progressively looser over time. This is probably related to the type of material used, implant location, geometry, stability of fixation, etc. Specific suggested causes for the failure of interfacial osteogenesis include (1) a surgical technique that was traumatic, leading to excessive thermal damage to the host bone site; (2) an implant placed in immediate function; (3) use of an implant material that contributed to a poor host response; and (4) a design that led to unfavorable stress concentrations in the surrounding bone.

Certainly the bulk of published evidence to date indicates that metallic endosseous implants are almost invariably surrounded by fibrous connective tissue, which is neither reminiscent of, nor analogous to, a periodontal ligament.

Anchorage via use of artificial fixatives

The apparent biomechanical incompatibility between reported metallic endosseous implants and host tissues suggested the use of a bone cement to simulate the stress distribution and attachment roles of the periodontal ligament. Acrylic cement has found a widespread use in orthopedic surgery. Very good five-year clinical results with a 90% or more success rate in cases of hip joint replacements have been reported by several investigators.[10,11] However, the reported clinical results are less compelling when examined radiologically, with a reported loosening in 70% or more of the cases.[12] Furthermore, strict testing of the clinical stability of the femoral component of cement-fixed hip arthroplasties revealed a 30% loosening frequency.[13] Actually, Johnston[14] stated that all cemented hip arthroplasties will loosen with time, but the relatively advanced age of the patient will, in most cases, make reoperations unnecessary. This eventual loosening of cemented implants is not very surprising because the interface between cement and bone consists of a layer of low differentiated fibrous tissue.[10,15,16] Figure 3-3 is a schematic representation of the outcome of implants anchored in fibrous tissue, with or without interposed acrylic cement in the interface. The favorable clinical results of cemented hip arthroplasties in relation to fibrous tissue anchored dental implants point to the importance of a correct interpretation of this figure. If n is large enough, the increased failure percentage over time may be a matter of academic interest only.

An attempt to cement endosseous metal implants was reported in 1979.[17] This animal study did not replicate the Charnley successes (qualified as they are). In fact, fibrous connective tissue encapsulation of each implant frequently led to early exfoliation or extensive implant mobility. These observations suggested a poor prognosis for the clinical application of such a technique to dentistry.

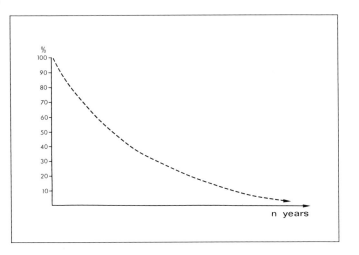

Fig. 3-3 The implant anchored in fibrous tissue is becoming loose with time, indicated by subsequently poor success figures with each year following the implantation procedure. If *n* is large enough, this may be primarily an academic problem. However, it seems that dental implants anchored in fibrous tissue are mostly lost within a 10-year period, indicating that this type of anchorage is not sufficient to carry the loads of the masticatory apparatus.

Direct anchorage in vital bone

Several authors have speculated that certain implant materials may have a dynamic surface chemistry that could induce histological changes at the implant interface, which normally would occur if the implant were not present. This suggests a situation akin to the creation of a partial surgical fracture (host implant site) with a biocompatible material (the implant or tooth root analogue) introduced into the site of predictable healing as demonstrated by the development of mature differentiated tissue. The clinical research objective would then be the introduction of an implant system that could reconcile (1) the predictable behavior of such a material in vivo with (2) a technique of host site preparation which would not compromise such an objective, and (3) with a design for the implant which would withstand clinical functional and nonfunctional forces in the long run. If induction of bone formation around such an implant were clinically feasible, then a secure method of attachment or anchorage could be predicted, and interfacial osteogenesis or "osseointegration" would take place. Such a direct

apposition of bone toward metallic implants, without any interposed fibrous tissue, has been experimentally verified with titanium,[18] stainless steel,[19] and Vitallium.[20] Brånemark coined the term osseointegration to describe the direct contact between living haversian bone and loaded implant surface, which he observed in clinical cases of dental implants.[21] A most interesting feature of the osseointegrated interface is that, contrary to low differentiated fibrous tissue interfaces, it seems to establish a stronger implant bond with increasing time. Since 1965, Brånemark and his colleagues at the University of Göteborg, Sweden, have inserted over 4,000 threaded, cylindrical pure titanium implants into mandibular and maxillary sites as well as in tibial, temporal, and iliac bones for various dental and orthopedic restorative procedures. All the titanium fixtures were implanted using a meticulous surgical technique aiming at a direct contact between living bone and implant. The interface zone between bone and implant was investigated using radiology, scanning electron microscopy (SEM), transmission electron microscopy (TEM), and histology. The SEM study showed a very

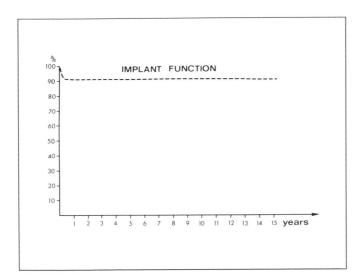

Fig. 3-4 A consecutive series of osseointegrated, mandibular implants show an initial loss of 6% during the first year after implantation. These losses depend on failure to achieve osseointegration for one reason or another. Thereafter, practically no implants are lost. This 96% plus success rate (with control for losses during the first year) indicates the unique feature of a proper direct bone anchorage—that functioning implants because of a bone condensation around them actually become more stable with longer times of clinical function.[21]

close spatial relationship between titanium and bone. No wear products were seen in the bone or soft tissues in spite of implant loading tissues up to 90 months.

Brånemark attributes the success of his method to the development of interfacial osteogenesis, osseointegration. This clinically documented fact makes Brånemark's work a dramatic improvement on the other implant systems currently used. While Brånemark's results do not preclude the possibility that other materials and/or systems could lead to similar osseointegration results, his is the only reported body of work supported by documented evidence. Figure 3-4 demonstrates long-term clinical results of consecutively inserted osseointegrated, mandibular dental implants. There is an initial 6% loss of the implants during the first year after insertion, but with control for these failures, the 10- to 15-year results demonstrate a 96% to 99% clinical success rate. This finding is, so far, a unique one, and it presents a challenge to apply osseointegrated implants in other cases of reconstruction, for instance, those of joint arthroplasty.

Gingival response

Some preliminary comments about the gingival response are relevant at this point, although this subject is discussed in chapter 5.

At the 1982 Toronto Conference on Osseointegration in Clinical Dentistry, Lindhe presented histological and microbiologic evidence from 20 patients who had been treated with osseointegrated dental prostheses for several years. He found a relatively sparse inflammatory infiltrate in the connective tissue, as well as reduced pathogenicity of the microorganisms in the plaque on the fixtures. His results seemed to suggest that the epithelial interface with the pure titanium surface may be a very adequate one and comparable in some ways to one with enamel or root surface of the natural tooth. It is tempting to conclude that the soft tissue/titanium relationship cannot and, perhaps, should not be assessed by conventional dental indices, and is *not* necessarily the "peri-implant" seal of consequence that implant literature suggests is necessary. In fact, Brånemark contends that osseointegration of the fixture into the host bone is adequate to ensure the ongoing viability of an abutment, even if an attachment apparatus coronally to the bone level does not occur.

In this context, Wennström's recent research suggests findings which may be extrapolated to the titanium-gingival unit.[22] His experimental observations with dogs and humans with natural teeth showed two very important features: *(1)* mechanical plaque control can be maintained without sign of recession or attachment loss, even in sites where attached or keratinized gingivae are lacking; and *(2)* a free gingiva supported by loosely attached alveolar mucosa is not more susceptible to bacterial plaque infection than a free gingiva supported by a wide zone of attached gingiva.

Conclusion

The pursuit of an analogue for the periodontal ligament has not led to a substitute that replicates its inseparable biological and mechanical roles.

It has, however, led to a clinical method that allows for interfacial osteogenesis or osseointegration. A great deal about the physical properties of the periodontal ligament attachment per se is unknown in both health and disease states. By the same token both the nature and the quality of osseointegration are still undergoing extensive investigation. But extensive clinical experiences in several countries and at least one comprehensive replication study endorse the clinical viability of the Brånemark method.

References

1. *Powell, R. N.*
   Tooth contact during sleep. Thesis, University of Rochester, 1963.

2. *Glickman, I., et al.*
   Functional occlusion as revealed by miniaturized radio transmitters. Dent. Clin. North Am. 13:667, 1969.

3. *Graf, H.*
   Bruxism. Dent. Clin. North Am. 13:659, 1969.

4. *Pilliar, R. M., et al.*
   Radiographic and morphologic studies of load-bearing porous-surfaced structured implants. Clin. Orthop. 156:249, 1981.

5. *Jacobs, H. G.*
   Implantologie und Zahnersatz. München: Hanser Verlag, 1976.

6. *Jacobs, H. G.*
   Formgestaltung und Materialfrage bei enossealen Implantaten zur Aufnahme von Zahnersatz. Dtsch. Zahnärztl. Z. 36:63, 1977.

7. *Muster, D., and Champy, M.*
   Le problème d'interface os-biomatériaux. Actual. Odontostomatol. 121:109, 1978.

8. *Osborn, J. F., and Newesly, H.*
   Dynamic aspects of the implant-bone-interface. In G. Heimke (ed.) Dental Implants, Materials and Systems. München: Hanser Verlag, 1980.

9. *Southam, J. C., and Selwyn, P.*
   Structural changes around screws used in the treatment of fractured human mandibles. Br. J. Oral Surg. 8:211, 1970.

10. *Charnley, J.*
    The nine and ten year results of low-friction hip arthroplasty of the hip. Clin. Orthop. 95:9, 1973.

11. *Ahnfeldt, L., Andersson, G., and Herberts, P.*
    Reoperated total hip prostheses in Sweden. Annual Meeting of the Swedish Orthopaedic Association, 1983, p. 14.

12. *Cotterill, P., Hunter, G., and Tile, M.*
    A radiographic analysis of 166 Charnley-Müller total hip arthroplasties. Clin. Orthop. 163:120, 1982.

13. *Stauffer, R. N.*
    A 10-year follow-up of Charnley total hip replacement with particular reference to loosening. J. Orthop. Res. 1:211, 1983.

14. *Johnston, R. C.*
    Long-term outcomes—Hip Society collective U. S. experience. J. Orthop. Res. 1:213, 1983.

15. *Feith, R.*
    Side effects of acrylic cement implanted into bone. Acta Orthop. Scand. 161 (Suppl.), 1975.

16. *Linder, L.*
    Bone cement monomer. Thesis, University of Göteborg, Sweden, 1976.

17. *Zarb, G., et. al.*
    The effects of cemented and uncemented endosseous implants. J. Prosthet. Dent. 42: 202, 1979.

18. *Brånemark, P.-I., et al.*
    Intraosseous anchorage of dental prostheses. I. Experimental studies. Scand. J. Plast. Reconstr. Surg. 3:81, 1969.

19. *Linder, L., and Lundskog, J.*
    Incorporation of stainless steel, titanium and Vitallium in bone. Injury 6:277, 1975.

20. *Klawitter, J. J., and Weinstein, A. M.*
    The status of porous materials to obtain direct skeletal attachment by tissue ingrowth. Acta Orthop. Belg. 40:755, 1974.

21. *Brånemark, P.-I., et al.*
    Osseointegrated implants in the treatment of the edentulous jaw. Scand. J. Plast. Reconstr. Surg. 11 (Suppl. 16), 1977.

22. *Wennström, J. L.*
    Keratinized and attached gingiva. Regenerative potential and significance for periodontal health. Thesis, University of Göteborg, Sweden, 1982.

Chapter 4

Metal Selection and Surface Characteristics

Bengt Kasemo and Jukka Lausmaa

Introduction

The choice of material for a particular implant application will ultimately be a compromise to meet many different required properties such as mechanical strength, machinability, elasticity, chemical properties, etc. Some properties may be more important than others. There is, however, one aspect that is always of prime importance: namely, how the tissue at the implant site responds to the biochemical disturbance that a foreign material presents. A closely related aspect is how the implant responds chemically to the living tissue environment.

Currently, there is no way to predict, a priori, how a particular material will react to or disturb its environment when positioned as an implant. However, choices based on general knowledge of chemical properties of materials, and on empirical knowledge from experiments with different implant materials, can be made. Such considerations have been, at best, the basis for experiments in the past, with many different materials such as polymers, ceramics, bioglasses, metals, and composite materials. The properties and applications of such materials in implant situations have been reviewed by several authors.[1,2]

In this chapter we focus on the physics and chemistry of solid surfaces as a basis for discussions of the biocompatibility of various inorganic materials, with special attention to titanium. Such an approach is highly relevant because all *primary interactions*, except long-range mechanical forces, take place over atomic dimensions at the implant-biotissue interface. The relative importance of the various types of interaction (van der Waal's interaction, strong chemical interaction, etc.) is dependent on the actual microstructure of the implant surface on an atomic scale. Thus, it is important to be able to prepare implant surfaces in a controlled way, and to analyze them.

This chapter's intention is to discuss the most important surface properties that may influence the biocompatibility of a particular implant material. An important ingredient in the study of implant surfaces, before and after implantation, is the possibility of surface composition control and composition analysis. In the Appendix an introduction is given to the principles and more general features (for example, sensitivity) of the most important surface sensitive spectroscopies.

The treatment deliberately focuses on the inorganic side of the implant-tissue interface. The use of titanium as a reference material in the explicit examples may appear to be a limitation. However, the discussion is general and valid for almost all metallic materials of interest, which are covered by a dense, protective oxide. Polymer materials, on the other hand, are beyond the scope of the present treatment.

Different classes of solid materials

Almost all inorganic materials that are of any interest as construction materials consist of very dense arrangements of their constituent atoms. They are penetrable (often very slowly) only by diffusion of single atoms, but do not allow passage of even the smallest molecules. Most of these materials are *crystalline* and are composed of a large number of small crystallites. Each crystallite is an ordered arrangement of atoms. Such materials are called *polycrystalline.* Most metals and many ceramics are polycrystalline.

In some materials the atoms are arranged in a less ordered way, almost as in a liquid but with much less mobility. Such materials are called *amorphous,* and in this context, the most important are glasses. Many materials can take different crystalline forms in different situations. One well-known example is carbon, which can be completely crystalline as in a diamond. Graphite, another form of carbon, is also crystalline. Carbon can also be amorphous. These different forms have very different properties, which originate from their differences in atomic arrangements.

Metals are special among the construction materials. They are single-element materials (composed of one kind of atom), many are easily machined, they are ductile, and they have advantageous mechanical properties. Metals, however, are also reactive (except the noble metals Au, Pt, Pd, etc.) and therefore usually exist in nature as chemical compounds. One important consequence of this reactivity is that most pure metals are covered by an oxide layer.

Sometimes two or more different metals are mixed in order to make better certain properties. Such metallic mixtures are called *alloys.* Well-known examples are brass (63% Cu, 27% Zn) and stainless steel (Fe plus small amounts of other metals such as Cr, Ni, V, Mo).

Many *nonmetallic* materials are formed as chemical compounds between metals and other elements such as oxides, nitrides, and carbides. Many of these materials are classified as *ceramics.* Examples include aluminum oxide (Al_2O_3), titanium oxide and titanium nitride, and tungsten carbide. Characteristic properties of ceramics are their great hardness (but usually high brittleness), good high-temperature properties, and chemical inertness. Usually, they are mechanically not as strong and advantageous as metals and they are much more difficult to machine.

Glasses are materials related to the ceramic materials (or they may be regarded as a particular class of ceramics) but have an amorphous structure. Glasses are often compounds of several elements and can usually be formed to particular geometric structures via their molten state or by machining.

Each class of materials mentioned above has its own virtues, and the choice for a particular construction detail or implant application will be a compromise between different requirements. Metals are the most versatile inorganic materials in view of their high strength and ductility, elasticity, and machinability, but sometimes it is advantageous to combine these properties with some of the superior properties of ceramics, for example. This combination has led to the development of composite materials and surface coating techniques, which combine the best characteristics of two or more different materials. For example, the mechanical strength may be obtained from a bulk metal whereas the corrosion or wear resistance is obtained from a layer of ceramic material. Metals are, in this respect, very special because they offer this kind of combination of properties. Stainless steel, for example, has enormous versatility due to its bulk metallic properties, but its corrosion resistance is the result of the very dense and chemically inert oxide (i.e., ceramic) of ~5 nm thickness that automatically forms on the surface of this alloy upon exposure to air. Independent of which material is chosen as an implant material, it will be its surface that comes into contact with the host tissue. Therefore, the following sections will deal with the surface properties of solid, inorganic materials in more detail.

Properties of solid surfaces

In the same way as three-dimensional solids, surfaces can be crystalline, polycrystalline, and amorphous. The outermost surface of 1-10 atomic distances in thickness, however, may be very different from the corresponding bulk material. Subtle differences that exist concern electronic structure, crystal structure, spacing of atomic layers, etc.[3] More dramatic differences of importance in materials science applications concern changes in chemical composition at surfaces due to segregation or formation of surface compounds via chemical interaction with the environment.[3] It is, for example, widely known that an alloy with a particular bulk composition may have a dramatically different composition in the outermost atomic layers due to preferential accumulation of one alloy constituent on the surface. The driving force for such segregation is usually of purely thermodynamic origin, but it may be enhanced or decreased by chemical interaction with the environment. Since the primary chemical interaction between an implant and its host tissue takes place over a few atomic radii (see following section on bonding forces), such compositional changes may have a strong influence on the biocompatibility of materials.

The chemical composition of a surface is particularly important for the tendency of a surface to *adsorb* foreign atoms or molecules. This phenomenon is discussed in the next section, but we want to underline here that different surfaces have very different adsorption properties, and that these differences are closely connected to the chemical aspects of biocompatibility.

Consider the case of a metal implant. Let us assume that the pure metal, while being machined, is suddenly exposed to the environment (air at room temperature). Because the fresh metal is not in thermal equilibrium with its surroundings, and because, in most cases, it is capable of dissociating the oxygen molecules in the air, a surface oxide will form very quickly.[4] Figures 4-1a and b illustrate schematically the continuous growth of the oxide. The first step is adsorption of O_2 molecules, which immediately dissociate to O atoms. After as little as 10 nanoseconds the first monoatomic layer of oxygen is formed. Within about a millisecond an oxide layer of 1 nm thickness may have grown, and within a few seconds the oxide growth may be virtually completed at an oxide thickness of a few nanometers. This holds approximately for most metals that are used as construction materials. (The noble metals gold and platinum are exceptional in that very high temperatures or other extreme conditions are required for surface oxides to form.) The surface oxide stops growing for kinetic reasons, i.e., due to slow transport of oxygen and metal atoms, and not because of thermodynamics. The latter would predict complete oxidation throughout the whole metal piece. Therefore, the oxide growth will increase in rate and thickness if the oxygen and/or metal atom transport is accelerated, for example, by an increase in temperature or by the presence of certain impurities.

From this oxidation behavior we learn that almost any metal chosen for use as an implant material will be covered by an oxide layer a few nanometers thick. On the metals

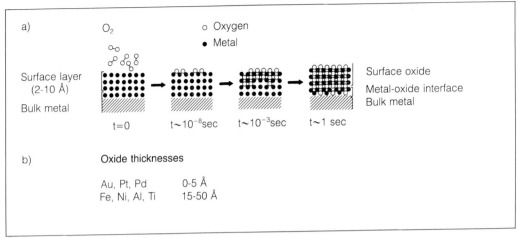

Figs. 4-1a and b   Short summary of some important aspects of metal oxidation.

Fig. 4-1a   Illustrates the time scale on which a fresh metallic surface oxidizes. The fresh metal ($t = 0$) can be prepared by a machining tool or a fracture. In less than one second (in air) a several angstrom-thick layer of oxide is formed on most metals. The resulting structure is a surface oxide plus a metal-oxide interface plus a bulk metal.

Fig. 4-1b   Indicates the oxide thicknesses that appear on various metals in air at about room temperature.

in question, and in not too aggressive environments, this oxide is highly protective and prevents direct contact between the environment and the metal itself. The importance of this cannot be overestimated. It means, in the context of implants, that *a contact is never established between the implant metal and the host tissue, but rather between the tissue and the surface oxide of the implant.*[5,6] Because the latter has completely different chemical properties than the metal itself, *it is the biocompatibility of the oxide that is the relevant parameter* in the discussion of biocompatibility from a chemical point of view. Thus, titanium implants biochemically resemble titanium oxides, and aluminum implants resemble alumina. Oxides on alloys will, in general, have a relative concentration of metal ions that differs considerably from that in the bulk metal.

A striking example of this is that 99.999% pure aluminum, with a small bulk impurity Mg-concentration, develops a surface oxide that predominantly contains MgO upon oxidation in air around 500°C.[7]

There are a few significant differences between surface oxides and bulk oxides that must be remembered. If the oxide on the metal is not fully protective it may start to grow or to corrode by metal dissolution, for example (see next section). A surface oxide may also contain a much larger number of defects and areas of nonstoichiometric composition than the corresponding bulk oxide. Such differences will in turn result in different chemical properties. In spite of these reservations we can safely say that an implant made from a metal which forms a very stable surface oxide such as Ti (TiO_2), Zr (ZrO_2), Al (Al_2O_3), Ta (Ta_2O_5), etc., can be

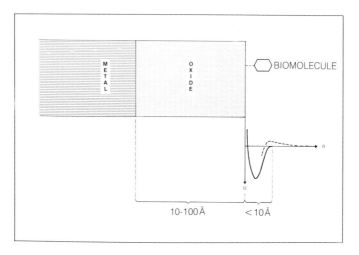

Fig. 4-2 Schematic of the length scales involved in the interaction between a small molecule and an implant surface. The full line shows the interaction potential, *U*, as a function of distance, *R*, between the biomolecule and the surface, in vacuum. The dashed curve shows the interaction in an aqueous medium, indicating a repulsive potential at distances beyond the short-range attractive potential.[9]

expected to have many chemical properties in common with implants made from the corresponding bulk oxides. By choosing the right metal as an implant material one can obtain the attractive combination of a mechanically strong nucleus (the metal) and a biochemically advantageous very thin surface coating (the oxide). This appears to be the case with titanium.

Bonding forces and chemical processes at surfaces

Bonding forces at the implant surface

There are several types of bonding by which biomolecules may be bound to solid surfaces.[3] Independent of the type of bonding the attractive interaction potential is of quite short range as illustrated in Fig. 4-2. The range of the interaction potential is considerably shorter than the oxide thickness on a metal implant, which underlines the argument that there is no direct interaction between the metal and the biomolecules.

The weakest type of bonding is the so-called *van der Waal's bonding* or *physisorption bonding* (Fig. 4-3a). Van der Waal's bonds have bond strengths of < 10 kcal/mole but may still dominate at distances ~1 nm from the surface, since they have a longer interaction range than the strong chemical forces. Bonds that are somewhat stronger are established between permanent electric dipoles that are frequently occurring both in biomolecules and at (polar) oxide surfaces. A third type of bonding important in biomolecule-surface interaction is *hydrogen bonding* (Fig. 4-3b) with bond strengths of ~1-10 kcal/mole. The strongest bonds are established by *covalent* and *ionic bonds* (Fig. 4-3c) which may give bond energies in the range of 10-100 kcal/mole. For the latter types of bonding the surface composition on an atomic scale will be important. Particularly strong bonds may be established at specific *defect sites* such as anion or cation *vacancies, impurity atoms, grain boundaries*, etc. (Fig. 4-4).

So far we have neglected the fact that the biological environment is aqueous, i.e., the most commonly occurring molecule is water. Water molecules can participate in the

103

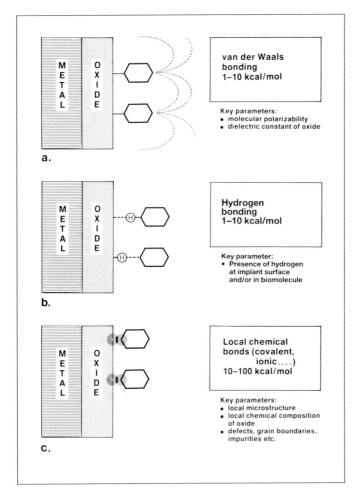

Figs. 4-3a to c Different types of bonding between a biomolecule and an implant surface.

Fig. 4-3a Van der Waal's bonding.

Fig. 4-3b Hydrogen bonding.

Fig. 4-3c Covalent and ionic bonding.

hydrogen bonding (see above), but will also modify, for instance, ionic bonding as the ions will be hydrated, that is, surrounded by a shell of water molecules. Furthermore, the presence of water may give rise to quite strong repulsive interaction[8, 9] at distances beyond the range of the short range attractive forces. In such cases, a more appropriate potential energy curve for a biomolecule at large distances from the surface is given by the dashed curve in Fig. 4-2. An excellent, short resume of the role of water in biomolecule-surface interaction is given by Parsegian.[9]

In a real situation all of the above-mentioned types of interactions are expected to compete and dominate on various parts of the heterogeneous implant surface. Some molecules will be weakly bound by van der Waal's or hydrogen bonds, others will be much more strongly bound, maybe at defect sites. Biomolecules with a high specificity for the implant surface are expected to build up the first monoatomic layer, on top of

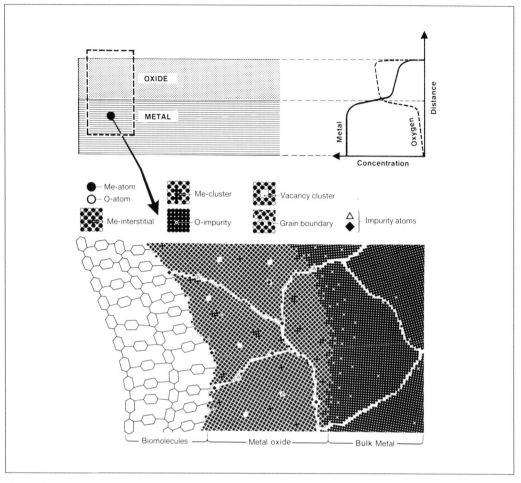

Fig. 4-4   Hypothetical picture of the implant biotissue interface. Shown are possible chemical bonding sites at the implant surface, such as vacancies, interstitials, impurities, and grain boundaries. The organic side of the interface is represented by a network of adsorbed biomolecules.[6]

which subsequent molecular layers build up. Eventually, at larger distances (> 1 nm), more organized biological complexes and cell structures are expected to appear. Figure 4-4 is an attempt to illustrate this rather hypothetical picture of the interface zone. Albrektsson et al. discuss this in more detail.[6]

One important consequence of the variety of bond strengths that can be established con-

cerns the *time scales* on which chemical processes may take place. If bonds stronger than ∼30 kcal/mole are formed, they may be regarded as essentially irreversible, as the exchange time of molecules in such bonds is several years. If, on the other hand, van der Waal's or hydrogen bonds prevail, the corresponding time scale is some microseconds or less at body temperature. Thus, the type of bonding de-

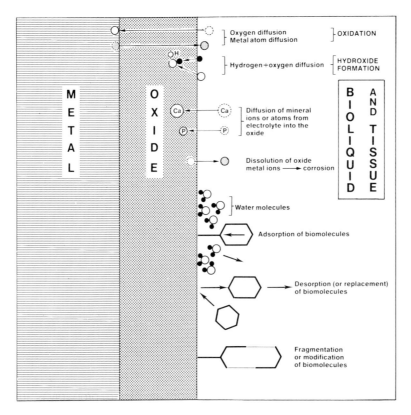

Fig. 4-5 Chemical processes that can take place at the interface at a molecular scale.[5]

termines whether the interface should be regarded as a *dynamic interface,* with continuous exchange of atoms, molecules, and radicals, or if a more *static* picture should be adopted. The experimental indications that there is a substantial in vivo growth in oxide thickness on titanium implants [10] supports a *dynamic picture.* It is thus relevant to discuss some of the chemical processes that may take place in the close proximity of the implant surface.

Processes at the implant surface

Figure 4-5 schematically illustrates some of the processes that may take place at the interface on an atomic scale. An investiga-

tion of the thickness of the surface oxide as a function of the implant period indicates that the oxide thickness increases much faster at the implant position in bone than when it is left in air.[10] This growth must take place by either or both of the mechanisms indicated at the top of Fig. 4-5, namely, metal atom/ion *diffusion* out to the oxide surface followed by oxidation, or oxygen diffusion from an oxygen-carrying species at the oxide surface to the metal oxide interface. As a result of participation of hydrogen atoms (or protons), the oxide can also grow by hydroxide formation, as indicated by the OH radical. Other components that can contribute to growth and modification of the oxide include the mineral ions of Ca and P.

The arrow labeled *corrosion* suggests the

possibility of dissolution of the protecting oxide layer, which may be a severe problem with some implant materials. The corrosion mechanism and the corrosion behavior of different implant materials have been reviewed by Williams.[11]

Figure 4-5 also illustrates the *adsorption* and *desorption* of molecules at the oxide surface. The bond strength between the biomolecule and the surface determines whether or not desorption (or replacement) of biomolecules takes place. Hydration of the oxide is another process that is likely to occur and that may be important in establishing a suitable chemical environment for the biomolecules.

So far we have only considered processes that influence the composition of the implant surface (oxide) layer. Ultimately, it is of course the influence of the implant surface on the surrounding biotissue and on the biological processes at the interface that determines the future success or failure of the implantation. It is, for example, important that the implant does not have a strong *denaturing* effect on proteins at the surface. Whether or not denaturing occurs depends critically on the type and strength of the bonds between the protein in question and the implant surface. If the internal bonds, which determine the protein conformation, are too strongly influenced, the protein will denature. On the other hand, if these bonds are only weakly effected, the protein will remain in its original conformation. (Since metal oxide surfaces are characterized by acidic and basic sites, one can in some respects use the analogy with acids and bases to understand how oxide surfaces can change protein conformation.) Another way by which denaturing may be prevented is if the implant surface selectively adsorbs biomolecules that form a separating layer between the implant surface and the proteins.

Finally, an even more active participation of the implant surface in the osseointegration process cannot be excluded. Most metal oxides are *catalytically active* for many inorganic chemical reactions and it is not unlikely that the implant surface oxide can catalyze some biological processes at the interface.[14,15]

In this context it is interesting to speculate how the implant zone develops with time after implantation.[6] From the first fractions of seconds the surface is exposed to an aqueous medium containing various biomolecules (blood). Some of them will rapidly be attached via formation of the bonds discussed above. Many or all of them will eventually be replaced due to appearance (for example, due to changes in the biochemistry) of more efficiently competing molecules. There is probably a continuous change in chemical environment during the entire healing period of a few months.[12] The oxide obviously starts to grow due to perhaps oxidizing radicals created in metabolic processes. We emphasize that the most appropriate picture probably is an interface that is dynamic on all time scales, from the first few seconds, over the first hours, days, and months, until more than a decade, when dental Ti implants at least still seem to function perfectly.[12]

This discussion has pointed out the variety of processes associated with implant surfaces that may influence the integration of an implant in the body. It should be obvious that the chemical properties of the outermost atomic layers of the implant are key factors in the integration process. Furthermore, there emerges no strong physical or chemical argument against, but rather for, the possibility of an integration between suitable implant surfaces and biotissue.

Surface roughness

Surface roughness of implants will have different roles depending on the different geometric dimensions involved. On the ~100 μm scale and upwards a rough or porous surface may sometimes be advantageous, from a mechanical point of view, because it can give a suitable stress distribution.[6, 13] The second region is below ~100 μm, but much above the nanometer region, where roughness may influence the interface biology, because a region is entered where the sizes of cells and large biomolecules are the same order of magnitude as the curvature of the roughness. The chemical bonding and the chemical processes discussed in the two preceding sections will in principle be the same, independent of the roughness on this scale. However, if for example metal ion dissolution occurs, it will be a disadvantage to have a very rough or porous surface, because the total exposed area, and thus the amount of dissolved metal, will be larger.

Surface roughness on the nanometer scale will influence the local electromagnetic fields close to the implant surface and may give changes in the bonding by van der Waal's interaction. Surface roughness on the atomic scale also introduces bonding sites of different bonding energies than on atomically flat surfaces. In practice, implant surfaces will almost always have considerable roughness on the nanometer scale.

The conclusion is that the basic chemical and physical properties discussed in this chapter are the same on a molecular scale, independent of whether or not the surface is rough. On the other hand, the adhesion of large aggregates such as cells and very large biomolecules are expected to be influenced by surface roughness far above the nanometer scale. The mechanical properties of the implant-host system will obviously also be influenced by the surface roughness on the coarser scale.

Titanium as an implant material

Selected properties

It should be clear that the proven high biocompatibility of titanium as an implant material is connected with the properties of its surface oxide. In air or water titanium quickly forms an oxide thickness of 3 to 5 nm at room temperature. Titanium can form several oxides of different stoichiometry— TiO, Ti_2O_3, TiO_2—of which TiO_2 is the most common. TiO_2 can have three different crystal structures—rutile, anatase, and brookite—but also can be amorphous. TiO_2 is very resistant against chemical attack, which makes titanium one of the most *corrosion resistant* metals, particularly in the chemical environment with which we are concerned. This is one contributing factor to its high biocompatibility. This property is also shared with several other metals such as Al which forms Al_2O_3 and Zr which forms ZrO_2 on their surfaces.

Another physical property that is unique for TiO_2 is its *high dielectric constant,* which ranges from 50 to 170 depending on crystal structure. This high dielectric constant would result in considerably stronger van der Waal's bonds on TiO_2 than on other oxides, a fact that may be important for the interface biochemistry.[6]

TiO_2, like many other transition metal oxides, is *catalytically active* for a number of inorganic and organic chemical reactions,[14, 15] which also may influence the interface chemistry.

Finally, the titanium metal itself is a construction material of more than sufficient strength for most implant applications. It is lighter

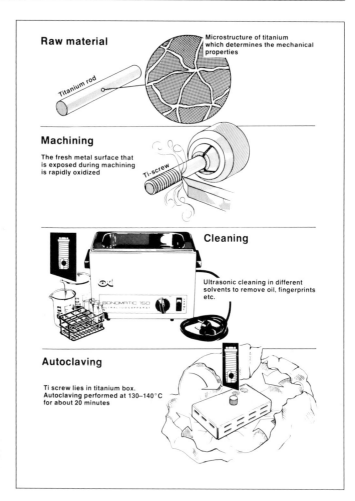

Raw material

Titanium rod

Microstructure of titanium which determines the mechanical properties

Machining

The fresh metal surface that is exposed during machining is rapidly oxidized

Ti-screw

Cleaning

Ultrasonic cleaning in different solvents to remove oil, fingerprints etc.

SONOMATIC 150

Autoclaving

Ti screw lies in titanium box. Autoclaving performed at 130–140°C for about 20 minutes

Fig. 4-6   The different steps in the preparation of titanium dental implants. During the different steps a surface oxide develops on the implant.[5]

than most construction metals due to its rather low density, which can be an advantage in some applications.

Preparation of titanium dental implants

The nature of the surface oxide on titanium (or any other metal) implants depends crucially on the conditions during the oxidation and the subsequent treatment of the implant. We will, therefore, briefly describe the preparation methods for the dental implants used by Brånemark as reported by Adell et al.,[12] and discuss how the various preparation steps may influence the implant surface (Fig. 4-6). The implants are made from pure titanium that is shaped by carefully controlled machining (lathing, threading, milling, etc.). During the machining procedure, the fresh metal is exposed to air (and lubricants or coolants) and oxidizes rapidly. The nature of the surface oxide will depend on the machining conditions (e.g., pressure and speed). During the subsequent preparation

109

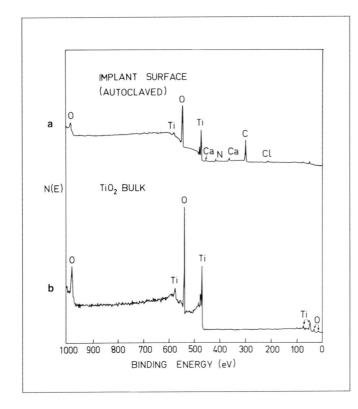

Fig. 4-7a XPS (ESCA) spectrum from the surface of a titanium sample, prepared according to the procedures described in the text and in Fig. 4-6.

Fig. 4-7b An XPS spectrum from a bulk TiO_2 sample. Comparison between the two spectra shows that the implant surface consists of mainly TiO_2, with small amounts of C, N, Cl, and Ca.[16]

steps (ultrasonic cleaning and sterilizing) the initial surface oxide will be modified. Especially during the sterilizing procedure (autoclaving) the oxide will undergo a slight growth in the elevated temperature and humid atmosphere. Autoclaving also might cause incorporation of OH radicals in the surface oxide.

Spectroscopic characterization and elemental composition of titanium implant surfaces

Considerable variations in the implant surface oxide are expected for different preparation conditions. The chemical composition of titanium surfaces prepared with the pro-

cedures just described is now quite well known[16] from studies using surface sensitive spectroscopies (see Appendix). Figure 4-7a shows a typical XPS (ESCA) spectrum from such a prepared pure titanium sample. As a reference a spectrum from a bulk TiO_2 sample is shown (Fig. 4-7b). From a comparison of the two spectra it is quite obvious that the oxide on the titanium surface is mainly TiO_2.[16] The thickness of the surface oxide is typically 3 to 5 nm, as determined by Mattsson and Lausmaa.[17]

There are several chemical elements present on the oxidized titanium surface that are absent on the reference TiO_2 sample. (The latter has been carefully cleaned in vacuum before analysis.) A large carbon signal ($\sim$40 atomic %) is always observed, as well as a smaller nitrogen one. Lower concentrations of chlorine, sulphur, and calcium are often detected. These impurities except Ca are confined to the outermost atomic layer, which means that their total concentrations are in the range of 0.001–0.01 µg per square centimeter implant surface. Ca, however, is found throughout the oxide layer.

The origin of these very small concentrations of contaminants is probably adsorption of C, N, S, and Cl containing molecules on the oxide surface during the preparation procedures. They can easily be removed by a slight ion etching in vacuum, but at least the C signal will reappear after air exposure. The Ca signal may originate from surface segregation of a low concentration of Ca in the titanium sample. Another type of analysis indicated that the oxide also contains relatively large amounts of hydrogen, probably bound as OH.[16]

Because the role of even small amounts of contaminants on the biocompatibility of implant materials is not well known, it is advisable to keep a high standard on the cleaning procedures. One recent example illustrates how an impurity of very low concentration can dramatically change the properties of the surface oxide.[18] Via the textile cloths wrapped around the container box for the titanium fixtures during autoclaving, a very minute amount of fluorine was deposited on the titanium surfaces. On the most exposed parts this resulted in the growth of more than 700-Å-thick oxide films, which is more than ten times the thickness usually found after autoclaving. The fluorine ions obviously accelerated the oxide growth considerably. Since the acceptance or nonacceptance of such changes by the body tissue are unknown, great care must be taken to avoid impurities. Particular attention should be paid to catalytically active elements, which can profoundly influence the chemical interface processes even at extremely low concentrations.

Alternative surface preparation methods

Although the present preparation procedures for dental titanium implants have been highly successful, it is unlikely that they are optimal from a biocompatibility point of view. It may therefore be desirable that new techniques are applied, by which the surface properties of titanium (or other metals) implants can be varied in a more controlled manner.

There exists today a large number of different methods for more or less sophisticated surface treatment,[19] including *anodic oxidation, plasma oxidation, plasma cleaning,* and *vapor deposition.*

Anodic oxidation

Anodic oxidation is an electrochemical method of treatment. The sample to be treated is made an anode in an electrolytic bath, and when a potential is applied on the sample, a current will flow through the electrolyte due to ion transport. The transport of oxygen ions through the electrolyte builds up a passivating oxide layer on the surface of the sample. The thickness of the surface oxide formed depends, often linearly, on the applied potential. Anodic oxidation thus offers a possibility to control the thickness of the surface oxide in a much wider range than thermal oxidation allows. By a proper choice of electrolytes, the chemical composition of the oxide can, to some extent, be controlled, for example, by incorporation of mineral ions. The crystal structure of the oxide can also be varied by using electrolyte, current density, and oxide thickness as parameters.

Plasma oxidation

In plasma oxidation, an oxygen plasma is used instead of a liquid electrolyte. Plasma oxidation offers essentially the same possibilities to control the surface oxide but is basically a cleaner method than anodic oxidation. Plasma cleaning is technically identical to plasma oxidation, but is used in order to increase the surface cleanliness, which usually results in an increase in the surface energy.[20]

Vapor deposition

Vapor deposition can be used to deposit desirable atoms or continuous films on surfaces. As the name implies, the method is based on the principle that the material to be deposited is heated until it evaporates. Alternatively, energetic ions can be used to vaporize the material. The vapor is then allowed to condense on the material to be covered. These techniques are often referred to as *physical vapor deposition (PVD)*. Deposition can also be made by chemical reactions and is then called *chemical vapor deposition (CVD)*. With PVD and CVD a wide range of composite materials and surface coatings can be produced.

Future development

It is likely that these techniques will play an increasingly important role in the future development of implant materials. The application of these and many other available surface preparation methods, however, requires knowledge of the parameters that are important for the biocompatibility in a certain application, and of which parameters are less crucial. One can safely say that the limitation lies in the methods by which biocompatibility can be "measured." The available tests that can decide whether one implant material is better than the other are inexact and time consuming. There is thus a great need for a combination of biochemical and medical tests that can specify relevant biocompatibility parameters. Once such tests are available, the state of the art of surface preparation and characterization techniques can be combined to tailor-make implant surfaces for optimal biocompatibility.

Summary and conclusions

On a molecular scale the basic physical and chemical interactions at implant-host interfaces are the same, independent of the type of inorganic material involved. Ceramic and metallic materials are, from a practical viewpoint, very closely related, because the chemical properties of metallic implants are governed by their surface oxides, which are ceramic materials (exceptions are the noble metals Au, Pt, Pd, etc.). This conclusion is based on the usually valid assumption that the surface oxides are stable and considerably thicker by several nanometers than the range of the chemical interaction forces at surfaces. The most important of the latter are van der Waal's interaction, hydrogen bonding, dipole interaction, and covalent and ionic interaction, with force fields of ≤ 1 nm. A large number of chemical processes that are expected to occur at implant interfaces are identified, such as ion transport, oxide dissolution (corrosion), adsorption and fragmentation of biomolecules, incorporation of mineral ions in the oxide, metabolically driven oxidation, denaturation of proteins, catalytic processes, etc. The relative importance of these various processes are expected to vary with time after the moment of implantation. The relevant time scales range from the first fractions of seconds to many years.

The more macroscopic interactions at implant interfaces, which take place mainly via mechanical forces, probably affect the chemical interface processes, but in a yet unknown way. Surface roughness does not influence the primary chemical interactions (i.e., on the nm scale), but is important on a macroscopic scale, e.g., for the strength of the implant-host system.

Analysis of titanium dental implants verifies that the surface is covered by a 3- to 5-nm-thick oxide. The oxide composition is mainly TiO_2. Small amounts ($\leq 10^{-8}$ g/cm^2) of contaminants (mainly carbon) on the outermost atomic layer of the implant surface probably originate from the preparation procedure.

Important properties that are expected to influence the biocompatibility of implants are the corrosion resistance of the surface (of the surface oxide on metallic implants), the tendency for proteins to denature, the selective adsorption of biomolecules, the dielectric constant, and perhaps the catalytic activity.

The proven high biocompatibility of titanium is probably connected with the high corrosion resistance of the surface oxide, its high dielectric constant, and the preparation procedure that produces a relatively clean surface. Other factors that may be relevant are the defect density in the oxide, its crystalline structure, and incorporation of OH radicals. It is unlikely that the surface preparation used today optimizes the biocompatibility of implants. Alternative methods for implant preparation include electropolishing, anodic oxidation, plasma oxidation, plasma cleaning, and physical and chemical vapor deposition. These methods offer a higher flexibility in surface preparation than the methods used today. Spectroscopic methods that can be used to map out the implant surfaces and the implant-biotissue interface, on the molecular scale, are extremely important in this context.

With the large variety of implant surface preparation and characterization methods that are available, tailor-made surfaces that optimize healing-in periods, success rates, etc., could probably be made. Such a development is prevented, mainly because of the lack of reliable methods to measure the biocompatibility of an implant for a specific application. *The development of such methods for rapid in vitro and in vivo tests is thus one of the most urgent tasks for research in the field of biocompatibility.*

Appendix
Selected methods for spectroscopic characterization of implant surfaces

From the discussions in this chapter it is obvious that characterization of implant surfaces on the atomic scale is desirable. Fortunately, there are several methods available that allow a detailed mapping of chemical composition, depth profiles, crystal structure, bonding types, etc., at surfaces. For a more detailed description of these and other spectroscopic techniques refer to textbooks on the subject.[21, 22]

Most surface spectroscopies are based on the principle that the surface to be investigated is irradiated by a beam of particles (e.g., photons, electrons, or ions). The primary particles induce excitations in the surface, which responds by emitting secondary particles. Surface sensitivity is achieved if the primary (and/or secondary) particles have short penetration (or escape) depths in solids. By measuring some suitable physical property of the secondary particles, information about the surface may be derived.

The most important techniques for studying the chemical composition of surfaces are *x-ray photoemission spectroscopy (XPS)*, also called *ESCA (electron spectroscopy for chemical analysis), Auger electron spectroscopy (AES),* and *secondary ion mass spectroscopy (SIMS).*

In XPS the surface is irradiated by an x-ray beam which induces emission of secondary electrons (so-called photoelectrons) from the atoms in the sample. Each element present at the surface will emit photoelectrons with some characteristic energies. By measuring the energies of the photoelectrons, an energy distribution spectrum will be obtained. This spectrum exhibits peaks at energies corresponding to the elements present at the surface, thus giving a "fingerprint" of the surface chemical composition. The relative intensities of the peaks can be used to obtain quantitative values of the concentrations of each element. Because electrons have short escape depths in solids, most of the photoelectrons originate from the few outermost atomic layers of the surface, thus giving XPS a high surface sensitivity. All elements except hydrogen can be detected by XPS and the detection limit is typically ~0.5 atomic %. In addition to elemental analysis, XPS reveals the chemical bonding state (for example, oxidation number) of the detected elements. This ability is due to measurable energy shifts (chemical shifts) in the electron levels of atoms in different chemical environments.

In AES the surface is irradiated by a reasonably monoenergetic (1-10 keV) electron beam. The electron bombardment results in emission of secondary electrons from the surface atoms. Some of the secondary electrons, the so-called Auger electrons, will show up at energies that are characteristic for the element from which they originate. Element identification is made, analogously to XPS, by recording the energy spectrum of the Auger electrons. Since AES is based on more complex physical processes than XPS, AES spectra are more difficult to quantitate than are XPS. AES, however, is a faster

and more sensitive (~0.1 atomic %) technique than XPS. Often AES is combined with ion sputtering techniques, which involve removal of atomic layers from the surface so that concentration depth profiles can be measured.

SIMS is based on a controlled removal of particles (atoms, molecules, and fragments) from the surface by an energetic ion beam. Those particles that leave the surface in an ionized state are analyzed in a mass spectrometer. The secondary ion mass spectrum reflects (often in an indirect way) the chemical composition of the surface. By using low-intensity ion beams it is possible to analyze only the outermost atomic layer of the surface *(static SIMS).* If instead high-intensity ion beams are used the information will originate from a continuously increasing depth *(dynamic SIMS).* This latter application of SIMS is especially suited for measuring depth profiles. The depth resolution for such measurements is typically 1 to 10 nm. The main advantages with SIMS are that it is one of the few analytical techniques that can detect hydrogen and that it is extremely sensitive (concentrations $<10^{-4}$ atomic % can be detected). Interpretation of SIMS results, however, relies strongly on empirical background knowledge in form of reference samples and calibrations.

These three methods provide a powerful combination for studying the chemical composition of surfaces and surface layers. Other methods that should be mentioned in this context are the nuclear micro analysis *(NMA)* techniques. These include Rutherford backscattering *(RBS)* and methods based on *nuclear reaction resonances.* Molecules adsorbed on surfaces are best studied by *infrared absorption reflection spectroscopy (IRAS)* and *high-resolution electron energy loss spectroscopy (HREELS).*

We should also mention the electron microscopic techniques. With *transmission elec-*

tron microscopy (TEM), detailed information about the crystal structure of bulk material and surface oxides can be obtained. *Scanning electron microscopy (SEM)* is useful for studying the morphology of surfaces and for microstructural characterization of implant-biotissue interfaces. For these applications, SEM is superior to the optical microscope due to its high lateral resolution (~10 nm) and wide depth of focus. SEM is often combined with elemental analysis by x-ray fluorescence spectroscopy. It should be said, however, that such elemental analysis is not surface sensitive.

The above-mentioned methods are mainly directed toward identification of elements, their chemical bonding states and concentrations, or the microstructure of the sample surfaces. For studies of chemical interaction between implants and biomolecules other methods directed toward kinetic behavior, for example, are needed. One powerful method for such studies is *ellipsometry,*[23] which can be used for both kinetic studies and, in its most advanced form, for spectroscopic identification of adsorbed biomolecules. Development of methods for studies of implant-biomolecule interactions, in the complex biological environment that is the reality of practical implant situations, is strongly needed.

References

1. *Williams, D. F. (ed.)*
   Biocompatibility of clinical implant materials. *In* Fundamental Aspects of Biocompatibility. Vols. I-II. Boca Raton, Fla.: CRC Press Inc., 1981.

2. *Hench, L. L.*
   Biomaterials. Science 208:826, 1980.

3. *King, D. A., and Woodruff, P. (eds.)*
   The Chemical Physics of Solid Surfaces and Heterogeneous Catalysis. Vols. I-IV. Amsterdam: Elsevier Scientific Publishing Company, 1981.

4. *Fromhold, A. T., Jr.*
   Theory of Metal Oxidation. Vol. I. Amsterdam: North Holland Publishing Company, 1976, pp. 3-24.

5. *Kasemo, B.*
   Biocompatibility of titanium implants: Surface science aspects. J. Prosthet. Dent. 49:832, 1983.

6. *Albrektsson, T., et al.*
   The interface zone of inorganic implants in vivo: Titanium implants in bone. Ann. Biomed. Eng. 11:1, 1983.

7. *Rönnhult, T.*
   Personal communication.

8. *Lis, L. J., et al.*
   Interactions between neutral phospholipid bilayer membranes. Biophys. J. 37:657, 1982.

9. *Parsegian, J. A.*
   Molecular forces governing tight contact between cellular surfaces and substrates. J. Prosthet. Dent. 49:838, 1983.

10. *McQueen, D. H., et al.*
    Clinical applications of biomaterials. pp. 179-185 *In* A. J. C. Lee et al. (eds.) Advances in Biomaterials. Vol. 4. Clinical Applications of Biomaterials. New York: John Wiley & Sons, 1982.

11. *Williams, D. F. (ed.)*
    Fundamental Aspects of Biocompatibility. Vol. I. Boca Raton, Fla.: CRC Press Inc., 1981, pp. 11-42.

12. *Adell, R., et al.*
    A 15-year study of osseointegrated implants in the treatment of the edentulous jaw. Int. J. Oral Surg. 10:387, 1981.

13. *Skalak, R.*
    Biomechanical considerations in osseointegrated prostheses. J. Prosthet. Dent. 49:843, 1983.

14. *Voorhoeve, R. J. H., et al.*
    Perovskite oxides: Materials science in catalysis. Science 195:827-833, 1977.

15. *Samsonov, G. V. (ed.)*
    The Oxide Handbook. New York: IFI/Plenum Data Corporation, 1973, pp. 411-440.

16. *Lausmaa, J., and Kasemo, B.*
Unpublished work.

17. *Mattsson, H., and Lausmaa, J.*
Unpublished work.

18. *Lausmaa, J., and Hansson, S.*
Accelerated oxide growth on titanium implants during autoclaving, caused by fluorine contamination. Biomaterials 1985 (in press).

19. *Chapman, B. N., and Andersson, J. C. (eds.)*
Science and Technology of Surface Coatings. New York: Academic Press, 1974.

20. *Baier, R. E., and De Palma, V. A.*
Calspan Corporation, Report No. 176, Buffalo, N.Y., 1970.

21. *Czanderna, A. W. (ed.)*
Methods of Surface Analysis. Amsterdam: Elsevier Scientific Publishing Company, 1975.

22. *Kane, P. R., and Larrabee, G. B. (eds.)*
Characterization of Solid Surfaces. New York: Plenum Press, 1974.

23. *Poste, G., and Moss, C.*
The study of surface reactions in biological systems by ellipsometry. pp. 139-232 *In* G. Davidsson (ed.) Progress in Surface Science. Vol. 2, Part 3. New York: Pergamon Press, 1972.

Chapter 5

Aspects of Biomechanical Considerations

Richard Skalak

Introduction

This chapter reviews biomechanical considerations in the design and performance of prosthetic reconstructions on osseointegrated implants beginning with the nature of the osseointegrated fixture system of transmittance of stresses from the implant to the bone. At the microscopic scale, the close approximation of the osseointegrated bone with the surface of an implanted fixture allows the transmission of forces with little relative displacement of the bone and implant even in the absence of adhesive bone. This behavior on a microscale is comparable to the resistance of a screw to lateral or axial forces on a macroscopic scale. Such resistance does not require adhesive bond. The exception is the torque required to unscrew a screw. If the surface of the screw is perfectly smooth, bonding and/or frictional stresses are required to resist the torque. Since titanium is much stiffer than bone, a first approximation of the motion of an implant is that of a rigid body motion which must be accommodated by the appropriate stress and strain distribution in the bone. This may lead to stress concentrations at the surface of the bone and the end of the implant, particularly under lateral loading. The stiffness of the implant will be a function of the density of the surrounding bone, but no abrasive motion or progressive loosening will develop in an osseointegrated im-

plant as long as the stresses are below the failure stress of the bone. In a nonintegrated fixture, the progressive abrasion of bone due to fibrous tissue layer movement is possible.

Considerations of the stress and strain distribution in a prosthetic reconstruction on osseointegrated implants include the safe level of stresses and functionally satisfactory performance of the reconstruction itself and its effect in distributing loads to the several implanted fixtures. In general, a stiff reconstruction will distribute loading more widely to the several implanted fixtures. However, if a single implanted osseointegrated screw can safely carry the maximum applied loads directly, then no redistribution is strictly necessary and a lighter, more flexible reconstruction is feasible. A special problem arises if a reconstruction is to be connected to an integrated implant and a natural structure such as an existing tooth. If the implant is stiffer than the tooth, it will tend to carry more of the load. This may be compensated to some extent by the design of an appropriately flexible bridge or by a suitable flexible connection of the bridge to the implanted fixture to reduce its apparent stiffness.

When a load is applied to a dental prosthesis supported on osseointegrated implants, two stages of load transmission are important for the successful performance of the entire design. First is the consideration of the distribution of the load to the several osseointegrated screws supporting the prosthesis. Second, the load picked up by each screw must be safely transmitted to the bone without fracture, abrasion, or loosening of the screw. These two phases are interdependent in that the load picked up by a given screw depends on the stiffness of its connection to the bone. On the other hand, the manner of transmission of stresses from a screw to the bone depends on the nature of the connection of the screw to the prosthetic bridge as this may restrict its possible motion. This interaction problem is particularly important if the bridge is supported by osseointegrated screws and some natural teeth acting together. It is anticipated that the implanted screws will be stiffer than natural teeth and hence tend to carry most of the load. Some considerations of such partial edentulous designs will be discussed after consideration of the mechanisms of load transmission from an individual osseointegrated screw to the bone supporting it.

Load transfer from osseointegrated implants to bone

The fact that osseointegrated dental implants can perform successfully for many years[1, 2] indicates that such implants can transfer loads from the implanted screws to the bone without progressive failure or loosening. The magnitudes of the bite forces in patients with osseointegrated implants have been shown to be comparable to those in patients with natural dentition.[3] Although extensive data are not available on the failure loads of osseointegrated implants, the clinical experience indicates that the failure loads are well above the usual bite forces. The fact that there is not a progressive wear or loosening of an osseointegrated implant

may be attributed to the fact that the very close apposition of bone to titanium in osseointegrated implants is provided at a molecular level. In this situation, there can be a stress transfer without any relative motion of the titanium and bone.

Since titanium is generally stronger and stiffer than bone, any failure at the interface may be expected to be in the bone, or in the bone interface with the titanium, rather than in the titanium. The Young's modulus of titanium is about $1.1 \times 10^{11} N/m^2$ and it has a yield strength in tension of about $3 \times 10^8 N/m^2$.[4] The Young's modulus of cancellous bone is of the order of $10^{10} N/m^2$ and has a tensile failure stress of $5 \times 10^7 N/m^2$. In view of these relative magnitudes, it may be expected that when an osseointegrated implant is stressed the titanium will be deformed much less than the bone. In effect the titanium implant will move as a rigid body and the bone will be carried along and deformed according to the stresses induced.

The important aspect of the load transfer from implants to bone in an osseointegrated implant is the absence of relative movement between the implant and bone. An implant becomes osseointegrated when the bone is allowed to heal around it in the absence of loading so that a perfect fit of the growing bone to the implant is achieved without any stresses being developed in either material. The final situation is comparable to the case in which cement or plastic is poured against an implant and hardens without any curing or shrinkage stresses. As has been shown by microscopic examination, the bone follows any irregularities at the angstrom level in the surface of the titanium implant. Such a close interface is able to carry loads in any direction without relative motion of the two materials at the interface.

An osseointegrated implant in the form of a screw is able to transmit axial loads to the surrounding bone by compression on the

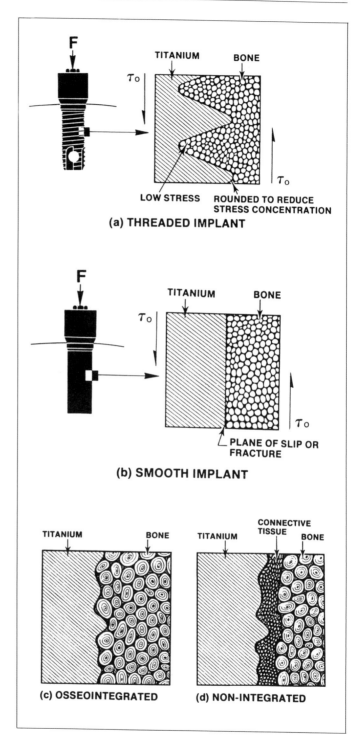

Fig. 5-1a Schematic sections of threaded implant showing detail of thread in close apposition to bone.

Fig. 5-1b Smooth implant indicating that a bond is required to prevent slippage.

Figs. 5-1c and d Microscopic schematic sections showing close ingrowth of bone (osseointegrated) and implant with a layer of fibrous connective tissue between implant and bone (nonintegrated). (Modified from Albrektsson et al.[4])

inclined faces of the screw threads. In view of the relative strengths and stiffnesses of the titanium and bone, the full strength of the bone may be developed prior to failure (Fig. 5-1a). No true bond is required on the surface of an osseointegrated screw to transmit such loads. The close interlocking at the microscopic plus the macroscopic form of the screw allows load transfer without any tendency for slippage. In contrast with a perfectly smooth implant such as that shown in Fig. 5-1b, a bond between the bone and titanium would be required in order to prevent slippage. For an implant in the form of a screw, bond is required only to resist torsion which tends to unscrew the implant along the threads. Fortunately, this type of stress does not usually occur under the normal loading of dental implants. Even in this case, the surface roughness of an osseointegrated implant can produce a beneficial interlocking effect similar to that of the screw threads at the macroscopic scale (Fig. 5-1c). The interlocking of bone and titanium asperities can transmit shear stresses in a manner similar to that of the screw threads. The beneficial effects of surface roughness requires that bone is closely integrated into the asperities of the implant surface. If a soft, connective tissue layer forms around the implant (Fig. 5-1d) loading may lead to some relative motion and gradual degradation of the bone. Osseointegration allows for a direct transfer of stress from the titanium to the bone so that no relative motion occurs at the interface.

Load distribution to several implants

A dental prosthesis supported by several screws results in a combined structure in which the distribution of applied loads depends on the relative stiffnesses of the several members involved, as well as on the geometry of their arrangement. The combined structure generally will be so complex that the equations of statics alone are insufficient to determine the distribution of the loads acting. The deformations of the prosthesis, the screws, and the jaw must be taken into account to determine the load distribution. Such a structure is called *statically indeterminate* and the analysis must treat the prosthesis as a curved elastic beam under bending and torsion. Such a complete analysis requires a knowledge of the stiffness of the connections of the screws to the prosthesis and to the bone, as well as the stiffness of the mandible itself. At present these variables are not known with sufficient accuracy to warrant an elaborate analysis. Some estimates of load distribution may be made by simplified models, and the general principles involved can be illustrated in simplified cases such as those discussed in the following paragraphs.

With a solid, stiff bridge, such as a gold casting, a first approximation to the load distribution may be obtained by assuming that the bridge itself behaves rigidly while the response of each screw is elastic. This means that the deflection of each screw is assumed to be proportional to the load applied to it. Under these assumptions, the analysis of load distribution is similar to that encountered in the design of bolted joints.[5] The assumption of a rigid bridge and elastic response of the screws may be utilized for both horizontal and vertical components of any load applied to the bridge.

For a load P in the horizontal plane (in the plane of the bridge) as shown in Fig. 5-2, the horizontal load F_i on the *ith* fixture may be estimated by the formula

$$F_i = \frac{P}{N}n_p + \frac{P_e}{\Sigma\ R_j^{\ 2}}R_i\ n_i \qquad (1)$$

where F_i is the vector force on the *ith* fixture and P is the magnitude of the horizontal load. The unit vector n_p is in the direction of

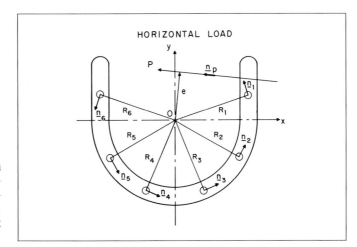

Fig. 5-2 Schematic plan of a fixed partial denture with horizontal load, P, in plane of prosthesis. Load P has eccentricity, e, with respect to center O, of six fixtures shown. (From Skalak[7])

the applied load P. As shown in Fig. 5-2, the radii R_j to each screw are measured from the center of gravity of the screws O, which is chosen as the origin of the coordinates x, y. The eccentricity of the load with respect to the origin is the distance e in Fig. 5-2. The summation in equation 1 is over the total number of screws, N. The unit vector n_i is defined to be perpendicular to each R_i for each i. Equation 1 holds that for each i, $i = 1$, 2, ..., N. The first term of equation represents an equal distribution of the load P and the second term represents the effect of the eccentricity of the load which causes a torsional moment about the point O. The end result of applying equation 1 to any particular prosthesis will generally be that the maximum load on any one screw will be less than the load P.

The reduction of the load per screw by the combined action of several screws connected by a stiff bridge will not be important clinically if each screw could carry the maximum load P directly without failure or loosening. In this case, a light and flexible bridge would be sufficient, as the maximum load will generally not exceed the applied load P unless there are long cantilevers.

For a vertical load P as shown in Fig. 5-3, the force F_i on each screw may be computed under the rigid bridge assumption and elastic deflection of screws by the following equation:

$$F_i = \frac{P}{N} + P(Ax_i + By_i) \tag{2}$$

where N is the number of screws, and x_i, y_i are the coordinates of the ith screw as shown in Fig. 5-3. The coefficients A and B in equation 2 depend on the location of the load x_p, y_p and are given by

$$A = (I_{xy}y_p - I_{xx}x_p)/(I^2_{xy} - I_{xx}I_{yy}) \tag{3}$$
$$B = (I_{xy}x_p - I_{yy}y_p)/(I^2_{xy} - I_{xx}I_{yy}) \tag{4}$$

where

$$I_{xx} = \Sigma y^2_i I_{yy} = \Sigma x^2_i \tag{5}$$

and

$$I_{xy} = \Sigma x_i y_i \tag{6}$$

The summations indicated in equations 5 and 6 are taken over by the N screws. The origin O in Fig. 5-3 is again the centroid of the set of screws. It follows that the fixtures near the load P will sustain larger forces F_i

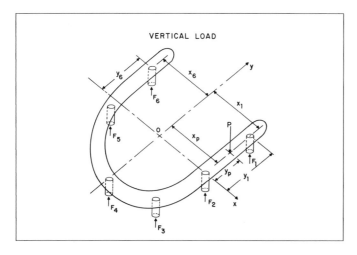

Fig. 5-3 Schematic sketch of a fixed partial denture with vertical load, P. Center of gravity of six fixtures shown is O. Eccentricity of load is x_p with respect to y axis and y_p with respect to x axis. (From Skalak[7])

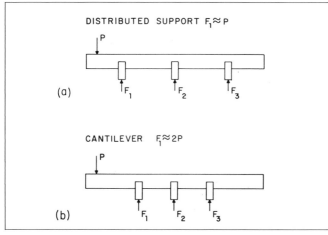

Fig. 5-4a Schematic load distribution with distributed supports (fixtures) and small overhang.

Fig. 5-4b Closely spaced supports (fixtures) with large overhang (cantilever). (From Skalak[7])

than on the opposite side. The results of using equation 2 for geometry such as shown in Fig. 5-3 will show that the load per screw F_i will generally be less than the applied load P. The exception is the case of the cantilever (unsupported overhangs) such as shown in Figs. 5-4a and b.

Equation 2 can be used to estimate the effect of cantilevers in cases as seen in Figs. 5-4a and b. In the case of a well-distributed support and a moderate cantilever (Fig. 5-4a), the maximum load per screw will be approximately equal to the applied load P.

In the case of a larger overhang (Fig. 5-4b) the maximum load per screw may reach one and a half to two times the applied load P. This may still be tolerable and safe if the capacity of a single screw is equal to or greater than the maximum force per screw. The experience to date, which includes several cantilever cases, indicates that a certain amount of cantilever is clinically tolerable. However, as indicated by equations 1 and 2, it is beneficial to spread out a given number of screws, N, as widely as is convenient because this will generally reduce the maximum load per screw due to a given applied load P.

Equations 1 and 2 deal with horizontal and vertical loads separately based on the same assumptions of a stiff bridge and elastic screws. A load applied in any direction can be resolved into horizontal and vertical components and the effects of each component computed separately by equations 1 and 2. The forces exerted on each screw can then be combined vectorially. In this way the most general case can be conveniently computed.

Load distribution to combinations of implants and natural teeth

In a partially edentulous case, the situation may often arise in which it is convenient to support a prosthesis partially on implanted screws and partially on natural teeth. This situation presents several possible hazards. If the natural teeth do not carry a fair share of loading, the implanted screw may be overloaded and fail. At the same time, teeth that are not sufficiently or properly loaded may undergo disuse atrophy of their supporting tissues more rapidly than under conditions of appropriate loading. It is also possible that the teeth become overloaded or improperly loaded, such as having a tension develop which may tend to extract the teeth. All of these hazards are, in effect, problems of proper load distribution to the several supporting elements.

Load distribution in general depends on the geometry and relative stiffness of the parts of any structure. In the case of a prosthetic bridge and support by screws and/or teeth, the stiffnesses involved concern displacements (lateral stiffness), torsion and bending of the bridge, and bending or rotation of the screws and/or teeth relative to the supporting bone. A complete analysis should consider all of these factors simultaneously and consider their interactions. At the present time, the various stiffnesses involved are not so well known as to permit an accurate analysis in a particular case, but the general principles can be illustrated by some consideration of one degree of freedom, namely, lateral stiffness.

The concept of lateral stiffness is illustrated in Figs. 5-5a and b. In Fig. 5-5a, the unit structure shown may represent an implanted screw or a tooth. In either case a lateral force F (horizontal force) applied to the structure causes a deflection δ_1. In Fig. 5-5b, the idealized elastic response of the deflection δ_1 as a function of the force F is shown as a straight line. The elastic constant of the unit in lateral stiffness is defined as $K = F/\delta_1$. The inverse of the stiffness constant K is defined as the compliance $C = 1/K$. Although no extensive quantitative data are available, it is clear from clinical experience that the stiffness of a typical implanted screw is much greater than that of a natural tooth. This is to be expected since the osseointegrated screw is in effect in direct contact with the bone whereas the natural tooth has the periodontal ligament between the tooth and the bone which allows a greater compliance. In terms of compliance, the natural tooth is expected to be much more compliant than the implanted screw.

For equitable load distribution it may be desirable to adjust the stiffness of the bridge to the screw by the insertion of a compliant material between the bridge and the screw. This might take the form of a plastic ring or cap between the screw and the bridge. Such an arrangement is shown schematically in Fig. 5-5c. When a lateral force F is applied to the bridge the deflection δ_1 will be greater than that of the screw itself due to the compliance of the connection. Figure 5-5e shows the steep curve of δ_1 versus F without a compliant connection and the more compliant connection giving δ'_1 versus the same

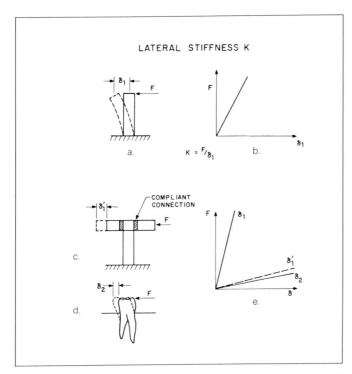

Figs. 5-5a to e Definition of lateral stiffness.

Fig. 5-5a Horizontal deflection δ, of implant under horizontal force F.

Fig. 5-5b Plot of δ_1 vs. F, idealized elastic response.

Fig. 5-5c Compliant connection with plastic or resin ring around metallic implant.

Fig. 5-5d Lateral deflection δ_2 of tooth under horizontal force F.

Fig. 5-5e Comparison of deflection of implant, δ, of tooth, δ_2, and of compliant connection to implant, δ_1.

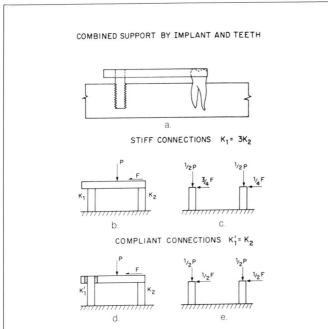

Figs. 5-6a to e Combined support by implant and teeth.

Fig. 5-6a Schematic sketch of implant and tooth connected by a fixed bridge.

Fig. 5-6b Vertical load P and horizontal force F applied to bridge.

Fig. 5-6c Distribution of loads with stiff connection between implant and bridge.

Fig. 5-6d Bridge with compliant connection to implant.

Fig. 5-6e Distribution of load with compliant connection between bridge and implant.

force F. The natural tooth under a similar lateral force F will have a lateral displacement δ_2 (Fig. 5-5d). If the compliant connection in Fig. 5-5c is appropriately adjusted the compliance of the unit in Fig. 5-5c and the tooth in Fig. 5-5d may be comparable as indicated by the similar slopes in Fig. 5-5e. The results to be expected in the case of a combined support by implanted screws and natural teeth in a simple situation (Fig. 5-6a) will depend on the type of connection and compliances of each supporting unit. In Figs. 5-6b and c the results for a stiff connection between the bridge and screw and the bridge and the natural tooth in Fig. 5-6a are shown for an assumed stiffness of the screw three times that of the tooth, i.e., $K_1 = 3K_2$. For the purposes of this discussion, it is assumed that the bending stiffness of the connection is not large. In this case a vertical load P applied midway between the two supports will be distributed more or less equally between them (Fig. 5-6b). On the other hand, a horizontal load F applied to the bridge at any point will be divided between the screw and the natural tooth in proportion to their lateral stiffnesses. The result (Fig. 5-6c) is that the screw will pick up $0.75F$ and the tooth will carry only $0.25F$. This may in itself be a satisfactory situation if the implanted screw is able to carry the larger share of the load. A more equitable distribution of the load occurs if a compliant connection is used between the bridge and the screw (Fig. 5-6e). In this case, a vertical load P applied midway between the two supports is more or less equally distributed between the screw and the tooth. The lateral load F is also equally distributed between the screw and the tooth on the assumption that the compliant connection at the screw gives a net stiffness, K_1, equal to the stiffness of the natural tooth, K_2. It may be anticipated that the compliant connection shown in Fig. 5-6d probably should be the safer and preferable design. It should avoid undue loading of the

screw and at the same time provide a stimulus loading to the natural tooth to maintain it in a healthy condition over a long period of time.

The same kind of considerations outlined above for lateral stiffness should apply also to torsional stiffness and bending stiffness. These stiffnesses are related to the torque and bending moments in the bridge and transferred to the screws or teeth supporting them. The analysis of these effects is more complex since it requires the consideration of the geometric curvature of the bridge as well as the rotational stiffnesses of the screws and teeth. However, the principles are the same in that a stiff connection to the relatively stiff screws will tend to increase the proportion of the moments and torques to be exerted on such a screw. Thus, even in the absence of a precise analysis, it can be stated qualitatively that a compliant connection in which the stiffnesses and screws and teeth are in balance should most likely produce satisfactory long-term results.

There is another general effect that may be important with respect to the design of prostheses to be supported by implanted screws and natural teeth. The flexibility of the prosthesis itself plays a role somewhat similar to the compliance of the connections to the screws and implants. Generally speaking, a very flexible bridge will tend to reduce the distribution in loading among units of support which have more or less equal stiffness. With a flexible bridge, the tendency is for any applied load to be transmitted primarily to the nearest support whether it be a natural tooth or an implanted screw. A very rigid prosthesis tends to distribute the load to all of the supports in the manner described earlier. An appropriate flexible support could be said to help prevent the overprotection of a natural tooth from being always underloaded. At the same time, a flexible bridge is unlikely to deliver to a particular implanted screw more

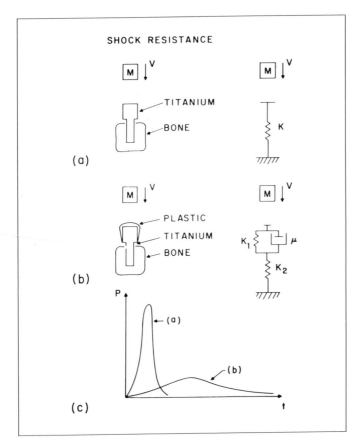

SHOCK RESISTANCE

(a)

(b)

(c)

Fig. 5-7a Schematic sketch showing impact of a mass, M, at velocity, V, onto a metallic fixed partial denture on fixtures that are osseointegrated with bone. System behaves like a stiff spring with modulus, K, as shown.

Fig. 5-7b Same scheme as in Fig. 5-7a except that an acrylic resin sheath (for example, acrylic resin teeth) is placed over metallic fixed partial denture. Theoretical model includes a softer spring, K_2, and dashpot, μ, representing acrylic resin.

Fig. 5-7c Qualitative sketch of force versus time resulting from impact in Figs. 5-7a and b. Impulse (area) for two cases is same, but peak force is much less in Fig. 5-7b (curve b). (From Skalak[7])

than the applied load (P or F). The precise interplay of the stiffness of a bridge and the compliance of the natural teeth, or of the implanted screws and their connections, is a matter of precise analysis using the theory of structures. This can be carried out with considerable precision when material properties, and stiffnesses of the supports and of each junction, are accurately known. The trends and general effects discussed above may be expected to have quantitative expression by such analysis, but must be qualitatively the same as indicated above.

Shock resistance

The close apposition of an osseointegrated implant to bone results in a stiff connection which transmits stresses with little relative motion or delay. This means that any force applied to the implant is transmitted to the bone without changes of magnitude or duration. Consequently, the bone may be overstressed or fractured if sudden large impact forces are applied to the fixture.

Large impact forces can be developed during chewing if a hard object is inadvertently encountered when the moving lower jaw and muscles are suddenly stopped by impacting on the obstruction. For purposes of illustrating the mechanical principles involved, the situation may be modeled as mass, M, impacting onto a bridge with velocity, V (Fig. 5-7a). An osseointegrated implant may be represented by a stiff spring (Fig. 5-7b), which will bring the mass, M, to rest in a very short time and generate a large peak force, illustrated by curve a in Fig. 5-7c. The impulse (the integral of force with respect to time) required to bring the mass, M, to rest is independent of the time history of the force. The mass can be brought to rest by a large force acting over a short time or a smaller force acting over a longer time. An osseointegrated implant supporting a metallic bridge with no softer materials interspersed can result in a sufficiently large peak force to cause fracture of the supporting bone. To reduce the peak force, the pulse needs to be spread out in time. This can be accomplished by placing a layer of softer material in the path of the force transmission.

A soft layer to reduce peak impact forces can be provided by a plastic sheath, molded in the form of teeth as shown schematically in Fig. 5-7b. Plastics generally have a much lower modulus of elasticity than metals and also provide some internal damping. Such a material is represented by a spring, K_1, in parallel with a dashpot with viscous coefficient μ (Fig. 5-7b). Such a unit is known as a Kelvin body[6] and is the basic unit of a shock absorber. This unit is mechanically in series with the spring, K_2, representing the implant and its connection to the bone. The spring constant, K_1, associated with the plastic is assumed to be much smaller (more compliant) than the spring constant, K_2, of the implant. Then the impact of the same mass, M, at the same initial velocity, V, as in Fig. 5-7a will result in pulse of longer duration and lower peak force when applied to the assembly shown in Fig. 5-7b. This is illustrated by the curve b in Fig.

5-7c. The reduction of the peak force is the basic shock-absorbing action which can protect the bone against fracture.

From a mechanical standpoint, the shock-absorbing action would be the same if the soft layer was located between the metallic implant and the bone in Fig. 5-7b instead of on the upper surface. In the natural tooth, the periodontium is between the tooth and the bone and provides a shock-absorbing function. It could as well be located on the outer surface of the teeth as far as shock resistance is concerned, but it would then be subject to wear and abrasion. The acrylic resin or other plastic used in prostheses can be replaced if subject to excessive wear, but clinical experience shows that this is not usually necessary at least for several years.[1]

Summary and conclusions

On the basis of the above discussion, several general conclusions may be drawn:

1. The close apposition of bone to a titanium implant—the essential feature of osseointegration—allows transmission of stresses from the implant to the bone without any appreciable relative motion or abrasion at the interface. The absence of any intermediate fibrotic layer allows stress to be transmitted without any progressive change in bond or degradation of the contact zone between the bone and implant.

2. The use of a threaded screw provides a form of interlocking with the bone that allows full development of the strength of the bone for any direction of loading. The close apposition of bone to an osseointegrated implant provides a similar transmission of load at the microscopic level at the interface of the bone and implant.

3. The distribution of loads applied to a fixed prosthesis to the supporting implants or teeth depends on the geometry and stiffness of the supports and the stiffness of the prosthesis. A stiff prosthesis will distribute loads to supporting abutments more effectively. A flexible prosthesis may be adequate if any one fixture can carry the full load applied. Cantilevered ends of a fixed prosthesis increase loading on the screw nearest to the cantilevered end. Moderate extensions may be tolerated if the fixtures are sufficiently strong.

4. If a fixed partial denture is to be supported on a combination of osseointegrated implants and natural teeth, a more uniform distribution of load can be achieved by use of a flexible connection of the prosthesis to the implanted screw. Otherwise loads tend to be concentrated on the implant, which is stiffer than natural teeth.

5. The osseointegrated implant provides direct contact with the surrounding bone and will transmit any stress waves or shocks applied to the fixture. For this reason, it is advisable to use a shock-absorbing material such as acrylic resin in the form of artificial teeth on the surface of the denture. Such a plastic layer can provide adequate shock protection to the stiff and close connection of an osseointegrated implant to the supporting bone.

References

1. *Brånemark, P.-I., et al.*
   Osseointegrated Implants in the Treatment of the Edentulous Jaw. Stockholm: Almqvist & Wiksell, 1977.

2. *Adell, R., et al.*
   A 15-year study of osseointegrated implants in the treatment of the edentulous jaw. Int. J. Oral Surg. 6:387, 1981.

3. *Haraldson, T., and Carlsson, G. E.*
   Bite force and oral function in patients with osseointegrated oral implants. Scand. J. Dent. Res. 85:200-208, 1977.

4. *Albrektsson, T., et al.*
   The interface zone of inorganic implants in vivo: Titanium implants in bone. Ann. Biomed. Eng. 11:1-27, 1983.

5. *McGuire, W.*
   Steel Structures. Englewood Cliffs, N. J.: Prentice-Hall, Inc., 1968.

6. *Flugge, W.*
   Viscoelasticity. Waltham, Mass.: Blaisdell Publishing Co., 1967.

7. *Skalak, R.*
   Biomechanical considerations in osseointegrated prostheses. J. Prosthet. Dent. 49:843-848, 1983.

Chapter 6

Bone Tissue Response

Tomas Albrektsson

Introduction

Bone tissue is highly cellular and richly vascularized. In rest, bone will receive about 11% of the cardiac output.[1] A predictable outcome of any implantation procedure will depend on (1) if the bone is truly recognized as living tissue, and (2) if this living and active state of the bone is maintained, as much as possible, through careful surgery and appropriate loading of the bone-implant complex.

No matter how careful the preparatory technique, a necrotic border zone will inevitably appear around any surgically created bone defect. The width of this necrotic zone around an implant site will primarily depend on the generated frictional heat at surgery, but other factors such as the degree of vascular perfusion, which may vary considerably even in different regions of the same bone,[2] are additional parameters of some significance for the extension of the necrosis. In principle, bone may react in three different ways as a response to the necrosis (Fig. 6-1):

1. Fibrous tissue formation may occur.
2. Dead bone may remain as a sequester without repair.
3. New bone healing will ensue.

Both bone and fibrous tissue belong to the connective tissues of the body. Bone will permanently heal with fibrous tissue as a response to severe trauma, whether it is of a physical, chemical, or other nature. If the

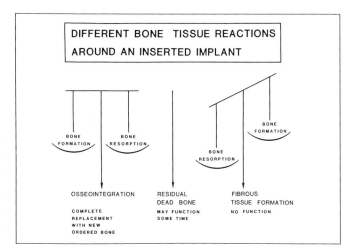

Fig. 6-1 Bone may react in three different ways as a response to the necrosis in the border zone: fibrous tissue healing resulting in no function, no healing with residual dead bone, or complete replacement with new bone resulting in osseointegration of an implanted device.

revascularization of the necrotic zone is prevented, there will be no healing. The dead bone will remain and, as with the dead branch of a tree, be capable of some load-bearing. Bone will heal with new bone only if certain local conditions are optimized.

The first section of this chapter deals with the background to bone healing around an inserted implant. In essence, because bone is differentiated higher than fibrous tissue,[3] proper bone healing around an implant is difficult to achieve, whereas it is simple to insert the same implant and have it anchored in fibrous tissue.

The adequate bone response after implant insertion is that of remodelling with a gradual functional adaptation to the loads at host site. The first stage in this bone response is replacement of the nonvital tissue which will border the implant immediately after insertion. Thereafter, the anchoring bone will become subsequently remodelled, usually over a period of several years, and preferably establish a bone condensation around the implanted device which in the ideal case will become more stable in the bone with longer times of implantation. This chapter gives an overview of factors that will govern the bone response to an implant. These factors are related to the bone tissue and its inherent healing capacity, to the implant material and configuration, and to the surgical technique and loading conditions at and after insertion of the foreign device.

Conditions for bone repair at an implant site

Bone repair of the necrotic implant cortex will depend on the presence of (1) adequate cells, (2) adequate nutrition to these cells, and (3) adequate stimulus for bone repair.

Adequate cells

The differentiated bone cells are the osteoblast, the osteocyte, and the osteoclast. The *osteoblast* is a cell of local origin[4] which on average has been described capable of producing 0.17 mm^3 of matrix daily.[5] The *osteocyte* is the cell of living bone which in addition may participate in the bone remodelling process as responsible for a direct perilacunar resorption[6] or as part of a coupled resorptive function with the osteoclast.[7] The origin of the *osteoclast* is mononuclear cells of blood.[8-11] The osteoclast is mulitnuclear because of a cell union in which presumably some cells of local origin may participate. The osteoclast may resorb bone at a pace of 100 μm per day,[12] and its action seems to depend on a coupled function with primarily osteoblasts or osteocytes. The repair of the cortical necrotic border zone around an implant will to a large extent depend on one particular type of coupled osteoclast/osteoblast action called creeping substitution,[13,14] indicating a simultaneous bone resorption and bone formation through the action of cutting cones. Vascular invasion into the necrotic cortex will depend on osteoclasts acting as burheads to resorb the necrotic bone while osteoblasts form new bone that will gradually replace the necrotic tissue. Such burheads have been demonstrated to propagate at a rate of around 50 μm per day.[12, 15]

Not only bone cells, which are differentiated at the time of injury, but also primitive, mesenchymal cells are important for bone repair of the necrotic implant bed. Such undifferentiated mesenchymal cells, which may be stimulated to transform into preosteoblasts and later osteoblasts, are responsible for a major part of the bone repair except for the first days after injury.[16] The mesenchymal cells need an adequate stimulus to become induced to bone-forming cells as they are pleuripotent and equal-

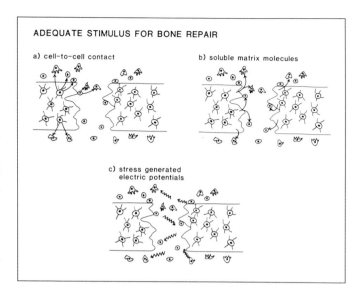

Fig. 6-2   The adequate stimulus for bone repair may be *(a)* cell-to-cell contact dependent on a cellular activity, *(b)* an action of soluble matrix molecules, or *(c)* an action dependent on stress-generated electric potentials. These various ways of triggering the bone response are probably combined in one way or another.

ly well may develop into fibroblasts, for example, instead of into bone-forming cells.

Adequate bone cell nutrition

For proper function the bone cells must be properly nourished. As has been discussed, cells may remain alive on some diffusion mechanism in the absence of vessels.[17] However, bone repair will not start before a regained local circulation has been established.[18] In cancellous bone the maximal vascular penetration rate has been established to 0.5 mm per day[15, 19] compared to 0.05 mm per day in cortical bone. Based on Rhinelander's [20] estimation of a 0.5-mm minimal necrotic border zone after bone preparation this would indicate that bone remodelling in the region adjacent to the implant would not start until at least 10 days after insertion and it would be several months before a major part of the necrotic bone has been replaced with newly formed hard tissue.

Adequate stimulus for bone repair (Fig. 6-2)

In general terms bone healing will be triggered by trauma. This, of course, is not a very subtle way of defining the adequate stimulus for bone repair, and it must be kept in mind that increasing the trauma will weaken the bone-healing response, not reinforce it. The minimal amount of surgical trauma inevitable in a bone preparation procedure seems to be more than what is optimal to trigger the bone-healing response, as increased trauma will kill more of the cells that are necessary for repair. A mild inflammatory response may be a stimulus for bone remodelling as suggested by Küntschner,[21] who stated that tissue proliferation arises and induces bone formation in a few days as a result of the inflammatory response.

Perhaps the signals to bone remodelling are mediated via *electrical stimuli* as demonstrated by Yasuda[22] in 1953 showing that piezoelectric forces acted over the fracture gap and stimulated the bone-healing response. Several authors[23-26] have experimentally demonstrated an improved implant incorporation after externally applied electrical stimulation. This may indicate that, even in the absence of external electrical stimulation, stress-generated "natural" electrical potentials are important to trigger the bone-healing response,[27, 28] for instance, after insertion of an implant.

The first authors to postulate a *bone-inductive capacity* of the bone ground substances were Levander[29] and Urist and McLean.[30] This bone-inductive substance is probably a protein[31] that will leak from injured bone and initiate the differentiation of the primitive mesenchymal cells into preosteoblasts. Hulth[32] presented a theory of "competing healing forces," which is based on the assumption that the same undifferentiated mesenchymal cells may either be induced to a bone-forming cell or transformed into a soft-tissue cell as a fibroblast. The outcome of this cell differentiation process would depend on the relative magnitudes of the soft-tissue and hard-tissue trauma, i.e., the more soft-tissue injury the more inductive stimulus for soft-tissue formation and vice versa. A surgical technique of minimal tissue violence should be used in the preparation of the soft tissues to avoid an undue stimulus for soft-tissue repair.

The *cell-to-cell* theory[33] puts an emphasis on the cellular stimulus to repair in contrast to or in addition to the theory of bone induction, which is based on the contributions from the noncellular ground substances. Injured or dying cells may stimulate surrounding undifferentiated cells to become osteogenic. There is experimental evidence from healing bone grafts that undue surgical trauma to the graft tissues will delay or prevent the bone repair.[18, 34] This bone-healing impairment may depend on denaturation of the inductive proteins or on some direct cellular disturbance, which will hamper the possibilities of a cell-to-cell contact. In the discussion on bone and bone graft healing, relevant for the discussion of implant incorporation as well, there has been some considerable controversy as to the importance of surviving differentiated bone cells and their possible direct bone-healing capacity.[35] Actually, the question of whether some differentiated bone cells may remain alive or not is slightly academic as dying cells may contribute also to repair through a cell-to-cell contact. Living cells, even if they are doomed to die because of an ischemic injury, for instance, will probably have a positive influence as bone stimulators in contrast to dead cells with denatured proteins. Boiling will reduce the capacity for ground substance inducement[36] but not much is known of the critical temperature that will disturb a cell-to-cell contact. Presumably, the cell-to-cell contact is more sensible to heat than is ground substance inducement. We know that the critical temperature for bone cells is as low as 47° at an exposure time of one minute,[37] but this does not at all imply that a cell-to-cell contact is prevented at this same temperature.

The so-called necrotic border zone around an implant, in fact, is composed of dead cells as well as a portion of slowly dying cells and, presumably, a few scattered differentiated bone cells that will survive the trauma, as they will be nutrified by new ingrowing vessels before ischemic death is definite. The relative importance of these latter cells in the incorporation of an implant is, however, unknown. In summary, the possible adequate stimuli for bone repair triggered by "trauma" has been presented as being either dependent on electrical phenomena, a ground substance induction, or a cell-to-cell mechanism. Of course, the theories may be combined in various ways. For example, one possible mode of an electrical action would be activation of a ground substance and/or a cellular-inductive factor.

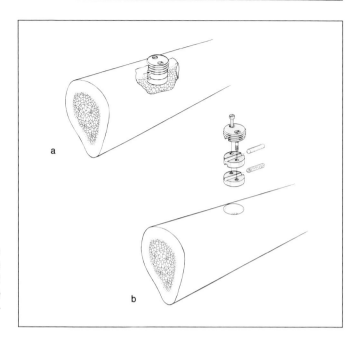

Figs. 6-3a and b The bone growth chamber is a dividable titanium implant which is used experimentally to assess the bone formation rate under various conditions.

Bone remodelling in porous, titanium implants

The *bone growth chamber* (Figs. 6-3a and b)[38] is a dividable implant of commercially pure titanium which in assembled form is inserted in the rabbit tibial metaphysis. Bone and vessels will grow through the implant. At a predetermined interval, usually three to four weeks after implant insertion, the chamber is removed and taken apart and the tissue that has grown into a 1 × 6 mm-long macropore (the "canal") is collected for microradiographic and histologic analyses. Three weeks after implant insertion, the bone tongues growing in from each end of the canal may have reached contact in the middle of the implant. The bone front in the titanium milieu may propagate as rapidly as around 150 µm per day, on average. This rapid propagation of bone is in contrast to the case where bone, when allowed to grow into similar implants manufactured from Delrein plastic, invaded the Delrein[26] in sparse amounts. When the bone ingrowth rate into pure titanium canals was compared with that into canals coated with polymerized bone cement, a significantly slower ingrowth rate was observed in the cemented case.[40] So far, the bone growth chamber has not been used in comparative studies of the bone ingrowth rate into various metallic materials.

The *optical titanium chamber* (Fig. 6-4)[35] permits direct microscopic investigations of living bone tissue through an optical system in the titanium framework. With this method it is possible to study bone remodelling as well as the bone vascular pattern and blood flow. Vascular ingrowth always precedes osteogenesis. The primary vessels appear as vascular loops that gradually invade the titanium implant at a rate of up to 0.5 mm per day. Bone formation occurs first when there is a fairly dense vascular network de-

133

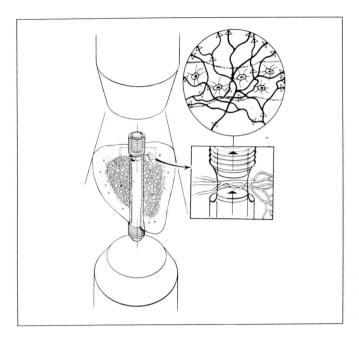

Fig. 6-4 The optical bone chamber permits in vivo and in situ analyses of bone remodelling and vascular topography in the experimental animal.

veloped. Initially, there is formation of woven bone which within a few weeks is replaced by mature, lamellar bone. The osteogenic front may move at a rate of 25 to 50 μm per day. Bone remodelling has been observed in the form of surface resorption or as creeping substitution; in the latter case cutter heads move at about 40 μm per day.[15] In a bone cement environment, a creeping substitution rate of only 12 μm per day has been recorded.[41]

In summary, the studies of bone remodelling performed with the bone growth chamber and the optical titanium chamber have demonstrated that vascular invasion and bone formation and resorption occur inside the porous titanium implants in a manner quantitatively and qualitatively not differing from vascular penetration and bone remodelling in bone tissue where no implant has been inserted. The titanium material seems to cause no adverse bone tissue reactions, in contrast to the findings in Delrein or cement

implants. This is an indication of pure titanium being accepted as "self" rather than "nonself" by the defense mechanisms of the body.

Theoretical possibilities to reinforce bone response at implant sites

Several approaches have been tried to accelerate the bone healing response after fracture, at repair of bone grafts, or after insertion of bone implants (Table 6-1). If the previously discussed morphogenic protein was identified, surely this may constitute such a potential bone-accelerating substance. However, to the knowledge of this author no one has been able to determine the composition of a morphogenic protein in humans. Hormonal stimulation would be another way of reinforcing the osteogenic response, because it is known that osteo-blastic function is stimulated by Growth Hormone (GH). However, administration of GH to healing bone grafts in a rabbit experimental model was not shown to have any beneficial effect.[41] Fibrin Adhesive System (FAS) has been suggested to reinforce the incorporation of experimental bone implants.[42] However, contradictory evidence has been presented by Albrektsson et al.[38] In addition, Zilch and Noffke[43] found no significant increase in bone formation after treatment with FAS. Electrical stimulation with direct current of magnitudes approximately 5 to 20 µA has been demonstrated to increase the interfacial strength of experimental implants by several groups.[23-25, 44] Buch et al.[26] used the previously described bone growth chamber and were able to demonstrate an increased bone formation in comparison to matched controls after electrical stimulation with 5 or 20 µA.

Even if there are some indications of a beneficial effect of electrical stimulation it seems premature to recommend this technique in clinical cases of implant insertion until more knowledge has been gained about the basic mechanisms behind the electrically induced osteogenesis.

Potential hazards disturbing proper bone integration

As mentioned in the previous section, the presence of adequate cells, adequate nutrition, and an adequate stimulus are necessary for proper bone repair at an implant site. However, even if these conditions are primarily fulfilled bone incorporation of an implant and permanent osseointegration[45] may not occur. The bone integration process may be prevented, first, by the use of traumatizing surgery or preoperative irradi-

Table 6-1 Theoretical possibilities to reinforce bone response at implant sites

Mode of stimulus	Reference Nr
Hormone administration (e.g., GH)	41
Drug influence (e.g., FAS, bone morphogenic protein)	38, 42, 43, 31
Electrical stimulation (e. g., DC, AC, pulsed electromagnetical fields)	22, 26, 27, 44

ation and, second, by implant movements or overloading interference, the latter leading to bone fracture. Implant factors such as poor biocompatibility or surface impurities may be a primary cause for failed bone integration if, for instance, an unsuitable material such as copper, which is toxic to cells, is used. As a rule, however, poor control of these latter factors represents secondary causes for failure.

Primary interference of bone integration

Traumatic surgery

The frictional heat generated at surgery will cause necrosis of surrounding differentiated and undifferentiated cells, thereby representing a primary cause for failed bone integration. Eriksson et al.[46] measured the temperature at a distance of 0.5 mm away from the drill periphery at preparation of holes for a Richard's plate in humans. In spite of generous saline cooling, the average temperature was 89°C. This temperature elevation is so severe that exposure times of only a few seconds will permanently prevent any bone healing of screws used for stabilizing the Richard's plate.[47] Eriksson and Albrektsson[48] inserted threaded titanium implants in the rabbit tibia and found that heating the implants to 50°C for one minute was enough to prevent implant incorporation over a follow-up period of four weeks. Heating to 47°C for one minute significantly reduced the amount of bone that grew into the porous implant, whereas heating to 44°C for one minute caused no demonstrable reduction in bone formation. Poor control of the surgical trauma is probably one of the most common reasons for permanent soft-tissue anchorage of an implant. For instance, cement-free implants as used in orthopedic surgery have become anchored in soft tissue instead of the desired bone integration,[49] to a large extent depending on difficulties to control the surgical trauma.

Surgical trauma is reduced with the use of well-sharpened drills run at a moderate (<2000 rpm) speed under flowing saline cooling. For a screw implant, a graded series of drill sizes should be used instead of one large drill. One stage through the bone preparation, without interruption, should be avoided.

Implant bed of low healing potential

There are some indications that various systemic diseases such as rheumatoid arthritis will negatively influence the bone incorporation of an implant. Hagert et al.[50] found a much more reliable bone integration of osseointegrated, metacarpophalangeal joint implants in clinical cases of osteoarthrosis in comparison to cases with rheumatoid arthritis. The possible relevance of these findings in jaw implant sites is, however, unknown. Neither is it known for certain whether severe osteoporosis is a relative contraindication for insertion of jawbone implants or not. Alveolar ridge resorption in the upper jaw may be so advanced that implant anchorage is disturbed in contrast to the situation for the lower jaw where, as a rule,

there is sufficient bone for insertion of osseointegrated dental implants without the need for previous grafting.[45, 52]

Irradiation may disturb the bone integration process, but cannot be regarded as an absolute contraindication for implant insertion.[52] There is experimental evidence from implantation in the rabbit tibia that irradiation at a dose between 5 and 15 Gy results in significantly impaired bone formation and thereby disturbed implant integration through interference with the cellular differentiation process.[53] However, it has been postulated that this negative influence of irradiation may become weaker with longer periods of times after irradiation.[53]

Secondary interference of bone integration

Implant movements

The early bone-healing process, called primary callus response by McKibbin,[16] is independent of mobility. However, it has been experimentally verified that the bone cell differentiation process will become disturbed of a prolonged (weeks) implant mobility.[54-57] Therefore, loading of a dental implant before it has been stabilized by a sufficient amount of bone is a potential hazard for its proper bone incorporation. Implant mobility and, as previously mentioned, poor surgery are the most probable reasons for the establishment of a fibrous tissue interface that occurs around most currently used dental implants.[60]

Overloading

As a rule, the weakest part of the osseointegrated bone-to-implant complex is the bone tissue itself. Brånemark et al.[59] measured the forces necessary for unscrewing an experimental osseointegrated implant from the canine jaw and found that, when applying forces around 100 kp, the anchoring bone tissue fractured while the bone-to-implant interface as well as the implant remained intact. In the clinical material, the use of heavy gold bridges on upper jaw implants caused implant fracture or bone fracture but, again, the actual interface remained intact. Therefore, overloading may be regarded only as a cause of secondary implant loss rather than reflecting an actual loss of the bone integration.

Poor implant biocompatibility and surface impurities

Primary osseointegration seems to be possible with many materials such as Al_2O_3, stainless steel, Vitallium, tantalum, niobium, and titanium.[60] The question is whether all these materials will stand the scrutiny of time when loaded in an implant site for the rest of the life span of the patient. Vitallium and stainless steel are corrosive in the body environment and probably will cause disturbances in the bone-implant complex with longer times of implantation. Already short-term implantation of 316 L stainless steel seems to indicate that, although a fibrous tissue-free interface may be established, there is a qualitative difference in the arrangement of the interfacial tissue between stainless steel and titanium. Albrektsson et al.[61] in an experimental study in the rabbit tibia found implants of commercially pure titanium to be surrounded by proteoglycan layers of a thickness of a few hundred angstroms, whereas 316 L stainless steel implants were bordered by much thicker proteoglycan coats in the range of a few thousand angstroms. The thickness of the proteoglycan coat around implants seems to be inversely related to the biocompatibility of the material.[62] Even if we can point at such potential negative characteristics of the 316 L stainless steel material when im-

planted in the bony bed, we are not certain of the time limit during which the stainless steel implant may function as a dental implant. However, to minimize the risks for secondary interference of the bone integration, it is recommended to avoid stainless steel as a dental implant material.

Even less is known of the potential hazards of alternating the surface conditions. It has been suggested[63] that surface microcrypts large enough to permit embedding of foreign proteins but too small (<1 µm) to allow for cellular defense could create a locus minoris resistentiae which may be responsible for secondary loss of the osseointegration. However, the practical relevance of this and other theoretically hazardous surface impurities as a secondary threat to the osseointegration over long periods of implantation are not known. The reason for this lack of knowledge is that any significant surface impurities may need several years to cause implant loss. Short-term animal experiments would teach us little about the possible importance of surface impurities. To identify the best tolerated surface we need data from large clinical materials in consecutively treated patients.

The response of bone to titanium implants

The very good biocompatibility of titanium is explained by the tightly adherent oxide layer that covers the implant and prevents a direct contact between the potentially harmful metallic ions and the tissue.

It must be emphasized that we do not know for certain if titanium is an implant material with unique characteristics. Among the metals, tantalum or niobium, for instance, may be equally well tolerated in the body,[64] but so far the only material with which we have long-term (more than 10 years) experience in a consecutive series of patients is commercially pure titanium.

It is important to define the titanium material. Many investigators would not specifically differ between Ti-6Al-4V alloy and commercially pure titanium. However, we have little detailed information of the bone-to-titanium alloy interface and it is not correct to assume that Ti-6Al-4V necessarily must be accepted in the bony bed equally as well as commercially pure titanium. The reason for preferring Ti-6Al-4V to pure titanium would be the better capacity of the former to carry loads. However, according to the very few reports on dental implant fractures, commercially pure titanium is of adequate strength.[45, 51] The exact composition of commercially pure titanium must always be defined by the investigator. For instance, the exact amount of iron present in a proportion of 0.05% in the titanium implants used by Brånemark et al.[45] is important for two reasons. Increasing the iron content to 0.5%, for example, would considerably increase the strength of the material but, at the same time, increase the risks for corrosion.[65]

There are frequent reports in the literature of a fibrous tissue interface demonstrated around titanium implants in bone. For instance, Harms and Mäusle[66] inserted semi-loaded cylinder-shaped implants of a.o. titanium and Ti-6Al-4V in long bones of rats and dogs and reported an interfacial soft-tissue layer with histiocytic cells over a follow-up period of as much as one year. Köhler et al.[67] described a fibrous tissue interface of 50 to 250 μm thick around titanium implants in canine bones. Similar observations were earlier reported by Manderson[68] and Meenaghan et al.[69] In addition, several papers claim a soft-tissue interface around titanium blade vent dental implants.[58, 70, 71] As mentioned previously, the finding of a fibrous tissue interface around bone implants of titanium is not very surprising as there are several parameters govern-

ing the outcome of any implantation procedure. Two of the most important factors for the establishment of a bone integration are the surgical technique and the prevention of implant movements by avoiding early loading. In none of the above cited studies claiming a fibrous tissue interface around titanium implants do these parameters seem to have been controlled. Actually, no matter what implant material is used, a fibrous tissue interface around a bone implant is unavoidable if these factors are poorly controlled.[39] Again, it is not difficult to establish a fibrous tissue interface around a titanium bone implant—the art is how to avoid it and how to maintain a direct bone anchorage over decades of clinical function (Fig. 6-5). There are many scientific reports that have demonstrated bone in direct contact with titanium implants without any intervening soft-tissue layers. Brånemark et al.[59] were the first to achieve what they later termed osseointegration in a study of dental implants in the canine jaw. Rüedi[72] inserted threaded titanium implants with an anodized (oxidized) surface in the sheep tibia and described a fibrous tissue–free interface. Linder and Lundskog[73] inserted cylindrical titanium implants in the rabbit tibia and were able to demonstrate a bone integration of these implants that may be regarded as "semiloaded." Karagianes et al.[74] inserted porous dental implants in miniature swine and also described a direct bone anchorage of the titanium material. Schroeder et al.[75, 76] and Juillerat and Küffer[77] inserted flame-sprayed porous titanium dental implants in the monkey jaw and described a direct bone anchorage without interposed soft tissue around the foreign devices. In the study by Schroeder et al.[76] the implants were subjected to masticatory forces. Young et al.[78, 79] inserted Ti-6Al-4V dental implants in the monkey mandible and demonstrated, by histology and microradiography, that bone tissue was in immediate ap-

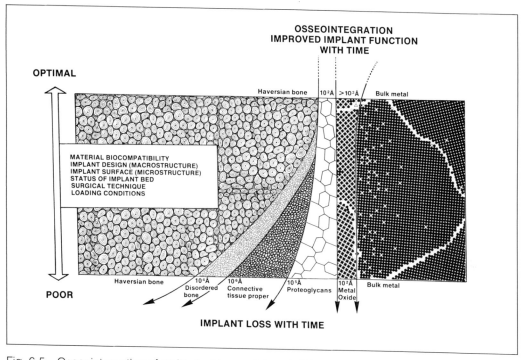

Fig. 6-5   Osseointegration of an implant is possible only if factors such as material biocompatibility, implant design, implant surface, status of the implant bed, surgical technique, and loading conditions are simultaneously controlled. In such a case, ordered bone may appear in close proximity (a few hundred angstroms) to the implant surface.

position to the titanium spheres of the implants. There were no discernible fibrous tissue interposed in the interface. These implants were not in occlusion, but in another paper[80] a bony integration was demonstrated of titanium dental implants which had been load-bearing more than three years. Brunski et al.[81] found experimental evidence of a direct bone-to-titanium contact in cases of canine dental implants that were not in occlusion. Albrektsson[35] described osseointegration of implants of commercially pure titanium that were inserted in the rabbit tibia, femur, or ulna. Apart from these experimental observations there are quite a few clinical reports of

a direct bone-to-titanium contact. Brånemark reported of the outcome of osseointegrated dental implants in several publications.[45, 51, 52, 82] Ledermann,[83] Ledermann et al.,[84] Grundschober et al.,[85] and Kirsch[86] published clinical reports with strong evidence of a direct bone anchorage of titanium implants.

Ultrastructural investigations of the interface between bone and titanium

Albrektsson et al.[60] studied the interface zone around bone-integrated dental implants that had to be removed after two and a half years of clinical function in spite of an undisturbed bone anchorage. It was possible to obtain intact bone-to-titanium sections by the use of an oblique cutting technique through the undecalcified bone and the outermost part of the implant. Scanning Electron Microscopy (SEM) and Trans Electron Microscopy revealed a fibrous tissue–free interface. The exact border zone between titanium and bone consisted of a proteoglycan layer, a few hundred angstroms thick, as indicated by staining reactions to lanthanum and Alcian blue.

Albrektsson et al.[87] described an experimental technique to permit an ultrastructural, high resolution analysis of the bone-to-titanium interface. The authors evaporated a thin (around 1000 Å) layer of titanium on the surface of a cylindrical plastic implant. After a three- to six-month insertion time in the rabbit tibia, the evaporated implants were removed together with the adjacent bone. Thereafter, the bone-implant complex was sectioned and intact bone-to-titanium specimens for TEM and SEM analyses were obtained. This technique has been used with titanium implants by Albrektsson et al.,[38] Hansson et al.,[88] Linder et al.,[89] and Albrektsson et al.[61] The general observations of the bone-to-titanium interface as described by these authors are as follows: The bone was *not* separated from the titanium surface by any fibrous tissue membrane. Collagen bundles were seen at a distance of 1 to 3 μm from the interface. Collagen filaments were observed closer to the interface, but always separated from the titanium surface by a proteoglycan layer of a minimal thickness of 200 Å. This proteoglycan layer was partly calcified, and calcified tissue was observed in direct continuity with the implant surface at a resolution level of the used equipment, i.e., 30 to 50 Å. Bone cells and processes from them were likewise separated from the titanium surface by a proteoglycan layer of a thickness of a few hundred angstroms.

References

1. Gross, P., Marcus, M., and Heistad, D.
   Measurements of blood flow to bone and marrow in experimental animals by means of the microsphere technique. J. Bone Joint Surg. 63A: 1028, 1981.

2. Töndevold, E., and Eliassen, P.
   Blood flow rates in canine cortical and cancellous bone measured with ^{99}Tc^m-labelled human albumin microspheres. Acta Orthop. Scand. 53:7, 1982.

3. Knese, K. H.
   Stützgewebe und Skelettsystem. In W. Bargman and K. H. Knese (eds.) Handbuch der microskopischen Anatomie des Menschen. Vol. 2, Part 5. Berlin: Springer-Verlag, 1979.

4. Young, R. W.
   Nucleic acids, protein synthesis and bone. Clin. Orthop. 26:147, 1963.

5. Baylink, D., Wergdal, J., and Rich, C.
   Bone formation by osteocytes. Clin. Res. 18:183, 1970.

6. Boyde, A.
   Scanning electron microscope studies of bone. In G. H. Bourne (ed.) The Biochemistry and Physiology of Bone. Vol. 1. 2nd ed. New York: Academic Press, 1972.

7. Jande, S. S., and Belanger, L. F.
   The life cycle of the osteocyte. Clin. Orthop. 94:281, 1973.

8. Göthlin, G., and Eriksson, L. E.
   On the histogenesis of the cells in the fracture callus. Virchows Arch. Abt. B. Zellpath. 12:318, 1973.

9. *Hanaoka, H.*
The origin of the osteoclast. Clin. Orthop. 145:242, 1979.

10. *Chambers, T. J.*
Cellular basis of bone resorption. Clin. Orthop. 151:283, 1980.

11. *Bonucci, E.*
New knowledge on the origin, function and fate of the osteoclasts. Clin. Orthop. 158:252, 1981.

12. *Schenk, R., and Willenegger, R.*
Morphological findings in primary fracture healing. Callus formation symposium on the biology of fracture healing. Symp. Biol. Hung. 7:75, 1967.

13. *Barth, A.*
Über histologische Befunde nach Knochenimplantationen. Arch. F. Klin. Chir. 46:409, 1893.

14. *Axhausen, G.*
Die Pathologisch-Anatomischen Grundlagen der Lehre von freien Knochentransplantationen beim Menschen und beim Tier. Med. Klin. (Suppl.) 2:23-58, 1908.

15. *Albrektsson, T.*
Repair of bone grafts. Scand. J. Plast. Reconstr. Surg. 14:1, 1980.

16. *McKibbin, B.*
The biology of fracture healing in long bones. J. Bone Joint Surg. 60B: 150, 1978.

17. *Hübscher, C.*
Beitr zur Klin Chir. 4:395. Cited in Transp. Bull. 4:154, 1888.

18. *Albrektsson, T.*
The healing of autologous bone grafts after varying degrees of surgical trauma. J. Bone Joint Surg. 62B: 403, 1980.

19. *Rhinelander, F. W.*
The normal circulation of bone and its response to surgical intervention. J. Biomed. Mater. Res. 8:87, 1974a.

20. *Rhinelander, F. W.*
Tibial blood supply in relation to fracture healing. Clin. Orthop. 105:34, 1974b.

21. *Küntschner, G.*
Experimental and clinical solution of the callus problem. Symp. Biol. Hung. 7:153, 1967.

22. *Yasuda, I.*
Fundamental aspects of fracture treatment. Clin. Orthop. 124:5, 1977.

23. *Park, J. B., and Kenner, K. H.*
Effects of electrical stimulation on the tensile strength of the porous implant and bone interface. Biomater. Med. Devices Artif. Organs 3:233, 1975.

24. *Weinstein, A. M., et al.*
Electrical stimulation of bone growth into porous Al_2O_3. J. Biomed. Mater. Res. 10:231, 1976.

25. *Colella, S. M., et al.*
Fixation of porous titanium implants in cortical bone enhanced by electrical stimulation. J. Biomed. Mater. Res. 15:37, 1981.

26. *Buch, F., Albrektsson, T., and Herbst, E.*
Direct current influence on bone formation in titanium implants. Biomaterials 1985 (in press).

27. *Bassett, C. A. L.*
Biological significance of piezoelectricity. Calcif. Tissue Res. 252:252, 1968.

28. *Elmessiery, M. A.*
Physical basis for piezoelectricity of bone matrix. IEEE Trans. Biomed. Eng. BME 28A:336, 1981.

29. *Levander, G.*
A study of bone regeneration. Surg. Gynecol. Obstet. 67:705, 1938.

30. *Urist, M. R., and McLean, F. C.*
Osteogenic potency and new bone formation by induction in transplants to the anterior chamber of the eye. J. Bone Joint Surg. 34A:443, 1952.

31. *Urist, M. R., et al.*
Inductive substrates for bone formation. Clin. Orthop. 59:59, 1968.

32. *Hulth, A.*
Fracture healing. A concept of competing healing factors. Acta Orthop. Scand. 51:5, 1980.

33. *Burwell, R. G.*
Studies in the transplantation of bone. VIII. Treated composite homograft-autografts of cancellous bone: An analysis of inductive mechanisms in bone transplantation. J. Bone Joint Surg. 48B:532, 1966.

34. *Albrektsson, T., and Linder, L.*
Intravital long-term follow-up of autologous experimental bone grafts. Arch. Orthop. Traumat. Surg. 98:189, 1981.

35. *Albrektsson, T.*
Healing of bone grafts. Thesis, University of Göteborg, Sweden, 1979.

36. *Buring, K., and Urist, M. R.*
Effects of ionizing radiation on the bone induction principle in the matrix of bone implants. Clin. Orthop. 55:225, 1967.

37. *Eriksson, R. A., and Albrektsson, T.*
Temperature threshold levels for heat-induced bone tissue injury. J. Prosthet. Dent. 50:101, 1983.

38. *Albrektsson, T., et al.*
Fibrin Adhesive System (FAS) influence on the bone healing rate. A microradiographical evaluation using the bone growth chamber. Acta Orthop. Scand. 53:757, 1982.

39. *Albrektsson, T.*
Osseous penetration rate into implants pretreated with bone cement. Arch. Orthop. Traumat. Surg. 102:141, 1984.

40. *Albrektsson, T., and Linder, L.*
Bone injury caused by curing bone cement. An in vivo study in the rabbit tibia. Clin. Orthop. 83:280, 1984.

41. *Wittbjer, J., Rohlin, M., and Thorngren, K.-G.*
Bone formation in demineralized bone transplants treated with biosynthetic human growth hormone. Scand. J. Plast. Reconstr. Surg. 17:109-118, 1983.

42. *Pflüger, G., et al.*
Untersuchungen über das Einwachsen von Knochengewebe in poröse Metallimplantate. Wien Klin. Wochenschr. 91: 482-487, 1979.

43. *Zilch, H., and Noffke, B.*
Beeinflusst der Fibrinkleber die Knochenneubildung? Unfallheilkunde 84:363, 1981.

44. *Park, J. B., et al.*
Dental implant fixation by electrically mediated process. Biomater. Med. Devices Artif. Organs 6:291, 1978.

45. *Brånemark, P.-I., et al.*
Osseointegrated implants in the treatment of the edentulous jaw. Experience from a 10-year period. Scand. J. Plast. Reconstr. Surg. 16 (Suppl.), 1977.

46. *Eriksson, R. A., Albrektsson, T., and Albrektsson, B.*
Temperature measurements at drilling in cortical bone in vivo. Acta Orthop. Scand. 1985 (in press).

47. *Eriksson, R. A.*
Heat-induced bone tissue injury. Thesis, University of Göteborg, Sweden, 1984.

48. *Eriksson, R. A., and Albrektsson, T.*
The effect of heat on bone regeneration. J. Oral Maxillofac. Surg. 1985 (in press).

49. *Lord, G. A., Hardy, J. R., and Kummer, F. J.*
An uncemented total hip replacement. Experimental study and review of 300 Madreporique arthroplasties. Clin. Orthop. 141:2, 1979.

50. *Hagert, C.-G., et al.*
Osseointegrated implants for metacarpophalangeal joint prostheses. 1985 (in press).

51. *Adell, R., et al.*
A 15-year study of osseointegrated implants in the treatment of the edentulous jaw. Int. J. Oral Surg. 10:387, 1981.

52. *Brånemark, P.-I., and Albrektsson, T.*
Osseointegrated dental implants in the treatment of the edentulous jaw. In H. Davis and R. Fonseca (eds.) Dental Implants. Philadelphia: W. B. Saunders Co. 1985 (in press).

53. *Jacobsson, M., et al.*
Short- and long-term effects of irradiation on bone regeneration. 1985 (in press).

54. *Uhthoff, K.*
Mechanical factors influencing the holding power of screws in compact bone. J. Bone Joint Surg. 55B:633, 1973.

55. *Schatzker, J. G., Horne, J. G., and Sumner-Smith, G.*
The effects of movement on the holding power of screws in bone. Clin. Orthop. 111:257, 1975.

56. *Pilliar, R. M., et al.*
Radiographic and morphologic studies of load-bearing porous-surfaced structured implants. Clin. Orthop. 156:249, 1981.

57. *Albrektsson, T.*
Direct bone anchorage of dental implants. J. Prosthet. Dent. 50:255, 1983.

58. *Linkow, L., Glassman, P. E., and Asnis, S. T.*
Macroscopic and microscopic studies of endosteal blade-vent implants (six-month dog study). Oral Implantol. 3:281, 1973.

59. *Brånemark, P.-I., et al.*
Intraosseous anchorage of dental prostheses. I. Experimental studies. Scand. J. Plast. Reconstr. Surg. 3:81, 1969.

60. *Albrektsson, T., et al.*
Osseointegrated titanium implants. Requirements for ensuring a long-lasting direct bone-to-implant anchorage in man. Acta Orthop. Scand. 52:155, 1981.

61. *Albrektsson, T., Hansson, H.-A., and Ivarsson, B.*
A comparative study of the interface zone between bone and various implant materials. In Biomaterials '84 Transactions Second World Congress on Biomaterials. 7:84, 1984.

62. *Albrektsson, T., et al.*
The interface zone of inorganic implants in vivo: Titanium implants in bone. Ann. Biomed. Eng. 11:1, 1983.

63. *Hansson, H.-A.*
Personal communication, 1982.

64. *Plenk, H., et al.*
Tantalum and niobium implants for high stress conditions. Transactions Seventh Annual Meeting of the Society for Biomaterials. IV: 40, 1981.

65. *Albrektsson, T.*
The response of bone to titanium implants. CRC critical reviews in biocompatibility. 1985 (in press).

66. *Harms, J., and Mäusle, E.*
Biokompatibilität von Implantaten in der Orthopädie. Hefte Unfallheilkd. 144:1, 1980.

67. *Köhler, S., et al.*
Untersuchungen der Grenzflächen zwischen Implantat und Knocken mit dem Elektronenstrahlmikroanalysator (ESMA). Zahn Mund Kieferheilkd. 69:4, 1981.

68. *Manderson, R. D.*
Experimental intra-osseous implantation in the jaws of pigs. Dent. Practit. 22:225, 1972.

69. *Meenaghan, M. A., et al.*
Evaluation of the crypt surface adjacent to metal endosseous implants: An electron microscopic study in clinically successful implants. J. Prosthet. Dent. 31:261, 1974.

70. *Babbush, C. A.*
Endosseous blade-vent implants: A research review. Oral Implantol. 3:261, 1973.

71. *Doms, P.*
The tissue response to endosteal blade implant—microradiographic and tetracycline marking. I. Oral Implantol. 4:470, 1974.

72. *Rüedi, Th.*
Titan und Stahl in der Knochenchirurgie. Hefte Unfallheilkd. 123:1, 1975.

73. *Linder, L., and Lundskog, J.*
Incorporation of stainless steel, titanium and Vitallium in bone. Injury 6:277, 1975.

74. *Karagianes, M. T., et al.*
Development and evaluation of porous dental implants in miniature swine. J. Dent. Res. 55:85, 1976.

75. *Schroeder, A., Pohler, O., and Sutter, F.*
Gewebsreaktion auf ein Titan-Hohlzylinder implantat mit Titan-Spritzoberfläche. Schweiz. Mschr. Zahnheilk. 86:713, 1976.

76. *Schroeder, A., et al.*
Über die Anlagerung von Osteozement an einen belasteten Implantatkörper. Schweiz. Mschr. Zahnheilk. 88:1051, 1978.

77. *Juillerat, D. A., and Küffer, F.*
Gewebsreaktionen auf Titan-Hohlzylinderimplantate mit verschiedenen Oberflächen. Thesis, University of Bern, Switzerland, 1977.

78. *Young, F. A., Spector, M., and Kresch, C. H.*
Porous titanium endosseous dental implants in rhesus monkeys: Microradiography and histological evaluation. J. Biomed. Mater. Res. 13:843, 1979a.

79. *Young, F. A., Kresch, C. H., and Spector, M.*
Porous titanium tooth roots: Clinical evaluation. J. Prosthet. Dent. 41:561, 1979b.

80. *Young, F. A., Keller, J. C., and Hanel, B. C.*
Histological and chemical analysis of tissues surrounding porous rooted titanium implants. IADR-abstracts. Sydney, Australia, 1983.

81. *Brunski, J., et al.*
The influence of functional use of endosseous dental implants on the tissue-implant interface. Histological aspects. J. Dent. Res. 58:1953, 1979.

82. *Brånemark, P.-I., et al.*
Reconstruction of the defective mandible. Scand. J. Plast. Reconstr. Surg. 9:116, 1975.

83. *Ledermann, Ph.*
Vollprotetische Versorgung des Zahnlosen Problemunterkiefers mit Hilfe von 4 titanplasmabeschichteten PDL-Schraubenimplantaten. Schweiz. Mschr. Zahnheilk. 89:1137, 1979.

84. *Ledermann, Ph., Schroeder, A., and Sutter, F.*
Der Einzelzahnersatz mit Hilfe des ITI-Hohlzylinderimplantates typ F (Spätimplantat). Schweiz. Mschr. Zahnheilk. 92:1087, 1982.

85. *Grundschober, F., et al.*
Long term osseous anchorage of endosseous dental implants made of tantalum and niobium. In G. D. Winter et al. (eds.) Biomaterials. Vol. 3. Chichester: John Wiley & Sons Ltd. 1980.

86. *Kirsch, A.*
Titan-spritzbeschichtetes Zahnwurzelimplantat unter physiolgischer Belastung beim Menschen. Dtsch. Zahnarztl. Z. 35:112, 1980.

87. *Albrektsson, T., et al.*
Ultrastructural analysis of the interface zone of titanium and gold implants. Adv. Biomater. 4:167-177, 1982.

88. *Hansson, H.-A., Albrektsson, T., and Brånemark, P.-I.*
Structural aspects of the interface between tissue and titanium implants. J. Prosthet. Dent. 50:108, 1983.

89. *Linder, L., et al.*
Electron microscopic analysis of bone-titanium interface. Acta Orthop. Scand. 54:45, 1983.

Chapter 7

The Gingival Junction

A. R. Ten Cate

Introduction

Teeth have a unique anatomical feature in that they are the only structures of the body that penetrate a lining or covering epithelium. Other appendages, such as nails, hair, and glands, are formed by epithelial invaginations, and therefore a continuous epithelial layer always exists. It is the degeneration of the dental lamina that divorces the developing tooth from the surface epithelium and causes a break in epithelial continuity, and this continuity is only reestablished when the tooth erupts and the dentogingival junction is formed. It is important to understand a number of basic biological phenomena involved in the establishment of this junction before considering the situation vis-à-vis dental implants.

Epithelial mesenchymal relationships

Connective tissue has an important role in determining the expression of the epithelium that it supports. Such a relationship is clearly seen in embryology, where it has been shown that mesenchyme dictates an epithelial response to determine (to use dental examples) where teeth will develop, what shape teeth will be, and where amelogenesis will occur. A most interesting

example of this relationship is the recent demonstration of the ability of mammalian mesenchyme to unmask the long-suppressed ability of avian epithelium to form teeth.[1] Examples may also be found in human adults; for instance, skin grafts placed in the mouth are unable to assume the characteristics of a mucosa (Fig. 7-1). The supporting connective tissue of the graft insists that the epithelium remains "skin." Changes in the epithelial expression can only be wrought if the supporting connective tissue is changed.

Ability of epithelial cells to stick to each other

Epithelial tissue is distinguished from connective tissue in that its constituent cells are closely packed together. All cells have charged surfaces which tend to repel each other so that specialized contacts are required to enable attachment to occur. These can be of several varieties; thus there are tight junctions (zonulae occludens), adhesive zones (zonulae adherens), and desmosomes (maculae adherens). In the formation of a tight junction the glycocalyx on the cell surface is lost and the two adjacent layers of the plasma membrane fuse with each other to seal the intercellular space. To prevent materials passing between cells tight junctions form a belt (zonula) surrounding the entire periphery of the contacting

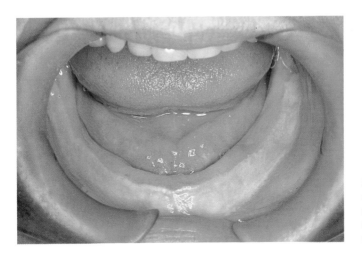

Fig. 7-1 Nine-year-old mandibular vestibuloplasty with a skin graft demonstrates a conspicuous demarcation between graft and mucosal boundaries.

cells. Zonulae adherens also form continuous belts around cells but in this instance the glycocalyx is maintained.

Desmosomes are specialized contacts studded around the cell. The gap between adjacent cell membranes is slightly widened and contains electron dense material. An attachment plaque, from which tonofilaments radiate, is found adjacent to the inner surface of the plasma membrane. The important feature of this junction is that the desmosome is a paired structure with a mirror image existing in the adjacent contacting cell.

Ability of epithelial cells to stick to supporting connective tissue

Epithelial cells, as well as sticking to each other, also have the ability to stick to their supporting connective tissue. This adherence is achieved, in part, by the desmosomal system described above except that, as adherence is not with another epithelial cell, only half the attachment unit is involved and this is therefore called the hemidesmosome. The epithelial cell also produces and rests upon a basal lamina which consists of two components, a lamina lucida (24 to 50 mm wide) and a lamina densa (30 to 60 mm wide). The lamina lucida consists of a glycoprotein (lamina) which is thought to function as a glue that causes the epithelial cells,[2] in association with the hemidesmosomes, to stick to the surface it covers. The lamina densa is constructed like a sandwich with the bread consisting of heparin sulphate,[3] which serves as a permeable membrane, and the filling being type IV collagen, which serves as a structural protein. The basal lamina is further firmly cemented to the connective tissue by anchoring fibrils (Fig. 7-2). These fibrils form closed loops which are incorporated into the lamina densa. Collagen fibers from the stoma pass through these loops.

Ability of epithelial cells to stick to nonbiological materials

It is well established that epithelial cells have the ability to stick to surfaces other than connective tissue and to nonbiological materials.[4, 5] Of particular interest in this connection is the report of Gould, Brunette, and Westbury, who demonstrated, in cul-

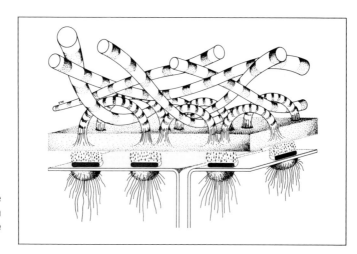

Fig. 7-2 Diagrams the fine structure of the junction between the epithelium and connective tissue. (From Squier et al.[23])

ture, that epithelial cells have the ability to attach to titanium surfaces by forming the hemidesmosomal, basal lamina system.[6] Although the importance of the hemidesmosome complex in this situation has been queried by Jansen et al.,[7] the ability of epithelial cells to adhere has not, so it may be assumed that epithelial cells can readily stick to most surfaces if they are able to secrete basal lamina.

Epithelial response to change in the nature of its supporting connective tissue

Most, if not all, epithelial cells behave in an identical manner when their supporting connective tissue is altered. Such similar responses have been described as occurring within epithelial cell rests of Malassez, oral epithelium and skin epithelium after wounding, and for gingival epithelium after experimental blockage of its nutritive supply.[8, 9] They involve (1) a change in the nuclear cytoplasmic ration of the cell with the development of increased amounts of cytoplasms, (2) a switch in cell metabolism from the Krebs cycle to pentose shunt, (3) a

synthesis of RNA, (4) an increased rate of cell division, and (5) loss of cell attachment with widening of intercellular spaces and eventual cell migration.

The following has been established:

1. There is a relationship between connective tissue and epithelium with the former determining the expression of the latter.
2. Epithelial cells have the ability to stick to each other, to connective tissue, and to a variety of nonbiological materials.
3. Epithelial cells, from a number of different sources, behave in a similar and characteristic manner when their supporting connective tissue is altered in some way.

Dentogingival junction

Anatomy

The dentogingival junction (Fig. 7-3) consists of keratinized gingival epithelium, nonkeratinized sulcular or crevicular epithelium, and junctional epithelium, all supported by connective tissue with that part of the connective tissue underlying the sulcular and

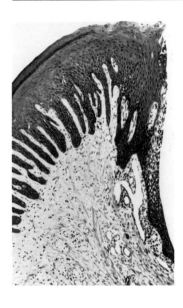

Fig. 7-3   Light photomicrograph of the completed dentogingival junction. It consists of two components, the junctional epithelium, which is attached to the enamel surface, and the sulcular epithelium, which lines the gingival sulcus. Note that the floor of the sulcus is formed by junctional epithelium.

junctional epithelium exhibiting inflammation. This inflammation in the connective tissue certainly determines the character of the sulcular epithelium and almost certainly helps, in part, in determining the anatomy of the junctional epithelium. In the case of the sulcular epithelium, if the inflammation is removed from the connective tissue supporting it, by transplantation[10] or by antibiotic therapy and rigid plaque removal,[11-14] the epithelium keratinizes. Junctional epithelium presents a slightly different situation. It is true that its cells possess all the characteristics of undifferentiated epithelial cells supported by an altered connective tissue[15] and widened intercellular spaces. But these epithelial cells are not permitted to differentiate to the same extent, as for example the basal cells of sulcular epithelium can, and this is probably because the junctional epithelial cells do not reach a free surface but, instead, come to be opposed to tooth surface. Indeed, as Squier has pointed out, the ability of epithelial cells to stick to surfaces other than other epithelial cells is inversely related to their degree of differenti-

ation.[16] For example, if an epithelium is disaggregated, it is only the basal cells that can subsequently attach to a substrate. In wound repair it is the basal cells that proliferate, migrate, and stick. Therefore, it is important that junctional epithelial cells, if they are to stick, remain relatively undifferentiated. As a result there is a layer of epithelial cells forming hemidesmosomes and basal lamina on their connective tissue face and on the face opposed to the tooth surface.

Development

The anatomy of the dentogingival junction can be explained in developmental terms. As the tooth erupts the connective tissue between it and the oral epithelium breaks down. This connective tissue supports both the dental epithelium covering the tooth surface and the oral epithelium overlying it. Both epithelia exhibit identical responses to this connective tissue change, which involves proliferation of the cells and a widening of intercellular spaces. The proliferative response helps to form an epithelial mass over the erupting tooth through which it erupts without exposing connective tissue. But the concomitant widening of the intercellular spaces permits ingress of antigens which evoke an acute inflammatory response in the connective tissue around the erupting tooth. It is over this inflamed connective tissue, and from a combination of dental and oral epithelium, that the dentogingival junction develops. This is the reason that the epithelium facing the tooth acquires the characteristics that it has, with junctional epithelium prevented from achieving maturation by its contact with the tooth surface. It has, however, been suggested that junctional epithelium differs from crevicular epithelium because of its origin from dental epithelium, but this is not a valid suggestion because, as will be discussed momentarily, junctional epithelium reforms after gingivectomy where the only available source of epithelium is oral epithelium.

Reformation

There have been a number of studies[17, 18] of the repair process following gingivectomy and they have all shown very clearly that (1) the dentogingival junction is reestablished with an anatomy similar in every respect to normal and (2) the epithelial component is derived from the migration and differentiation of basal oral epithelial cells.

It might be argued, and rightly so, that this negates the thesis just described that a determinant in the normal development of the dentogingival junction is the presence of inflamed connective tissue. It should be remembered, however, that the healing phase after gingivectomy involves an altered connective tissue so that a parallel situation does indeed exist. Furthermore, the tooth is covered with plaque flora which will also

help to maintain an inflammatory state in the connective tissue as the dentogingival junction reforms.

Epithelial migration

A fundamental property of epithelium is to cover any exposed connective tissue surface. This is well exemplified in wound healing where the epithelial cells bordering the wound margin proliferate and migrate across the defect until epithelial continuity is restored. Another example is seen in the development of the gingival pocket in relation to periodontally involved teeth. Here it can be demonstrated that as the connective tissue attachment is lost from the tooth surface, it is replaced by a downgrowth of epithelium.

So far a number of basic biological events have been described. These have been utilized to explain how the anatomy of the dentogingival junction is created, an important factor being the presence of inflamed connective tissue, and it has been established that this junctional apparatus can be, and indeed is, recreated after the surgical procedure of gingivectomy. We are now in a position to examine, in theoretical terms at least, what the situation should be in relation to dental implants. It is interesting that, when pieces of masticatory mucosa are grown in culture in contact with inert microporous filters, it is possible to show that an epithelium somewhat similar to junctional epithelium forms in contact with the filter.[19] Furthermore, these cells form hemidesmosomes and secrete a structure morphologically resembling basal lamina.

Theoretical considerations for the establishment of a gingival-implant junction

It would seem from gingivectomy and in vitro studies that the oral mucosa possesses all the necessary qualities to form a junction with any structure piercing it, be it tooth or dental implant. Clearly the epithelial cells are coded to proliferate, migrate, and cover any breach established within it. When they meet any surface they also have the ability to stick to it in that they can synthesize basal lamina and form hemidesmosomes. Consider the situation that occurs with the placement of an implant. In many instances this involves extensive manipulation of the oral mucosa, yet repair and healing is, initially, clinically satisfactory. In the case of the two-step process demanded by the osseointegrated technique the trauma inflicted on the oral mucosa at the time of insertion of the transmucosal post is minimal, and, again, the initial clinical result is very satisfactory. This would seem to indicate that, together with the evidence of experimental studies, a satisfactory epithelial attachment can be established between oral mucosa and dental implant; on theoretical grounds there is no reason to suppose that this cannot be the case.

Clinical and histological observations

In chapter 3 the point is made that with the majority of implant techniques a successful response is regarded as one where a fibrous encapsulation around the implant takes place—largely because this mimics a periodontal ligament. But the point is also made that this connective tissue is neither reminiscent of, nor analogous to, a periodontal ligament. Nor can this ever be expected, as an understanding of early tooth development clearly indicates that the

tooth-supporting tissues have a precise embryological origin from dental follicle[20]; therefore, these determined cells are required to regenerate a periodontal ligament. One of the unique features of a periodontal ligament is its ability to adapt to constant tooth movements, achieved in part by its fibroblast population, which constantly remodels the collagen, and probably ground substance too, at a surprisingly fast rate (the half-life of collagen in the periodontal ligament of a mouse, for example, is 24 hours). The fibrous capsule that forms around metallic implants is not derived from dental follicle and, therefore, does not have this ability to remodel in response to the movements an implant must make to accommodate the stresses placed upon it. Without such an ability the stresses placed upon it are translated as trauma, and subsequently inflammation occurs within the fibrous capsule. In this event the gingival epithelium will respond—in the only way it can—by migration as the connective tissue below it is destroyed.

The long-term clinical evaluation of osseointegrated implants suggests that the marginal mucosal reaction is better than with other forms of implants (see chapter 10). For instance, Adell has undertaken a longitudinal and cross-sectional study of the tissues in the marginal zone of osseointegrated fixtures and their abutments.[21] The histological results of the longitudinal study indicate that about 65% of soft-tissue biopsies had "no inflammatory infiltrates or had minimal inflammation." Furthermore, in the cross-sectional study "60% of the biopsies were free of inflammatory changes and a further 35% had minimal inflammation." These are important findings and, if substantiated, indicate that (1) there is minimal or no trauma inflicted on the marginal connective tissue and (2) the epithelial attachment is viable and functioning.

Both these observations can be related in the sense that, because there is no, or minimal, inflammation in the connective tissue, there is no corresponding epithelial proliferation as seen in other implants. But if there is no inflammation in the marginal connective tissue surrounding the implant, the nature of the implant gingival junction should be different from the dentogingival junction in the sense that the junctional epithelium in the former should not exhibit widened intercellular spaces, increased mitotic activity, and the other features associated with epithelial cells supported by inflamed connective tissue. Instead it should be anticipated that the junctional epithelium in the implant situation should resemble a layer of undifferentiated basal epithelial cells very similar to that described by Solomen and Santti in the culture situation.[19] Unfortunately, the ability to demonstrate the histological nature of the implant epithelial junction is beset by severe, difficult technical problems. Although the occurrence of hemidesmosomes and basal lamina is demonstrable, the only report of the tissue anatomy of such an attachment is a brief unpublished report given by Lindhe at the Toronto conference in 1983,[22] which indicated that implant junctional epithelium is slightly different to dental junctional epithelium, and these differences support the thesis presented here.

Conclusion

In any event, the debate and curiosity concerning the nature of the epithelium may be an academic issue. Past thinking about the reasons for implant success and failure has focused very much on the idea that failure is the result of an inability of epithelium to provide an adequate seal between the oral environment and the implant transgressing the epithelial barrier. This failure, in turn, leads to inflammation of the marginal connective tissue, with its subsequent loss and final exfoliation of the implant.

But all the available data indicates that this focus is erroneous. Undifferentiated epithelial cells can attach with remarkable facility to a wide variety of biological and nonbiological materials. Given that attachment is not the fundamental problem, the next issue is whether epithelium forms an adequate seal. Here again the issue is complicated by somewhat confused thinking. The assumption is made that a keratinized epithelium is less permeable than a nonkeratinized one; but, again, as indicated by Squier,[16] this is not the issue, as permeability is determined by the nature of cell contacts and the contents of intercellular spaces rather than the presence or absence of keratinization.

What the available evidence does indicate is a major role for connective tissue in determining the success or failure of dental implants. If the connective tissue is sound (a relative term), then so also will be the epithelial attachment. If the connective tissue is inflamed to an excessive degree, this prejudices both dentogingival and implant-gingival junctions. In the case of the former this is achieved by plaque accumulation, marginal gingivitis, connective tissue loss, and pocket formation, and not by mobility of the tooth, as the periodontal ligament, of specific embryological origin, is adapted to cope with movement. In this instance, the implant mobility exerts a traumatic effect on a connective tissue not adapted to cope with movement, and, therefore, inflammation occurs with subsequent connective tissue loss, epithelial migration, and isolation of the implant. The documented clinical success of many osseointegrated implants reflects their immobility and consequent lack of coincident connective tissue inflammation. It would be interesting to examine the marginal periodontal status of ankylosed teeth.

It seems then, on the basis of available biological evidence, that implants of any sort are not doomed to failure because of any inability of the epithelial component of the oral mucosa either to attach to the implant or to create a normal biological seal. Rather the connective tissue response in association with any implant is more likely to be the critical factor. This connective tissue is not, nor ever can be, derived from the same source as periodontal ligament and therefore does not have that tissue's ability to cope with constant movement, however minor. Mobility of any implant needs to be restricted to prevent an exuberent connective tissue response. This is likely one of the major reasons why osseointegration exhibits the clinical success it does, at least with respect to overcoming the biological problems associated with creating a transmucosal structure.

References

1. Kollar, E. J., and Fisher, C.
   Tooth induction in chick epithelium: Expression of quiescent genes for enamel synthesis. Science 207:993, 1980.

2. Terranova, V. P., Rohrbach, D. H., and Martin, G. R.
   Role of laminium in the attachment of P.A.M. 212 (epithelial) cells to basement membrane collagen. Cell 22, 1980.

3. Hassell, J. R., et al.
   Isolation of a heparin sulfate-containing proteoglycan from basement membrane. Proc. Natl. Acad. Sci. 77:4494-4498, 1980.

4. Taylor, A. C.
   Adhesion of cells to surfaces. In R. C. Marley (ed.) Adhesion in Biological Systems. New York: Academic Press, 1970.

5. Listgarten, M. A., and Lai, C. H.
   Ultrastructure of intact interface between an endosseous epoxy-resin dental implant and host tissues. Biol. Buccale 3(1):13-28, 1975.

6. Gould, T. R. I., Brunette, D. M., and Westbury, L.
   The attachment mechanism of epithelial cells to titanium in vitro. J. Periodont. Res. 16:611, 1981.

7. Jansen, J. A., et al.
   In-vitro experiments with epithelial cell cultures on metallic implant materials. In A. J. Lee et al. (eds.) Clinical Application of Biomaterials. London: John Wiley and Sons, Ltd., 1982.

8. Ten Cate, A. R.
   The epithelial cell rests of Malassez and the genesis of the dental cyst. Oral Surg. 34:956-964, 1972.

9. Ten Cate, A. R.
   The dentogingival junction. A review of the literature. J. Periodontol. 46:475-477, 1975.

10. Gelfand, H. B., Ten Cate, A. R., and Freeman, E.
    The keratinization potential of crevicular epithelium. An experimental study. J. Periodontol. 49:113, 1978.

11. Caffesse, R. G., Karring, T., and Nasjleti, C. E.
    Keratinizing potential of sulcular epithelium. J. Periodontol. 48:140, 1977.

12. Caffesse, R. G., Nasjleti, C. E., and Castelli, W. A.
    The role of sulcular environment in controlling epithelial keratinization. J. Periodontol. 50:1, 1979.

13. Caffesse, R. G., Kornman, K. S., and Nasjleti, C. E.
    The effect of intensive antibacterial therapy on the sulcular environment in monkeys. II. Inflammation, mitotic activity and keratinization of the sulcular epithelium. J. Periodontol. 51:155, 1980.

14. Bye, F. L., Caffesse, R. G., and Nasjleti, C. E.
    The effects of differential plaque control modalities on the keratinizing potential of the sulcular epithelium in monkeys. J. Periodontol. 51:632-641, 1980.

15. Schroeder, H. E., and Munzel-Pedrazolli, S.
    Morphometric analysis comparing junctional and oral epithelium of normal human gingiva. Helv. Odontol. Acta 14:53, 1970.

16. Squier, C. A.
    Keratinization of the sulcular epithelium—a pointless pursuit? J. Periodontol. 52:426-429, 1981.

17. *Listgarten, M. A.*
Ultrastructure of the dento-gingival junction after gingivectomy. J. Periodont. Res. 7:151, 1972.

18. *Braga, A. M., and Squier, C. A.*
Ultrastructure of regenerating junctional epithelium in the monkey. J. Periodontol. 51:386, 1980.

19. *Solomen, J., and Santti, R.*
An attempt to stimulate junctional epithelium of human gingiva in vitro. J. Periodont. Res. 18:311-317, 1983.

20. *Ten Cate, A. R., Mills, C., and Solomon, G.*
The development of the periodontium. Autoradiographic and transplantation study. Anat. Rec. 170:365-380, 1971.

21. *Adell, R.*
Paper presented at the Göteborg Conference on Osseointegrated Dental Implants, Göteborg, Sweden, Sept. 1983.

22. *Lindhe, J.*
In G. Zarb (ed.) The edentulous milieu. Proc. of Toronto Conf. on Osseointegration in Clinical Dentistry. J. Prosthet. Dent. 49 (6) and 50:1-3, 1983.

23. *Squier, C. A., et al.*
Human Oral Mucosa: Development, Structure, and Function. Oxford: Blackwell Scientific Publ., 1976.

Chapter 8

Functional Response

Gunnar E. Carlsson and Torgny Haraldson

Loss of teeth can usually be compensated for by prosthetic methods both in partially and completely edentulous patients. If routine clinical procedures are unsuccessful there are many modifications available to improve the efficacy of treatment.[1, 2] With such an escalation of conventional therapeutic modalities the great majority of patients who have lost teeth are supposed to function well with fixed, removable partial or complete dentures. An increasing amount of evidence has verified, however, the existence of a large number of patients with varying degrees of adaptation difficulties to removable dentures, and a smaller number who are unable to accept dentures at all.[3,4] This may be explained by a combination of anatomical, physiological, psychological, and prosthetic factors.[5]

Many functional tests demonstrate inferior performances in subjects with removable dentures in comparison with dentate controls.[6, 7] Even with optimal dentures, many oral functions appear impaired.[8] It has therefore been concluded that a great number of edentulous people are oral invalids, even when they are treated with the best possible complete dentures.[9, 10] The proportion of patients with removable dentures having adaptation difficulties is not well known, but figures taken from published studies indicate that the problems are frequent (Table 8-1).

With this background, it is easy to understand why the concept of oral implants for retention of dental prostheses is exciting for both dentists and patients. The many clinical problems encountered with earlier implant methods[12] probably account for the very few functional studies performed up to the end of the 1970s.[9] As the biological problems of predictable forms of implant attachment—for example, osseointegration—appear to have been solved[12, 13] interest has also focused on evaluation of functional effects of oral rehabilitation by means of implants. It is the aim of this chapter to review studies on the functional response to treatment with bridges on osseointegrated oral implants (OIB).

Table 8-1 Adaptation difficulties with removable dentures

Removable partial dentures

Dentures no longer used	31%[3]

Complete denture wearers

Can chew only soft or mashed food	29%[4]
(2% of the 70-year-old edentulous subjects did not wear any dentures, 11% did not wear lower dentures[4])	
Cannot chew all types of food	24%[11]
Assess their chewing ability as poor	9%[11]

Functional evaluation of the restored masticatory system

Patients' own assessment of oral functions

A useful way of evaluating functional capacity of the masticatory system is by means of questionnaires. Even if answers to questions on oral function give so-called "soft data," the method is valuable as it will—if the questions are appropriate—represent the patients' own judgment. This includes an amalgamation of many factors, some of which are impossible or difficult to evaluate singly.

Several studies using similar questionnaires have shown that the great majority of patients treated with OIBs were very satisfied with their oral function. This was true for the first cross-sectional studies,[9] as well as for the longitudinal investigations which directly compared pretreatment and posttreatment evaluations.[14-16] Positive answers were recorded for the stability of the OIB and improved chewing ability. Only a few patients found *some* foods difficult to chew, whereas the majority of patients had to avoid *many* foods before treatment. These findings corresponded well with the fact that practically all treated patients reported that they experienced the OIB as an integral part of themselves, and not as a "foreign body," which was the case with the complete denture. In an extensive survey of long-term treated patients, several remarks were noted in response to questions on the esthetic result of the bridges, phonetic adaptation, and acceptance of details of the bridges, but the total assessment was extremely favorable.[17] The subjective experience of functional improvement also appeared to affect the patients in a much wider sense, e.g., increased self-confidence,[15] and improved general psychological outlook (Table 8-2).[16,17]

Mandibular dysfunction

Patients treated with OIBs have in general reported few and mainly mild symptoms of mandibular dysfunction. Retrospective symptoms appeared to diminish after treatment,[9] an observation that was also noted in a longitudinal study with reports both before and after OIB treatment.[15] The recorded signs of dysfunction at clinical examination were generally mild, and they tended to diminish in frequency after treatment. The question of how temporomandibular joints and masticatory muscles may respond to OIB treatment can therefore be answered in a very positive way: the prognosis seems to be favorable. This question has been asked partly because of the relatively rigid contact between the implant and the jawbone in contrast to the resilient periodontal ligament, and partly because of the anterior location of occlusal contacts in OIB patients, usually with shortened dental arches and without molar support (Fig. 8-1).

Bite force

Few measuring methods have been developed for routine clinical use in spite of the recognized importance of maintaining or restoring acceptable masticatory function. Bite force measurements may be used as an indicator of masticatory function. In healthy subjects with a good dentition, the maximal bite force in the molar region averages 300 to 500 N but with great individual variation according to several studies.[6,7] Removable dentures are generally associated with a reduction of bite force which is most pronounced for complete dentures,[8] whereas fixed prostheses are not usually associated with such a reduction. In a comparison of bite force between a group of women treated with OIBs and a dentate group matched with respect to age and occlusal surface

Table 8-2 Questionnaire study of 152 responding OIB patients*

	Response	Male (N=55)	Female (N=97)
1. Do you think your jawbone-anchored bridge is stable?	yes	98%	92%
	no	2	5
	not answered	–	3
2. Is the bridge made so that you can chew satisfactorily?	yes	93	88
	no	7	8
	not answered	–	4
3. Have you any phonetic problems now due to the bridge?	yes	14	18
	no	86	77
	not answered	–	5
4. Had you any phonetic problems previously due to the dentures?	yes	34	35
	no	64	61
	not answered	2	4
5. Do you experience your bridge as a "foreign body" in your mouth (a) or as a part of yourself (b)?	a	–	1
	b	89	80
	both a and b	11	18
	not answered	–	2

* From Blomberg et al.[17]

extension of the dentition, there were no statistically significant differences. The maximal bite force in the OIB group, measured with a bite fork between opposing teeth, varied between 42 and 412 N, with a median value of 143 N. This wide range can partly be explained by the generally great variability in bite force (the range was 103 to 368 N in the control group), but some OIB patients reported a fear of breaking their bridges, which restricted their maximal forces. Another factor to consider is that the theoretically maximal bite force—that which is exerted on the molars—can usually not be obtained in the implant patients because of the shortened dental arches in the restored dentition. With the same measuring method, the mean maximal bite force in complete denture wearers was 69 N,[8] i.e., less than 50% of the OIB patients. In a longitudinal study of complete denture wearers the maximal bite force had increased by 85% two months after insertion of an OIB in the lower jaw.[14] At a three-year follow-up without further treatment the mean force was almost three times the pretreatment value (Fig. 8-2). This is probably due to an ongoing adaptation to the new prosthetic situation.[18]

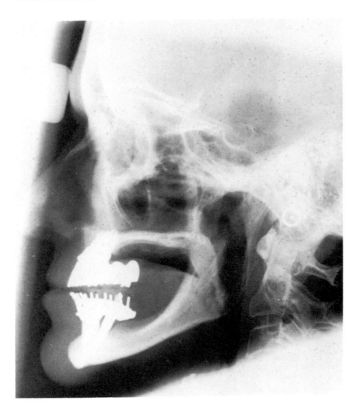

Fig. 8-1 Cephalometric radiogram showing the anterior location in the jaws of the fixed prostheses on the osseointegrated implants.

The use of a more sophisticated measuring method that employed six strain gauge transducers enabled the investigators to simultaneously analyze the force pattern in different regions during biting and chewing.[19] The functional forces recorded in OIB patients were close to those in patients with fixed bridges on teeth with reduced periodontal support.

Chewing efficiency

The most common tests for direct measurement of the capacity to reduce a test food to small particles are the so-called comminution tests. They are usually based on a system of sieves,[10] and the results of such tests have shown that chewing efficiency decreases as the natural occlusion deteriorates, and is worse for subjects with complete dentures. In patients treated with OIBs the chewing efficiency was comparable with that in a matched dentate group.[20] Neither the chewing rate nor the chewing time for the test food differed significantly between the OIB and the control group.

In a longitudinal study of completely edentulous patients,[18] optimal conventional treatment with complete dentures did not significantly change the chewing efficiency. Two months after insertion of an OIB in the

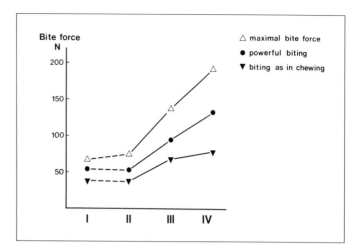

Fig. 8-2 Bite force measurements on three force levels in 24 edentulous subjects at four occasions: I = with old dentures; II = after denture treatment; III = two months; and IV = three years after insertion of a mandibular fixed bridge on osseointegrated dental implants.

mandible, a significant improvement had occurred, and this was substantiated by reduction in both the chewing time and the number of chewing strokes necessary for completing the test food. Three years post-treatment, the index value for chewing efficiency was still better, indicating a gradually improved adaptation.

Chewing pattern

The obvious improvement of the OIB patients' subjective assessment of masticatory function could also be verified in changes in chewing pattern. This has been studied in complete denture wearers by recording mandibular movements with the Selspot system.[21] The general chewing pattern was not changed to any great extent after OIB treatment in the mandible. However, some of the studied parameters did show apparent alteration with a registered increase in mandibular displacement and velocity, especially during the opening phase. The duration of the chewing cycle tended to decrease with a significant reduction of the occlusion phase. This was interpreted as a consequence of the stabilization of the occlusion following the insertion of the fixed mandibular implant bridge.

Neurophysiological studies

The loss of teeth is followed by the loss of periodontal receptors, which are considered to be of great importance for mastication and mandibular function. It is therefore logical to study OIB patients neurophysiologically. Such studies have been performed by means of (1) electromyography, (2) reflex activity, and (3) occlusal tactility.

Electromyography

Muscle function in OIB subjects was investigated according to a standardized program by means of EMG. Results were compared to those obtained in a control group with a natural but reduced dentition.[22, 23] The mean voltage amplitude was practically the same in both tested groups at postural activity and during biting, chewing, and swallowing. The order of the amplitude between the different muscles was also the same in both groups.

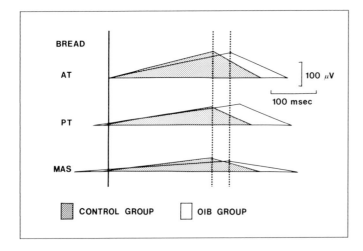

Fig. 8-3 Idealized electromyogram of the muscle activity during chewing of bread in a group of subjects treated with OIB and in a matched control group. AT = anterior part of the temporal muscle; PT = posterior part of the temporal muscle; MAS = masseter muscle.

The duration of activity during a chewing cycle was, however, significantly longer in the OIB than in the control group for all three tested elevator muscles during chewing of all three test foods (Fig. 8-3). During chewing of bread and peanuts the onset of activity was earlier in the OIB subjects than in the controls. The duration of the act of chewing, the number of chewing cycles, and the chewing rate were practically the same for both groups, however. In a more recent study[24] subjects with OIB seem to chew with approximately the same muscle activity during the whole chewing sequence, whereas control subjects with a natural but reduced dentition demonstrated reduced muscle activity at the end of the chewing act.

Reflex activity

The silent period in the masseter muscle and in the anterior portion of the temporal muscle during tooth tapping, the rate of tooth tapping, and the jaw jerk reflex evoked by a tap of the chin were the same in both groups of patients.[25] In tooth tapping rate, there was no difference between subjects with OIB and those with natural teeth. Nor was there a difference in occurrence, latency, or duration of the jaw jerk reflex. A silent period during tooth tapping was found in 12 of the 13 tested subjects with OIB. The latency of the SP was the same in both groups, but the duration tended to be somewhat longer in the OIB subjects. The SP and the jaw jerk was not measurably effected regardless of whether the OIB subjects had an implant bridge in one jaw or in both jaws.

Occlusal tactile sensibility tests

A study on oral tactile perception in patients with OIB in one jaw or in both jaws has also been performed.[26] Tests were made in complete denture wearers and in subjects with natural dentitions as reference groups. Subjects with natural dentitions had the lowest thresholds on the 20 μm level. Among the OIB subjects the corresponding perception value was found at 50 μm. This was the same for those with OIB in one jaw, and natural teeth in the opposite jaw, or OIBs in both jaws (Fig. 8-4). The subjects with complete dentures in one or both jaws reached that level of perception at a thickness of 100 μm of the test material.

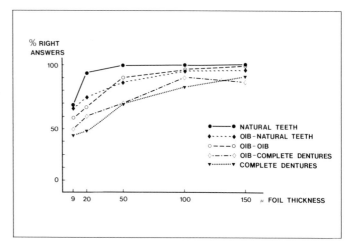

Fig. 8-4 Results from a test of occlusal perception in patients with natural teeth, complete dentures, and with OIB with different dentitions or dental treatments in the opposite jaw. The mean percentages of correct answers from the tested groups for different thicknesses of test foils are given.

It may be concluded that partial or complete lack of periodontal receptors is compensated for by other perceptive organs, and that implant bridge therapy according to the osseointegration method contributes to the restoration of occlusal sensibility.

Summary of functional results

The main finding from the reviewed studies is that substantial functional improvement results from treatment with OIB in edentulous patients. This is so even if they were provided with the best possible conventional complete dentures. Masticatory function following OIB rehabilitation is equal to, or very close to, that found in patients of the same age with a natural dentition, but with shortened dental arches (of the same extent as the OIB patients, i.e., those usually without molars). This improvement is a consistent finding from patients' assessments, from clinical examinations, and from different forms of clinical experimental studies. The

decisive factor that accounts for these results is the stability of the bridgework supported on the firmly osseointegrated implants, in contrast to complete dentures with their comparatively poor retention and stability. This enables patients to revert to a more normal physiologic situation which is similar to that enjoyed with natural teeth. This functional improvement is fundamental for overall recovery, including psychosocial reactions and life quality, which appear to be enhanced as reported by patients following OIB treatment.

Current studies aim at evaluating treatment effects as a result of alternative prosthodontic procedures performed in several centers. For example, preliminary results on patients with overdentures designed over two or three osseointegrated implants are very encouraging, at least at the subjective psychological and functional level. The same probably holds true also for implant therapy in partially edentulous patients who have difficulties adapting to removable partial dentures.

References

1. *Hickey, J. C., and Zarb, G. A.*
   Boucher's Prosthodontic Treatment for Edentulous Patients. 8th ed. St. Louis: The C. V. Mosby Co., 1980.

2. *Zarb, G. A., et al.*
   Prosthodontic Treatment for Partially Edentulous Patients. St. Louis: The C. V. Mosby Co., 1978.

3. *Carlsson, G. E., Hedegård, B., and Koivumaa, K. K.*
   Late results of treatment with partial dentures. An investigation by questionnaire and clinical examination 13 years after treatment. J. Oral Rehabil. 3:267, 1976.

4. *Österberg, T.*
   Odontologic studies in 70-year-old people in Göteborg. Thesis, University of Göteborg, Sweden, 1981.

5. *Laine, P.*
   Adaptation to denture-wearing. An opinion survey and experimental investigation. Proc. Finn. Dent. Soc. 78 (Suppl. II), 1982.

6. *Carlsson, G. E.*
   Bite force and chewing efficiency. pp. 265-292 In Y. Kawamura (ed.) Frontiers of Oral Physiology. 1. Physiology of Mastication. Basel: Karger, 1974.

7. *Bates, J. F., Stafford, G. D., and Harrison, A.*
   Masticatory function—a review of the literature. III. Masticatory performance and efficiency. J. Oral Rehabil. 3:57, 1976.

8. *Haraldson, T., Karlsson, U., and Carlsson, G. E.*
   Bite force and oral function in complete denture wearers. J. Oral Rehabil. 6:41, 1979.

9. *Haraldson, T.*
   Functional evaluation of bridges on osseointegrated implants in the edentulous jaw. Thesis, University of Göteborg , Sweden, 1979.

10. *Carlsson, G. E.*
    Masticatory efficiency: The effect of age, the loss of teeth and prosthetic rehabilitation. Int. Dent. J. 34:93, 1984.

11. *Agerberg, G., and Carlsson, G. E.*
    Chewing ability in relation to dental and general health. Analyses of data obtained from a questionnaire. Acta Odontol. Scand. 39:147, 1981.

12. *Schnitman, P. A., and Schulman, L. B.*
    Recommendations of the consensus development conference on dental implants. J. Am. Dent. Assoc. 98:373, 1979.

13. *Brånemark, P.-I., et al.*
    Osseointegrated implants in the treatment of the edentulous jaw. Experience from a 10-year period. Stockholm: Almqvist & Wiksell, 1977.

14. *Lindquist, L. W., and Carlsson, G. E.*
    Changes in masticatory function in complete denture wearers after insertion of bridges on osseointegrated implants in the lower jaw. Adv. Biomater. 4:151, 1982.

15. *Lundqvist, S., and Carlsson, G. E.*
    Maxillary fixed prostheses on osseointegrated dental implants. J. Prosthet. Dent. 50:262, 1983.

16. *Blomberg, S., and Lindquist, L. W.*
    Psychological reactions to edentulousness and treatment with jawbone-anchored bridges. Acta Psychiatr. Scand. 68:251, 1983.

17. *Blomberg, S., Brånemark, P.-I., and Carlsson, G. E.*
    Patientreaktioner vid långtidsuppföljning efter behandling med käkbensförankrad bro. Läkartidningen 81:2430, 1984.

18. *Lindquist, L. W., and Carlsson, G. E.*
    Long-term effects on chewing efficiency and bite force of treatment with osseointegrated implants in the lower jaw in complete denture wearers. Report Series No. 14, Department of Stomatognathic Physiology, Universities of Göteborg and Lund, Sweden, 1984.

19. *Lundgren, D., Laurell, L., and Bergendal, T.*
    Occlusal force pattern in dentitions restored with mandibular bridges supported on osseointegrated implants. Paper presented at the Symposium on Prosthetic Reconstructions on Osseointegrated Implants, Göteborg, Sweden, 1983.

20. *Haraldson, T., and Carlsson, G. E.*
    Chewing efficiency in patients with osseointegrated oral implant bridges. Swed. Dent. J. 3:183, 1979.

21. *Jemt, T., Lindquist, L., and Hedegård, B.*
    Changes of the general chewing pattern in complete denture wearers after insertion of bridges on osseointegrated oral implants in the lower jaw. Paper presented at the Symposium on Prosthetic Reconstructions on Osseointegrated Implants, Göteborg, Sweden, 1983.

22. *Haraldson, T., Carlsson, G. E., and Ingervall, B.*
    Functional state, bite force and postural muscle activity in patients with osseointegrated oral implant bridges. Acta Odontol. Scand. 37:195, 1979.

23. *Haraldson, T., and Ingervall, B.*
Muscle function during chewing and swallowing in patients with osseointegrated oral implant bridges. An electromyographic study. Acta Odontol. Scand. 37:207, 1979.

24. *Haraldson, T.*
Comparisons of chewing patterns in patients with bridges supported on osseointegrated implants and subjects with natural dentitions. Acta Odontol. Scand. 41:203, 1983.

25. *Haraldson, T., and Ingervall, B.*
Silent period and jaw jerk reflex in patients with osseointegrated oral implant bridges. Scand. J. Dent. Res. 87:365, 1979.

26. *Lundqvist, S., and Haraldson, T.*
Occlusal perception of sickness in patients with bridges on osseointegrated oral implants. Scand. J. Dent. Res. 92:88, 1984.

Chapter 9

Psychological Response

Stig Blomberg

Interest has focused for a long time on psychological reactions to various forms of loss of bodily organs. Such reactions have been systematically studied in patients undergoing a hysterectomy[1] or a mastectomy.[2] However, not much interest has been shown in the psychological response to total loss of teeth. Several reasons account for this relative lack of information:

1. Edentulism in one or both jaws is a common condition in most Western countries. For example, there are more than one million edentulous people in Sweden with a 70% frequency[3] in persons over the age of 70.

2. The edentulous state is neither fatal nor a condition that elicits particular sympathy. However, there are many people with feelings of inferiority and shame who do their best to conceal their denture-wearing status.

3. Most of those who lack teeth adapt relatively well to a removable prosthesis. In many patients, however, such treatment causes problems that may be primarily of a psychological nature, i.e., fear that the denture may loosen during meals or speech, which results in a state of tension and insecurity.

The observed and reported psychological difficulties in accepting a removable complete denture are influenced by several circumstances:

1. *Individual factors* such as psychological makeup, the circumstances of the extraction (for example, trauma or the rapid onset of periodontal disease), or if the extraction was carried out without the patient really being prepared for it.

2. *Interpersonal factors* such as reactions of spouse, relatives, and friends toward the wearing of a denture.

3. *Esthetic perceptions* as expressed in the ideals portrayed in the mass media—"beautiful white teeth"—or the opposite—jokes and comical situations involving loss of teeth and denture wearing.

4. *The symbolic significance of tooth loss* indicating aging and weakness, with subsequent loss of potency and sexual problems.[4]

Questions to patients as to whether wearing a denture has caused psychological problems and influenced their quality of life as a whole have hardly been very practical in a clinical therapeutic sense when the only realistic solution has been treatment with a removable denture. Regardless of the patient's possible negative reaction, adaptation to a denture is a necessity because the alternative would be unacceptable.

The psychological indication for treatment with osseointegrated implants is the patient's inability to adapt to and to function with a conventional denture, which results in psychosocial impairment with avoidance

165

behavior, phobic reactions, and contact problems.

The authors' extensive clinical experience with osseointegration has led them to regard the following conditions as psychiatric contraindications to treatment:

1. Psychotic syndromes, i.e., schizophrenia or paranoia
2. Alcohol or drug abuse, if not diagnosed with great certainty as secondary to the oral problem
3. Severe character disorders and neurotic syndromes, i.e., hysteroid and borderline personality
4. Dysmorphophobia, and patients with extreme and unrealistic expectations and demands regarding the cosmetic results of the operation, rather than the effects of the retention problems
5. Syndromes of cerebral lesions, and presenile dementia

The osseointegration method has made available a clinically scientifically accepted treatment as an alternative to conventional removable dentures. It is now possible to help patients who for anatomical or psychological reasons have been unable to cope with conventional prosthetic treatment.

Psychological studies

In a preliminary study on 49 patients who had undergone treatment,[5] psychological background factors and reactions were reported. The postoperative reaction was favorable and the patients reported that their jawbone-anchored bridges were on a par with their own teeth (Table 9-1).

In a controlled study[6] 26 patients were randomly chosen for treatment (probands), and matched against 26 control patients with regard to sex, age (± five years), and the

Table 9-1 Psychosocial function

Psychosocial function in 49 patients with osseointegration in the upper jaw (30), in the lower jaw (16), and both jaws (3), compared to the conventional denture

Significant improvement	42
Moderate improvement	4
Unchanged	2
Worse (due to dysmorphoparanoia)	1

degree of resorption of the alveolar crest in the lower jaw. All patients were completely edentulous, and wore conventional dentures in their upper and lower jaws or had no denture at all.

The psychiatric examination consisted of a semistructured clinical examination of about 30 minutes duration, Eysenck's personality inventory (EPI), and a questionnaire concerning the reactions to having dentures and a jawbone-anchored bridge, respectively. The patients in both groups received either new or optimized complete dentures in their upper and lower jaws from an experienced prosthodontist so as to achieve the best treatment from the start. After about two months they were again assessed psychiatrically with regard to adaptation and possible changes in motivation for treatment. Only two patients experienced good functional improvement to the extent that they would probably not have applied for an operation. At this stage of the study, however, all of the patients were willing to turn down an operation and complete the course of treatment as planned.

The probands were treated with an osseointegrated bridge in the lower jaw, and kept their removable dentures in the upper jaw. The probands were assessed postoperatively in psychiatric interviews, and also completed self-assessment forms three months (Postop I in the tables) and two

Table 9-2   Social and odontological background

Social background	Control group n = 26		Proband group n = 26	
	Men n = 9	Women n = 17	Men n = 9	Women n =17
Age				
Mean	51	53	53	52
Range	37	65	36	64
Marital status				
Married/cohabitating		14		20
Single		1		–
Divorced		8		5
Widow/widower		3		1
Occupation				
In employment		19		26
Housewife		3		–
Retired due to ill health		4		–

Odontological background	Control group n = 26	Proband group n = 26
Edentulous in upper jaw (years)		
1-5	1	1
6-10	2	–
11-20	11	9
>20	12	16
Edentulous in lower jaw (years)		
1-5	3	1
6-10	3	2
11-20	10	10
>20	10	13
Use of complete denture in upper jaw		
Always	24	24
Sometimes	2	1
Never	–	1
Use of complete denture in lower jaw		
Always	18	21
Sometimes	2	2
Never	6	3

Table 9-3 Reactions to conventional denture

	Control group n = 26	Proband group n = 26
Occupational problems due to denture		
None	11	13
Some	9	13
Great	6	—
Nervous disorders caused by edentulousness		
Yes	19	20
No	7	6
Treatment for other nervous disorders		
Yes	11	5
No	15	21

Table 9-4 Comparison of preoperative conditions and result of operation

	Control group n = 26	Proband group		
Retention problems		Preop n = 26	Postop I n = 26	Postop II n = 25
How good a fit is your denture in the upper jaw?				
Good	7	10	5	5
Acceptable	15	13	15	13
Bad	4	3	4	6
No answer	—	—	2	*
	N.S.	N.S.		
How good a fit is your denture/ bridge in the lower jaw?				
Good	—	1	25	23
Acceptable	7	2	1	2
Bad	18	22	—	—
No answer	1	1	—	—
	N.S.	P <0.01		
Must you be careful about what you eat and drink?				
No	2	1	17	17
Yes, sometimes	9	8	7	7
Yes, often	15	17	2	1
	N.S.	P <0.01		

* Has jawbone-anchored bridge in upper jaw.

Table 9-5   Feeling of the denture as a foreign element in the body

	Control group n = 26	Proband group		
		Preop n = 26	Postop I n = 26	Postop II n = 25
Do you feel any discomfort in having to take out your denture/bridge to clean it?				
No	12	7	22	20
Some	7	12	4	5
Much	7	7	–	–
	N.S.	P <0.01		
Do you experience your denture/bridge as a "foreign body" in your mouth or as part of yourself?				
Accepted	3	2	21	24
Both	8	9	5	1
Foreign	14	14	–	–
No answer	1	1	–	–
	N.S.	P <0.01		
Changed appearance due to having denture/bridge?				
Much worse	12	4	–	–
Somewhat worse	9	16	–	–
Unchanged	4	4	6	6
Somewhat better	–	–	11	11
Much better	–	–	8	8
No answer	1	2	1	–
	N.S.	P <0.01		

years (Postop II) after they had received a jawbone-anchored bridge in their upper jaws as well. The majority of these patients had worn conventional dentures in both upper and lower jaws for more than 10 years, and therefore had experience with denture adaptation (Table 9-2). However, eight patients in the control group and five of the probands seldom or never used their lower jaw dentures. A majority of the patients, 19 from the control group and 20 from the proband group, stated that they had nervous disorders secondary to their edentulous state, and in most cases had developed

social problems that required treatment (Table 9-3).

The postoperative reactions of the proband group were definitely positive for all of the variables studied. Retention problems show a significant change for the better (Table 9-4). The patients felt that the bridges stayed in position enabling them to eat and drink relatively freely. The jawbone-anchored bridges were also felt to be an integral part of each patient's own body in quite a different way than in the case of a removable denture. Fourteen patients in both the control group and the proband group felt that

Table 9-6 Social contact problems

	Control group n = 26	Proband group		
		Preop n = 26	Postop I n = 26	Postop II n = 25
Do you decline invitations to other people's homes?				
No	11	7	23	19
Sometimes	6	14	3	5
Often	9	5	–	1
	N.S.	P <0.01		
Do you avoid speaking to people?				
No	9	9	21	20
Sometimes	11	13	5	4
Often	6	4	–	1
	N.S.	P <0.01		
Do you notice other people's teeth?				
No	2	1	5	1
Sometimes	5	7	6	9
Often	19	18	15	15
	N.S.	N.S.		
Do you think that other people notice your denture/bridge?				
No	2	1	23	23
Sometimes	13	15	2	2
Often	11	10	–	–
No answer	–	–	1	–
	N.S.	P <0.01		
Do you try to hide your denture/bridge?				
No	6	8	20	21
Sometimes	13	11	5	3
Often	7	6	1	1
No answer	–	1	–	–
	N.S.	P <0.01		
Do you feel hurt by cartoons and "funny stories" about dentures and toothlessness?				
No	8	5	12	7
Somewhat	7	8	4	7
Much	11	13	10	11
	N.S.	N.S.		
Do your relatives know that you wear a denture?				
All	15	12	14	14
Some	9	13	11	10
None	1	1	1	1
No answer	1	–	–	–
	N.S.	N.S.		

Table 9-6 (continued)

	Control group n = 26	Proband group		
		Preop n = 26	Postop I n = 26	Postop II n = 25
Do you think that your contact with the opposite sex and your sex life have been affected?				
Much worse	8	6	–	–
Somewhat worse	7	13	–	–
Unchanged	8	6	16	13
Somewhat better	–	–	6	6
Much better	–	–	3	4
No answer	3	1	1	2
	N.S.	P <0.01		
Does your upper jaw denture cause you any general problems?				
No	7	10	6	10*
Moderate	16	10	16	9
Great	3	6	4	6
	N.S.	N.S.		
Does your lower denture/bridge cause you any general problems?				
No	–	–	25	24
Moderate	8	3	1	1
Great	16	23	–	–
No answer	2	–	–	–
	N.S.	P <0.01		
Are you afraid an accident might happen with your denture/bridge?				
No	3	2	23	22
Sometimes	9	9	2	3
Often	14	14	–	–
No answer	–	1	1	–
	N.S.	P <0.01		
Do you think that your denture/ bridge has affected your ability to speak clearly?				
Much worse	8	4	–	–
Somewhat worse	11	13	–	–
Unchanged	6	7	4	5
Somewhat better	–	–	11	10
Much better	–	–	11	10
No answer	1	2	–	–
	N.S.	P <0.01		

* One proband has jawbone-anchored bridge.

Table 9-7   Global assessment

	Control group n = 26		Proband group	
		Preop n = 26	Postop I n = 26	Postop II n = 25
Do you think that your confidence and self-esteem are affected by having a denture/jawbone-anchored bridge?				
Much worse	12	13	–	–
Somewhat worse	12	10	–	–
Unchanged	2	2	–	–
Somewhat better	–	–	5	3
Much better	–	–	21	22
No answer	–	1	–	–
	N.S.	P <0.01		
Has your denture/bridge caused any change in your way of life?				
Much worse	11	12	–	–
Somewhat worse	12	11	–	–
Unchanged	3	2	1	–
Somewhat better	–	–	4	4
Much better	–	–	21	21
No answer	–	1	–	–
	N.S.	P <0.01		
Has having a jawbone-anchored bridge affected you psychologically?				
Worse	–	–	–	–
No difference	–	–	2	1
Somewhat better	–	–	10	6
Much better	–	–	14	18

their dentures were foreign to their bodies, whereas postoperatively, 21 of the 26 probands felt that their bridge was "part of themselves" (Table 9-5).

Such improved retention and adaptation also led to a regression of the psychosocial problems. This suggested that the patients developed increased postoperative confidence which led to their making social contacts in quite another way than before treatment (Table 9-6). This was reflected in sexu-al relationships where 10 out of 25 probands indicated improvement. In the global assessment, 12 of the control group and 11 of the probands stated that before the operation their denture situation had caused a great deterioration in their way of life, while postoperatively 21 patients indicated a considerable improvement. Twenty-four out of 26 probands stated an improved postoperative general psychological situation (Table 9-7). It is interesting to note that the

Table 9-8 Patient responses

		Male n = 25 20-59	n = 30 over 60	Female n = 49 20-59	n = 48 over 60
				%	
1. Do you experience your bridge as a "foreign body" in your mouth or as part of yourself?	Accepted	88	90	76	83
	Both	12	10	22	13
	Foreign	–	–	–	2
	No answer	–	–	2	2
2. Has having a jawbone-anchored bridge affected your working ability compared with your previous denture?	Much worse	–	–	–	–
	Somewhat worse	–	–	–	–
	Unchanged	28	20	17	29
	Somewhat better	12	7	12	8
	Much better	56	63	59	58
	No answer	4	10	12	4
3. Has having a jawbone-anchored bridge affected your contact with other people?	Much worse	–	–	–	–
	Somewhat worse	–	–	–	–
	Unchanged	28	20	17	29
	Somewhat better	12	7	12	8
	Much better	56	63	59	58
	No answer	4	10	12	4
4. Do you think your confidence and self-esteem are affected by having a jawbone-anchored bridge?	Much worse	–	–	–	–
	Somewhat worse	–	–	–	2
	Unchanged	8	–	8	13
	Somewhat better	16	10	12	10
	Much better	76	90	72	73
	No answer	–	–	8	2
5. Has having a jawbone-anchored bridge affected you psychologically?	Worse	–	–	–	–
	Unchanged	8	10	2	17
	Better	92	83	86	75
	No answer	–	–	2	2

postoperative improvement in the probands was not temporary—it persisted throughout the two follow-up years.

In 1978[7] a questionnaire was mailed to all 189 patients treated during 1965 to 1978 so as to evaluate the long-term adaptation to the fixed prostheses and psychosocial function three to 13 years after the operation. The inquiry was answered by 152 (80%) of the patients. The majority of the patients perceived the jawbone-anchored bridge as an integral part of their own body. They reported a marked and lasting improvement in security and self-esteem, with a resolution of their previous psychosocial problems due to their oral invalidity. More than 80% judged that their psychic health improved overall as a result of wearing a jawbone-anchored bridge (Table 9-8).

Conclusion

The edentulous predicament which is poorly compensated for by means of a conventional removable denture is a handicap for many people. Their psychological security, their ability to make social contacts, and their general sense of well-being are undermined. The insertion of an osseointegrated bridge results in a marked functional improvement, both psychologically and so-cially. This is an outgrowth of restored security which accompanies the acceptance of, and faith in, the function of the jawbone-anchored bridge.

Patients expressed their deep gratitude for the treatment they had received and its aftereffects. They repeatedly stated that the fixed bridge is comparable to their own natural dentition, and that they have been fully restored to health both dentally and psychologically.

References

1. *Drellich, M.*
   Adaption to hysterectomy. Cancer 9:1120, 1956.

2. *Gyllensköld, K.*
   Cancerpatienters uppleverlse av och anpassning till sin sjukdom. Thesis, University of Stockholm, Sweden, 1973.

3. *Österberg, T.*
   Odontologic studies in 70-year-old people in Göteborg. Thesis, University of Göteborg, Sweden, 1981.

4. *Mellgren, A.*
   Zahnersatz und Psyche. Sexualmedizin 7:420, 1978.

5. *Blomberg, S.*
   Käkbensförankrad bettersättning. Kliniskt/psykiatriska aspekter. Läkartidningen 69:4819, 1972.

6. *Blomberg, S., and Lindquist, L. W.*
   Psychological reactions to edentulousness and treatment with jawbone-anchored bridges. Acta Psychiatr. Scand. 68:251, 1983.

7. *Blomberg, S., Brånemark, P.-I., and Carlsson, G. E.*
   Patientreaktioner vid långtidsuppföljning efter behandling med käkbensförankrad bro. Läkartidningen, 1984.

Chapter 10

Long-term Treatment Results

Ragnar Adell

Introduction and definitions

The overall success of dental rehabilitation of the edentulous patient with a fixture-supported bridge depends on the continuous stability of the bridge, which in turn is dependent on the long-term function of the individual fixtures. Any mobility of an implant-anchored prosthesis is liable to undermine a patient's confidence, with unhappy memories of the consequences of wearing the previous removable denture.

The statistical basis for ascertaining the long-term prognosis of a fixture-supported prosthesis depends on two factors: *(1) continuous bridge stability,* defined as the quotient of jaws, where the patients enjoy a continuous bridge stability in relation to the total number of jaws treated; and *(2) fixture anchorage function,* which is the percentage of clinically stable and/or radiographically osseointegrated fixtures that support fixed bridges in relation to the total number of fixtures installed.

The observation times for continuous bridge stability start on the date the bridge is inserted. Corresponding times for fixture anchorage function are always related to the individual fixture from the time of its installation, irrespective of whether it was an original fixture or was later included as an additional support.

Continuous bridge stability

Continuous bridge stability (Table 10-1) was achieved in almost 100% of lower jaws and 90% of upper jaws. These figures reflect both the positive long-term clinical results as well as the importance of careful patient evaluation in the treatment of upper jaws.

The definition of continuous bridge stability does not exclude the indication for additional support, although in these cases the remaining fixtures can function while the new fixtures are healing. In an earlier report[1] one additional fixture installation was required in 6% and 16% of different groups of upper jaws. Two supplementary operations were needed in 3% of these jaws. One extra fixture-installation had to be undertaken in 3% to 4%, and two in 6% of the lower jaws. Loss of bridge stability necessitates a temporary return to a removable denture. In a very few cases, fixtures supporting the original bridge after a period of function are found to be incapable of carrying the applied load and are either left for future use or exchanged, and some extra fixtures may be added. During the healing of the second

Table 10-1   Continuous bridge stability (Total)

Observation period	Upper jaws 99 jaws	Lower jaws 101 jaws
5-12 years	90%	100%

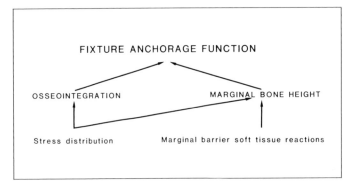

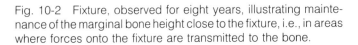

Fig. 10-1 Factors influencing fixture anchorage function.

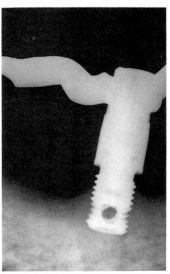

Fig. 10-2 Fixture, observed for eight years, illustrating maintenance of the marginal bone height close to the fixture, i.e., in areas where forces onto the fixture are transmitted to the bone.

generation of fixtures, the patient wears a denture but later on is provided with another fixture-supported bridge.

Fourteen out of about 1,000 treated patients had to revert to wearing a removable denture. This outcome involved upper jaws exclusively. Nine of these patients had severely resorbed jaws, three patients were not reoperated on for psychiatric reasons, one had extremely soft bone, and one died. Only two patients experienced loss of continuous bridge stability in their lower jaws. One of these patients suffered from Crohn's disease, which might have affected her osseous metabolism.

Fixture anchorage function

Two main factors influence long-term fixture anchorage function: a *maintained osseointegration* along the entire fixture surface, and a *maintained marginal bone height* along the vertical extent of the fixture (Fig. 10-1). Both factors depend on local *stress* concentrations, with the marginal bone height also being influenced by reactions in the *marginal soft tissues,* bordering the fixture site versus the oral cavity.

Stress distribution

Stress distribution in the *marginal* parts of the fixture sites was investigated in an in vitro photoelastic study.[2] Marginal stress concentrations resulted from forced tightening of the fixture, probably due to the wedge effect by its conical coronal part. This was designed so as to make a distinct stop against the marginal cortical bone and avoid damage of the more fragile threaded cancellous bone at tightening of the fixtures. A forced tightening of a fixture into dense marginal bone of low vascularity or an overextended cantilever may lead to a zone of marginal anemia.[2, 3] This creates unfavorable circumstances for proper marginal

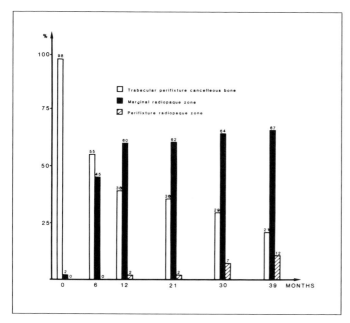

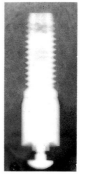

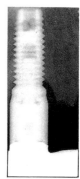

Fig. 10-3b Increase in marginal radiopacity over a three-year period mesially at a fixture in an upper jaw.

Fig. 10-3a Increase in marginal and perifixtural radiopacity at maxillary fixtures, observed through serial-identical radiography for more than three years. (From Adell et al.[4])

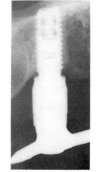

Fig. 10-3c Perifixtural radiopacity. (From Adell et al.[4])

bone remodelling. Such an effect may possibly be one of the reasons for the greater bone loss that occurs throughout the first year. On the other hand, adequate tightening of the fixture is of utmost importance for achieving the primary stabilization of the implant and subsequent osseointegration. Correct surgical judgment regarding installation force vis-à-vis mechanical properties and vascularity of the individual fixture site is therefore decisive. Adequate stress distribution may well contribute to the maintenance of marginal bone close to the fixture. In Fig. 10-2 the bone height has receded from the fixture in areas not significantly influenced by transmitted stresses.

Total fixture site surface stress distribution depends on functional and parafunctional loads, the accuracy of fit of the bridge, the cantilever extensions of the bridge, the mechanical properties, and the vascularity of the circumfixtural bone. It appears that any undue force—in relation to the local bone properties—may lead to bone microfractures which may heal with non-mineralized connective tissue. This is likely to occur if the excessive load is of a repetitive nature as are occlusal forces. The requirement for impeccable prosthodontics—to optimize stress distribution via the prosthesis to the supporting bone—cannot be overemphasized.

177

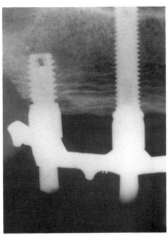

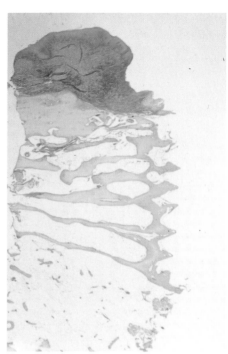

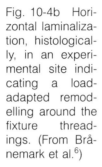

Fig. 10-4a Horizontal laminalization, radiographically, in an autologous graft to the upper jaw. (From Breine and Brånemark.[17])

Fig. 10-4b Horizontal laminalization, histologically, in an experimental site indicating a load-adapted remodelling around the fixture threadings. (From Brånemark et al.[6])

There are a number of radiographic indications that a circumfixtural osseous remodelling occurs regularly. Such a reaction was reported by Brånemark et al.[3] as an increasing perifixtural radiopacity through the years. Adell et al.[4] later observed marginal and perifixtural radiopaque zones to occur at significantly higher rates, when final serial-identical stereo-pair radiograms in a three-year longitudinal study were independently evaluated versus originals taken of the same fixtures (Figs. 10-3a to c). Moreover, they observed that the most distal fixtures frequently demonstrated a more radiopaque bone than those situated closer to the midline. This is probably due to the fact that the fixtures supporting distal cantilevers are subjected to greater forces than the remaining fixtures.[5]

A horizontal laminalization extending from the fixture edges after some years of loading was frequently observed in both radiograms and in experimental histologic sections (Figs. 10-4a and b). The threads are believed to distribute stress effectively over a large area of bone.[7] The observed changes of bone architecture corresponded to the fringe load pattern at horizontal loading in the experiments by Haraldson,[2] and suggest a load-adapted perifixtural bone remodelling.

Reactions in the marginal soft tissues

Two studies using identical periodontal investigative methods were undertaken to analyze marginal soft-tissue response to osseointegrated implants.[4, 8]

Clinical results

In the longitudinal investigation, 70% to

75% of *all the abutments* were not affected by any plaque, and 80% to 85% of *all the abutments* were surrounded by clinically healthy gingiva. These observations were constant throughout the study. The corresponding figures for the cross-sectional investigation were 46% and 20%, respectively. Expressed as percentages of affected *surfaces per jaw,* plaque occurred to 17% (S.D. 25) in the prospective study and to 37% (S.D. 37) in the retrospective study. The incidence of gingivitis-affected *surfaces per jaw* was 7% (S.D. 10) and 44% (S.D. 29), respectively. The mean probing depths in the two studies were 2.9 mm (S.D. 0.8) and 3.8 mm (S.D. 1.1), respectively. In the longitudinal investigation about 75% of the probing depths were 3 mm or less and no probing depths exceeded 5 mm. In the cross-sectional study 40% of the probing depths were 3 mm or less and 15% exceeded 6 mm, with higher mean values in upper than in lower jaws. In both studies the mean distance between the bridge and the marginal gingiva was 3.2 mm.

Attached gingiva surrounded 67% (S.D. 24) and 51% (S.D. 31) of the buccal and lingual *surfaces per jaw* in the prospective and the retrospective studies, respectively. Wennström's observations[9] that attached gingiva around natural teeth was not a necessary prerequisite for gingival health suggests that movable mucosa around the fixture-abutment's transepithelial part is not necessarily a vulnerable situation[10] (Figs. 10-5a and b). Of course a surrounding attached gingiva is preferable (Fig. 10-5c) because it is less susceptible to mechanical trauma such as chewing and toothbrushing.

Significant correlations between plaque and gingivitis and between gingivitis and probing depths were observed only in the retrospective study, whereas no such relationships were found in the prospective investigation. Observed differences were for two reasons: less plaque accumulation due to better patient monitoring in the latter study, as well as inter-observer and methodological differences.

Microbiological results

Two microbiological samples from abutment gingival pockets in each jaw were analyzed through dark-field microscopy in the studies by Adell et al.[4] and Lekholm et al.[8] The results were almost identical with regard to composition of the microbiota. About 94% of the microorganisms were coccoid cells and nonmotile rods, and spirochetes comprised only a few percent. Corresponding findings in the natural dentition are regarded as reflecting healthy conditions.[11] In order to expand the basis for the statistical analysis, the microbiologic results of the two investigations were combined. Only then could the occurrence of small spirochetes be related to gingivitis and deep pockets. Such a relationship was not present in the longitudinal study with its low values of plaque, gingivitis, and probing depths, nor in the cross-sectional investigation.

Histological results

One biopsy for histologic analysis was removed from each jaw in the two studies reviewed. The combined results demonstrated healthy gingiva in about half the number of biopsies according to Tagge et al.[12] It is interesting to note that inflammatory cells were also absent in the biopsies made for a scanning and transmission electron microscopic analysis by Albrektsson et al.[13] Another third of the biopsies revealed only mildly inflamed gingiva according to Tagge et al.[12] Plasma cells and lymphocytes were observed in superficial layers of the biopsies, but were seldom found in the deeper parts. The epithelium facing the abutments was thinner in the mid-portions of the biop-

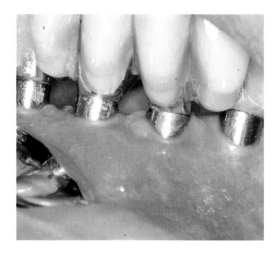

Fig. 10-5a Mobile, clinically healthy gingiva at fixture abutments after 10 years.

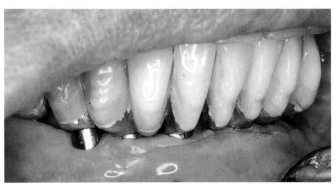

Fig. 10-5b Clinically healthy gingiva, both mobile and attached, in a lower jaw with short abutments and good oral hygiene after five years.

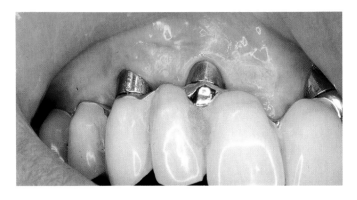

Fig. 10-5c Attached, clinically healthy gingiva at fixture abutments after five years.

sies than in their deeper parts, and its apical extension could not be established with certainty.

Evaluation of examination methods

It was clear in both studies that no correlation was observed between a periodontal type of clinical evaluation[10] on the one hand and radiographical, microbiological, and histological findings on the other. The examiner consequently has to rely more upon individual fixture stability and/or radiographic evaluation.

Marginal bone height variations

It has been claimed repeatedly[1, 3] that *if* the marginal mucoperiosteal reactions influence the marginal bone height changes, they have a clinical significance, but *if not,* they are more of an academic interest.

It appears that 1 to 1.5 mm of marginal bone was lost during the *first year* after bridge connection, mainly as a response to the surgical trauma, i.e., interference with periosteal vascularization at the raising of flaps, and marginal bone preparation.[3] The latter was made at a higher speed than the final cutting of the deeper parts of the fixture sites. Adell et al.[4] showed a first-year marginal bone loss of less than 1 mm. With further refinement of the marginal bone cutting technique this figure could possibly become even smaller.

Subsequent annual marginal bone loss through *follow-up years,* i.e., *after* the first year marginal bone remodelling is in the region of 0.05 to 0.1 mm.[1, 4, 8] Therefore, a bone loss of between 0.05 and 0.1 mm per year appears to be the probable outcome of routine treatment. These values may well be compared with the annual loss of bone height around teeth and in edentulous jaws.

This means a loss of about 2 mm vertical bone support or probably even less during the first 10-year period, which suggests a very favorable prognosis.

Longevity of fixture function

To date more than 6,000 fixtures have been inserted in 1,000 jaws of more than 1,000 patients in at least 70 different university centers, regional hospital clinics, and private dental offices in several countries around the world. The ages of the patients at the time of fixture installation has varied between 13 and 82 years, with a mean of 53 years. Presently, the oldest patient is 85 years old, and the longest time with continuous bridge function is 19 years.

The net effect of all the discussed factors is reflected in the fixture anchorage function. A proper evaluation of this parameter requires the establishment of routine techniques followed by a sufficiently long period of observation. These requirements were fulfilled for the material presented in Table 10-2. A five-year observation period is common in the medical literature for comparison of results, and this figure was specifically recommended at the 1978 Harvard Conference on dental implants.[15] It can be concluded from Table 10-2 that approximately 95% and 85% fixture survival rates were achieved for lower and upper jaws, respectively. These results indicate that it is more difficult to achieve and maintain osseointegration in upper jaws than in lower jaws. Factors influencing this outcome include *(1)* minimal available bone volume due to the very frequent occurrence of narrow buccopalatal width of the residual bone in spite of considerable vertical height; *(2)* anteriorly expanded maxillary sinuses or wide nasal cavities; and *(3)* a low mechanical density of the maxillary bone, which is generally de-

Figs. 10-6a to d   Patient with fixture-supported permanent bridges for 12 and 13 years in the upper jaw and lower jaw, respectively. The time interval between the radiograms of each fixture is 11 years. The bridges have been exchanged but the fixtures remain the original ones.

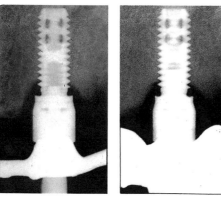 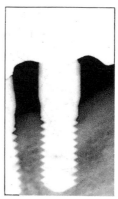 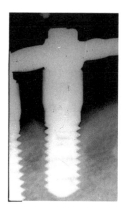

Fig. 10-6a   Upper right fixture.   Fig. 10-6b   Lower left fixture.

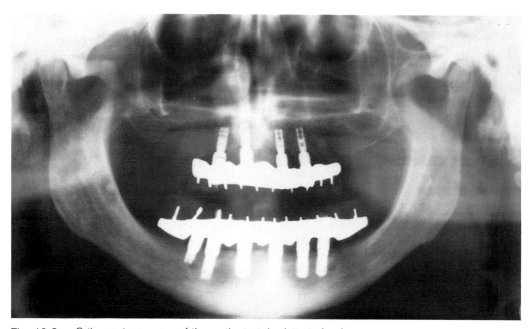

Fig. 10-6c   Orthopantomogram of the patient at the latest checkup.

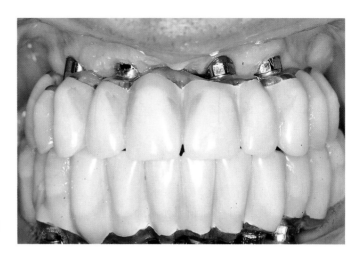

Fig. 10-6d Routine type of bridges in this patient.

Table 10-2 Fixture anchorage function (Total)

Observation period	Upper jaws 734 fixtures	Lower jaws 721 fixtures
1 year	88%	94%
5-12 years	84%	93%

Table 10-3 Fixture anchorage function (Four fixtures per jaw)

Observation period	Upper jaws 52 fixtures	Lower jaws 52 fixtures
5-12 years	88%	91%

Table 10-4 Continuous bridge stability (Four fixtures per jaw)

Observation period	Upper jaws 13 jaws	Lower jaws 13 jaws
5-12 years	95%	100%

Table 10-5 Fixture anchorage function (Fixtures penetrating the nasal cavity and the maxillary sinus*)

Obser-vation period	Sinus penetrating 44 fixtures	Nose penetrating 47 fixtures	Total 91 fixtures
5-10 years	70%	72%	71%

* From Brånemark et al.[16]

void of a defined outer cortical lining. Under these circumstances the stress distribution in upper jaws appeared to be a most crucial factor. It is also clear from Table 10-2 that the majority of fixture losses did occur during the first year.

Although the installation of six fixtures in each jaw is the recommended routine procedure, local bone anatomy—especially in upper jaws—did not always lend itself to this approach. Such patients were treated by installation of four fixtures only. A separate analysis of jaws with four fixtures (Tables 10-3 and 10-4) revealed that almost identical results were obtained, in spite of the fact that the stress distribution in such jaws was even more critical.

A separate analysis of fixtures that pene-

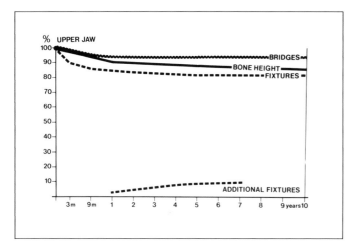

Fig. 10-7a and b Longevity of bridges, marginal bone heights, and fixtures as important prognosis-determining factors, which do not much change after the first year. (From Adell et al.[1])

Fig. 10-7a   In upper jaws.

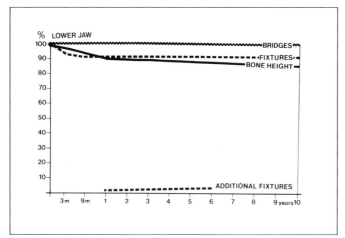

Fig. 10-7b   In lower jaws.

trated the nasal cavity and the maxillary sinus was made by Brånemark et al.[16] The experimental part of this study did not reveal any adverse signs of tissue reactions as judged radiographically or histologically. There was no radiographic evidence of untoward mucosal or bone reactions in the human material either. The fixture anchorage function observed over five to 10 years was about 10% below that of upper jaws in the total patient material (Table 10-5). Sinus-

penetrating fixtures, which functioned as terminal abutments and therefore sustained severe cantilever loads, were found to be vulnerable and were the ones most frequently removed. In recent years refinement in surgical techniques has led to an anchorage function of sinus- and nasal cavity-penetrating fixtures which is as good as that of nonpenetrating fixtures.

The method of using four fixtures only and penetrating the nasal cavity and maxillary sinus has reduced the indications for bone grafts in severely resorbed upper jaws. While the latter procedure[17] is a most helpful approach, it is time consuming and more traumatic for the patient.

Prognosis

The fate of individual fixtures and ultimately of the bridge they support depends on a maintained marginal bone height and osseointegration (Figs. 10-6a to d). Since most of the small amount of marginal bone loss

disappears during the first year after bridge connection and since most of the small number of mobile, nonosseointegrated fixtures also occur during the same period of time (Figs. 10-7a and b), it seems reasonable to postpone a prognosis in each individual patient until this first year has passed.[1, 18] Meanwhile the postsurgical load-related remodelling can take place and an evaluation of the patient's hygiene efforts can be made. After the first year of wearing a bridge, a well-founded prognosis can be made based on the reviewed statistical results, which generally are as good as or even better than those of bridges on natural teeth.[19]

References

1. *Adell, R., et al.*
   A 15-year study of osseointegrated implants in the treatment of the edentulous jaw. Int. J. Oral Surg. 6:387, 1981.

2. *Haraldson, T.*
   A photoelastic study of some biomechanical factors affecting the anchorage of osseointegrated implants in the jaw. Scand. J. Plast. Reconstr. Surg. 14:209, 1980.

3. *Brånemark, P.-I., et al.*
   Osseointegrated implants in the treatment of the edentulous jaw. Experience from a 10-year period. Scand. J. Plast. Reconstr. Surg. 16 (Suppl.), 1977.

4. *Adell, R., et al.*
   Marginal tissue reactions at osseointegrated titanium fixtures. I. A three-year longitudinal prospective study. Int. J. Oral Surg. 1985 (in press).

5. *Skalak, R.*
   Biomechanical considerations in osseointegrated prostheses. J. Prosthet. Dent. 49:843, 1983.

6. *Brånemark, P.-I., et al.*
   Intra-osseous anchorage of dental prostheses. I. Experimental studies. Scand. J. Plast. Reconstr. Surg. 3:81, 1969.

7. *Albrektsson, T., et al.*
   The interface zone of inorganic implants in vivo: Titanium implants in bone. Ann. Biomed. Eng. 11:1, 1983.

8. *Lekholm, U., et al.*
   Marginal tissue reactions at osseointegrated titanium fixtures. II. A cross-sectional retrospective study. Int. J. Oral Surg. 1985 (in press).

9. *Wennström, J.*
   Keratinized and attached gingiva. Regenerative potential and significance for periodontal health. Thesis, University of Göteborg, Sweden, 1982.

10. *Zarb, G. A., and Symington, J. M.*
    Osseointegrated dental implants: Preliminary report on a replication study. J. Prosthet. Dent. 50:271, 1983.

11. *Listgarten, M. A., and Helldén, L.*
    Relative distribution of bacteria at clinically healthy and periodontally diseased sites in humans. J. Clin. Periodontol. 5:115, 1978.

12. *Tagge, D. L., O'Leary, T. J., and El-Kafrawy, A. H.*
    The clinical and histological response of periodontal pockets to root planing and oral hygiene. J. Periodontol. 46:527, 1975.

13. *Albrektsson, T., et al.*
Osseointegrated titanium implants. Requirements for ensuring a long-lasting direct bone-to-implant anchorage in man. Acta Orthop. Scand. 52:155, 1981.

14. *Lekholm, U.*
Clinical procedures for treatment with osseointegrated dental implants. J. Prosthet. Dent. 50:116, 1983.

15. *Schnitman, P. A., and Shulman, L. B.*
Recommendations on the consensus development conference on dental implants. J. Am. Dent. Assoc. 98:373, 1979.

16. *Brånemark, P.-I., et al.*
An experimental and clinical study of osseointegrated implants penetrating the nasal cavity and maxillary sinus. J. Oral Maxillofac. Surg. 42:497, 1984.

17. *Breine, U., and Brånemark, P.-J.*
Reconstruction of alveolar jaw bone. Scand. J. Plast. Reconstr. Surg. 14:23, 1980.

18. *Adell, R.*
Clinical results of osseointegrated implants supporting fixed prostheses in edentulous jaws. J. Prosthet. Dent. 50:251, 1983.

19. *Karlsson, S., and Hedegård, B.*
Efterundersökning av patienter med större brokonstruktioner. Tandlakartidningen 76:935, 1984.

Chapter 11

Radiographic Results

Karl-Gustav Strid

All patients treated with jawbone-anchored prostheses since 1965 have been followed regularly by radiological examinations[1-3] which formed part of both preoperative routines and postoperative checkup schedules. During the healing and early remodelling phases, radiographic procedures have been rarely applied, due to the possibility of detrimental effects of ionizing radiation on healing and remodelling bone tissue. The interface between tissue and metal, where boundary-zone dose buildup may be expected,[4] is particularly vulnerable.

Methods

Recording techniques

Preoperative radiography of the jaw skeleton included a panoramic survey recording, a profile roentgenogram, and intraoral roentgenograms. In addition, in upper jaw cases, frontal tomograms of the maxilla were produced as indicated by the clinical examination.

Postoperatively the patients of the initial series of reconstructions were radiographed at two, five, and 12 months after bridge connection and subsequently once or twice annually.[1] Later, the schedule was changed to comprise radiography one week after abutment surgery, six and 12 months postoperatively, and then once every 12 months.[2] The postoperative examinations were based on intraoral recordings employing the orthonormal projection technique. To facilitate the comparison of roentgenograms obtained at different dates, a serial identical technique, using the Eggen[5] film holder was introduced in approximately 1973. The procedures were later extended by Hollender and Rockler[6] to include stereoscopic recording and viewing. The standardized radiographic techniques used at present are described in chapter 18.

Evaluation of roentgenograms

The intraoral roentgenograms were inspected with regard to density and architecture of perifixtural bone. The height of the anchorage zone (the marginal bone height) of each fixture was measured mesially and distally using the fixture threads as an internal dimensional reference.

The roentgenograms were assessed with due respect to the preoperative situation, which is usually characterized by advanced or even extreme resorption of alveolar bone. Indeed, the quality and quantity of bone tissue can vary considerably within different regions of the same jaw.[1] The surgical trauma inflicted at raising the periosteum, and the removal of bone tissue necessary in preparation of the fixture site, produce unavoidable tissue injury. During the healing phase, this will result in reduction of the marginal bone height. This phenomenon

187

appears to be more pronounced in cases of low tissue vitality caused by a long-standing preoperative edentulous state or by granulation tissue inadvertently left at extraction of teeth.

In the radiological assessment of jawbone reactions, special regard was given to cases with more than three years' observation period with bridge connected. This time limit was chosen because it was considered that the jawbone would then have disclosed its reaction to the implant—whether to keep it integrated or to reject it. Only roentgenograms of good contrast and with clearly depicted fixture threads and bone margins were examined.

Computer-aided assessment

Whereas visual examination of roentgenograms will, in general, yield the desired information on topographic details, such as outlines of bone and soft tissue, or qualitative features, such as the internal structure of bone, quantitative data relating to the density of tissues are not readily acquired. In order to assess the development of bone density, the intraoral roentgenograms were subjected to measurements by means of a computer-based interactive image-analysis system (IBAS I/II, Kontron Bildanalyse GmbH). By means of a television camera of good geometrical and densitometrical linearity, the radiographic recordings were translated into a standard 625-line video signal, which was subsequently analog-to-digital converted to a numerical array of 512 × 512 picture elements in computer memory, suitable for further manipulations or measurements. Density profiles were measured through the individual fixtures and the surrounding bone at different levels along the fixtures. The measurements were performed according to a standard protocol so that roentgenograms recorded on differ-

ent occasions could be compared. Moreover, geometrical quantities such as marginal bone height could be measured in the numerical representation, using the fixture as a dimensional reference.

Material

The total material of the Göteborg clinics at present amounts to about 4,500 fixtures, inserted into the jaws of some 600 patients, with a maximum observation time of 19 years. All pertinent findings from clinical and radiological examinations are continuously added to a computer-handled patient data base at The Institute for Applied Biotechnology.

An account of the performance of 1,618 fixtures, consecutively installed into 235 jaws from 1965 to 1975, was given in 1977 by Hansson,[7] and a further analysis of 2,768 fixtures, installed consecutively from 1965 to 1980 into 410 edentulous jaws of 371 patients, was presented in 1981 by Adell and co-workers.[2] The materials of these studies comprise both experimental and developmental cases and cases treated by routine procedures. In the latter study, the material was accordingly divided into a developmental group (fixtures installed from 1965 to 1971) and two routine groups, I (fixtures installed from 1971 to 1976) and II (fixtures installed from 1976 to 1980). In this study, the earlier roentgenograms were reexamined, and where stereoscopic pairs were available, these were used for bone-height measurements.

For a proper evaluation of changes in marginal bone height to be carried out (1) the roentgenograms should meet the technical requirements outlined above, (2) the patients should return at regular intervals, and (3) the clinical data should be appropriately documented. Some of the collected

Figs. 11-1a to c   Male patient born in 1916, lower jaw fixture surgery in 1979, bridge connected five and a half months postoperatively. Roentgenogram 14 months after fixture surgery displays normal bone tissue in intimate contact with the fixture surfaces at the resolution of radiography. The fixture is clinically stable. Densitometry by means of the computer-aided image analysis system substantiates this observation.

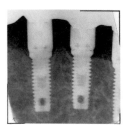 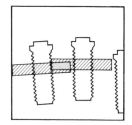 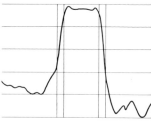

Fig. 11-1a   Roentgenogram.

Fig. 11-1b   Shaded areas indicate the zones of densitometry.

Fig. 11-1c   Densitometric profiles through fixtures and surrounding tissue. The locations of crests and roots of the thread are indicated by vertical bars.

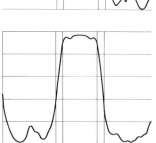

material did not meet one or more of these criteria and was accordingly excluded from the analysis.

Results

With regard to the changes occurring in the perifixtural bone, the time after successful fixture installation can be divided into three phases. During the *healing phase,* which lasts for about three months, osseointegration is established. During the subsequent *remodelling phase,* which lasts for 12 to 18 months, changes in bone density and architecture take place under the influence of the altered pattern of force transmission in the tissue. Finally, an *equilibrium phase* is reached, which is characterized by the absence of any major changes in bone anatomy. In some cases, changes in bone anatomy and marginal bone height may be observed during the first few years, but equilibrium will nevertheless be established at a later stage.

Radiographic signs of osseointegration and of fixture loss

A clinically stable fixture is invariably associated with the radiographic appearance of normal bone tissue in intimate contact with the fixture surface at the resolution level of radiography (Fig. 11-1a). On the other hand, a close relationship has been found to exist between the mobility of a fixture and the presence of a thin, radiolucent perifixtural

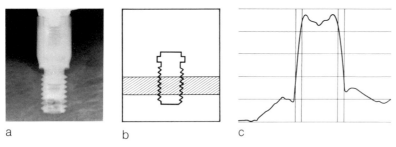

a   b   c

Figs. 11-2a to c   Female patient born in 1919, fixture implanted into lower jaw in 1971. Roentgeno-gram five and a half years postoperatively reveals a thin radiolucent perifixtural space, of about the width of a normal periodontal space; the fixture is clinically mobile. Computer-aided densitometry substantiates this observation (see Fig. 11-1).

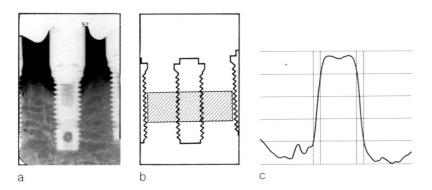

a   b   c

Figs. 11-3a to c   Male patient born in 1912, lower jaw fixture surgery in 1974, bridge connected six and a half months postoperatively. Roentgenogram four years and three months after fixture surgery demonstrates successful implantation. Note the characteristic horizontal architecture of perifixtural trabeculae, individually approaching the titanium surface and radiating predominantly from the edges of the fixture threads (see Fig. 11-1).

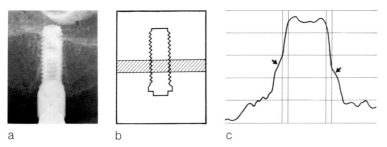

a   b   c

Figs. 11-4a to c   Male patient born in 1915, fixture implanted into upper jaw in 1973, bridge connected five and a half months postoperatively. Roentgenogram four and a half years after fixture surgery displays a sheath of cortical bone, about 1 mm thick, enclosing the implant, as seen in about one tenth of the cases. The cortical zone is clearly seen in the densitometric profile (arrows) (see Fig. 11-1).

space, of approximately the width of a normal periodontal ligament space (Fig. 11-2a). Thus, every fixture observed to be surrounded by a radiolucent zone also was found clinically to be mobile at removal of the bridge. The radiolucent space closely follows the outline of the fixture. Densitometry by means of the computer-aided analysis system substantiates these observations (Figs. 11-1b and c and Figs. 11-2b and c). The presence or absence of a radiolucent perifixtural space is of decisive importance in establishing a prognosis for an individual fixture.[1]

A minority of the originally osseointegrated fixtures showed a progressive loss of bordering bone to such an extent that the anchorage was lost within a few years, suggesting that equilibrium was never developing. This is the case of insidious fixture loss described by Hansson.[7] In some of these cases, however, renewed inspection of early roentgenograms demonstrated the presence of a thin soft-tissue layer interspersed between fixture and perifixtural bone.

Architecture and density of bone

The bone tissue in most cases of successful implants is radiologically characterized by a horizontal architecture of perifixtural trabeculae, individually related to the titanium surface and radiating predominantly from the edges of the fixture threads (Figs. 11-3a to c). For about one tenth of the fixtures, however, the roentgenograms demonstrate a thin layer of cortical bone, typically about 1 mm thick, enclosing the implant (Figs. 11-4a to c). In both cases, increased density of bone tissue is observed in a zone extending several millimeters perifixturally. From longitudinal radiographic examinations it has been observed that the bordering zone remodels throughout the years, a change that results in increasing bone density. Computer-aided densitometry provides a quantitative assessment of bone condensation, indicating that the major changes in density take place during the first two years following fixture implantation (Fig. 11-5).

In fixture-loss cases, a thorough reexamination of the roentgenograms has shown that it is doubtful whether the fixtures later found to be mobile were ever integrated into the bone (Fig. 11-6).

Marginal bone height

Marginal bone was lost both during the healing phase, with the fixtures covered by mucoperiosteal tissue, and, later, after abutment connection. During the healing phase, bone loss was more extensive in upper than in lower jaws, whereas the reverse was true for the remodelling phase (Table 11-1). This might be due to differences in remodelling capacity and remodelling rate between maxillary and mandibular bone. Because of the rich vascular supply and the cancellous character of the maxillary bone, much of the necessary remodelling after fixture installation could take place during the healing period, while the slower reacting mandibular bone would demand an extended period of time for the same purpose. The decrease in the rate of marginal bone loss during the healing period (Table 11-1) between the three different groups is probably explained by successive refinement of the surgical technique. The higher values for bone loss in the remodelling period might be explained by the higher torque applied at installation of fixtures in the routine groups.[8] The total reduction in marginal bone height from fixture installation to the end of the first year after abutment connection was, however, almost equal in all the three groups, that is, about 1.2 mm. During the follow-up period—the observation time after the first

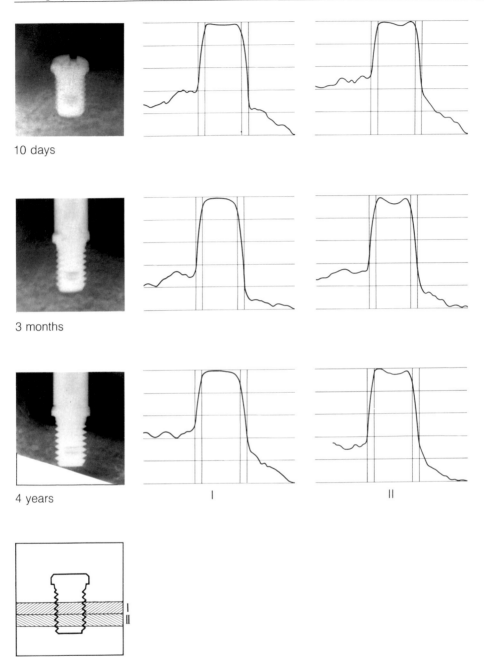

10 days

3 months

4 years

I   II

Fig. 11-5 Male patient born in 1931, lower jaw fixture surgery in 1965, bridge connected one year and nine months postoperatively. Densitometry seems to indicate that the bone density decreases during the first three postoperative months. Subsequently, the bordering zone remodels throughout

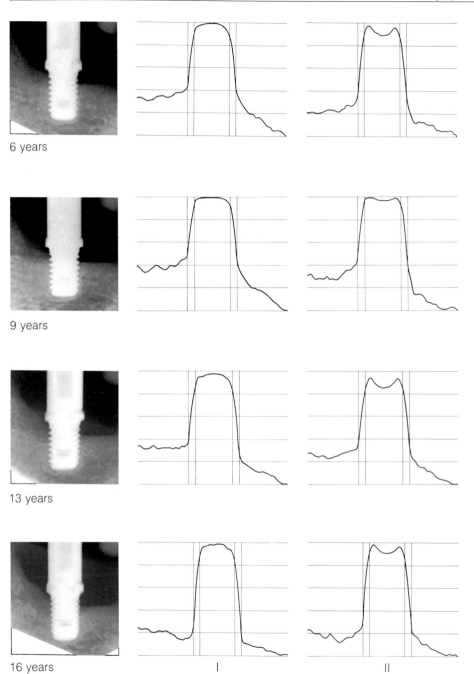

6 years

9 years

13 years

16 years

I   II

the years, with increasing bone density as a result. Computer-aided densitometry, giving quantitative assessment of bone condensation, proves that the major changes in density take place during the first two years following fixture implantation.

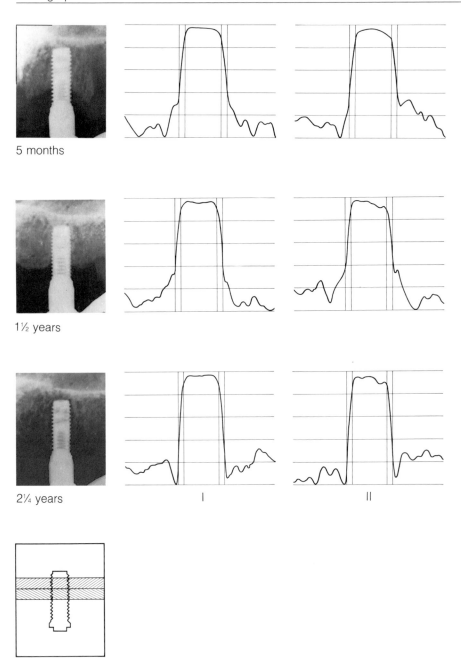

5 months

1½ years

2¼ years   I   II

Fig. 11-6 Female patient born in 1923, upper jaw fixture surgery in 1973, bridge connected five months postoperatively. This patient had a very thin buccal wall. The radiologist reported this fixture to be loose after one and a half years, which is clinically confirmed. However, already after five months densitometry of the roentgenogram gives some indication of fixture mobility.

194

Table 11-1   Marginal bone loss during the healing and remodelling phases*

(For the development group and the early cases of routine group I, there is a great variation in the duration of the healing period, implying that most of the bone remodelling in many cases did actually take place during the healing period.)**

	Upper jaw		Lower jaw	
	healing	remodelling	healing	remodelling
	mm			
Development group	1.2 ± 0.9 (207)***	0.1 ± 0.8 (43)	0.7 ± 0.9 (147)	0.1 ± 0.4 (58)
Routine group I	1.3 ± 1.1 (358)	0.2 ± 0.9 (153)	1.0 ± 1.0 (211)	0.4 ± 0.6 (86)
Routine group II	0.7 ± 1.0 (431)	0.6 ± 0.8 (227)	0.3 ± 0.5 (1,006)	0.8 ± 0.8 (358)

* Mean values ± standard deviations.
** From Adell et al.[2]
*** Number of observed fixtures.

year with the fixtures loaded by the bridge—the mean annual bone-height loss amounted to 0.1 mm for the routine groups (Table 11-2). This period, however, includes the late remodelling phase, and if statistics are confined to the equilibrium phase, virtually no additional loss of marginal bone is observed, in accordance with the statement of Brånemark and co-workers.[1] This suggests that a reliable long-term prognosis can be established after one year, at least with regard to marginal bone height.

The annual decrease in marginal bone height in the follow-up periods is comparable with or even less than the loss of attachment level or marginal bone height at teeth as reported for patients after treatment for severe periodontitis with the same postoperative checkup intervals of six to 12 months.[2] Provided that the periabutment and perifixtural tissues react in the same way as periodontium to the presence of microbial plaque, even better results than those observed might be expected with more frequent oral hygiene checkups for

Table 11-2   Rate of marginal bone loss during follow-up periods*,***

	Upper jaw	Lower jaw
	mm/year	
Development group	0.1 ± 0.4 (179)***	0.1 ± 0.8 (184)
Routine group I	0.1 ± 0.6 (1,145)	0.1 ± 0.5 (963)
Routine group II	0.1 ± 0.6 (69)	0.1 ± 0.6 (130)

* Mean values ± standard deviations.
** From Adell et al.[2]
*** Number of observed fixtures.

patients with bone-anchored bridges.[9] This would require the present checkup system to be reorganized to incorporate referral of patients with jawbone-anchored bridges for appropriate hygiene therapy.

When interpreting postoperative variations in marginal bone height perifixturally, it is important to keep in mind the varying preoperative topography of the marginal bone. In many cases, the residual alveolar

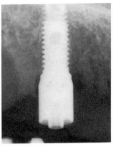
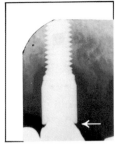
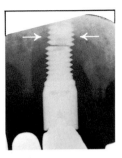

a 6 months   b 9 months   c 1½ years

Figs. 11-7a to c   Female patient born in 1926, upper jaw fixture surgery in 1977, bridge connected eight months postoperatively.

Fig. 11-7a   Radiographic appearance of fixture after abutment surgery, prior to bridge connection.

Fig. 11-7b   Roentgenogram nine months after fixture surgery demonstrates improper abutment-bridge contact *(arrow)*.

Fig. 11-7c   After 10 months with the bridge (one and a half years postoperatively) excessive bone loss and fixture fracture have resulted; the marginal bone level *(arrows)* has retracted 6 mm (see Fig. 18-15).

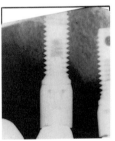
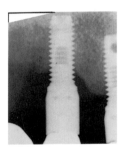
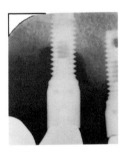
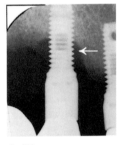

a 1½ years   b 2½ years   c 3¾ years   d 4¾ years

Figs. 11-8a to d   Female patient born in 1913, upper jaw fixture surgery in 1975, bridge connected 16 months postoperatively.

Figs. 11-8a and b   No marginal bone loss is displayed in the roentgenograms of one and a half and two and a half years.

Fig. 11-8c   Radiography three years and nine months after fixture surgery disclosed marginal bone loss amounting to 1.5 mm in 15 months.

Fig. 11-8d   One year later, the bridge was found loose, and on bridge removal a fixture fracture was discovered at the level of the apical end of the abutment screw *(arrow)*. Note that this fracture is not visible in the roentgenogram.

196

crest is extremely thin in the buccolingual direction, a condition that, with no apparent relation to the clinical width or height of the gingival crest, will not always be fully revealed by radiography. In order to provide complete osseous enclosure of the fixture it is in such cases necessary to resect the marginal alveolar bone locally until sufficient buccolingual width is achieved.

The amount of marginal bone loss also agrees with the annual loss of bone height reported[10, 11] for edentulous jaws in patients wearing removable dentures.[2] It is interesting to note that the marginal bone level can even remain at a more coronal level close to the fixtures rather than farther away.[2] This could be interpreted as though the fixtures exert a stimulating influence on the remodelling perifixtural bone. The same view is suggested by model studies[8] and by histological findings from experimental series[12] that demonstrate the horizontal architecture of bone trabeculae described above.

Mechanical failure

In some cases an abnormal rate of marginal bone loss (about 3 mm per year) was observed. Radiological reexamination of these cases invariably revealed mechanical failures associated with irregular stress distribution, such as misfit between the components or component fracture (Figs. 11-7a to c). Thus, in 2,757 consecutively installed fixtures, fractures at different levels were observed in 90 fixtures, 75% to 80% of them occurring in maxillary implants. Fractures were only occasionally observed later than six years after fixture installation, and most of these occurred with mechanically rigid bridges employed in the early routine series. Extensive loss of marginal bone demands an examination of the functional relations of the prosthesis components. In some cases, reexamination of roentgenograms may reveal a previously undetected fixture or screw fracture (Figs. 11-8a to d).

After adequate treatment, even fractured fixtures can remain integrated, with a favorable prognosis.

Conclusions

Radiography offers the sole method of noninvasive analysis of the perifixtural anchorage zone. A clinically stable fixture is radiologically characterized by normal bone in intimate contact with the metal surface, whereas the presence of a radiolucent perifixtural space is indicative of implant mobility. Marginal bone loss in successful cases takes place during the first 18 to 24 months following fixture implantation. A reliable long-term prognosis with regard to marginal bone height can be established one year after bridge connection.

Extensive loss of marginal bone is a sign of mechanical failure and should always give rise to a careful scrutiny of the components and their functional relationships.

References

1. *Brånemark, P.-I., et al.*
   Osseointegrated implants in the treatment of the edentulous jaw. Experience from a 10-year period. Scand. J. Plast. Reconstr. Surg. Suppl. 16, 1977.

2. *Adell, R., et al.*
   A 15-year study of osseointegrated implants in the treatment of the edentulous jaw. Int. J. Oral Surg. 10:387-416, 1981.

3. *Brånemark, P.-I., et al.*
   Osseointegrated titanium fixtures in the treatment of edentulousness. Biomaterials 4:25-28, 1983.

4. *Alm Carlsson, G.*
   Dosimetry at interfaces: Theoretical analysis and measurements by means of thermoluminescent LiF. Acta Radiol. Suppl. 332, 1973.

5. *Eggen, S.*
   Standardiserad intraoral röntgenteknik. Sveriges Tandläkarförb. Tidn. 61:867-872, 1969.

6. *Hollender, L., and Rockler, B.*
   Radiographic evaluation of osseointegrated implants of the jaws. Dento-Maxillo-Fac. Radiol. 9:91-95, 1980.

7. *Hansson, B.-O.*
   Success and failure of osseointegrated implants in the edentulous jaw. Swed. Dent. J. Suppl. 1, 1977.

8. *Haraldson, T.*
   Functional evaluation of bridges on osseointegrated implants in the edentulous jaw. Thesis, University of Göteborg, Sweden, 1979.

9. *Axelsson, P., and Lindhe, J.*
   Effect of controlled oral hygiene procedures on caries and periodontal disease in adults. J. Clin. Periodontol. 5:133-151, 1978.

10. *Wictorin, L.*
    Bone resorption in cases with complete upper denture. Acta Radiol. Suppl. 228, 1964.

11. *Crum, R. J., and Rooney, G. E.*
    Alveolar bone loss in overdentures. A 5-year study. J. Prosthet. Dent. 40:610-613, 1978.

12. *Brånemark, P.-I., et al.*
    Intra-osseous anchorage of dental prostheses. I. Experimental studies. Scand. J. Plast. Reconstr. Surg. 3:81-100, 1969.

Chapter 12

Patient Selection and Preparation

Ulf Lekholm and George A. Zarb

The biological and functional implications of being edentulous[1] were reviewed in chapter 2. It was suggested that a predictable method for long-term host acceptance of an alloplastic tooth root analogue would dramatically improve preprosthetic surgical therapy. It is tempting, therefore, to regard the osseointegration procedure as one that can be universally prescribed. This would imply that every partially and completely edentulous patient would be a candidate for this technique. In fact, the ongoing development of diverse systems of predictably integrated tissue prostheses could very well evolve into a practical, cost-effective, and routine clinical procedure. However, at this stage of clinical development, other conventional prosthetic procedures must also be considered, since they represent viable, time-proven treatment strategies. It is therefore important for the clinical specialist to evaluate thoroughly which method would be most beneficial in each individual situation.

Patient selection

The selection of patients for the osseointegration procedure can be based on the treatment indications listed in Table 12-1. Patients with one or more of these criteria are usually incapable of comfortably wearing a removable prosthesis, and may therefore be referred to the oral surgeon for a presurgical examination.[2] Two main questions are of special interest: *(1)* can the proposed surgical procedure be undertaken, and *(2)* how can the surgery be carried out? Both questions are answered by conventional preoperative assessments, which are performed to establish:

1. *General health condition* of the patient
2. *Local health conditions* of mucous membranes and jaws
3. *Morphological features* of the area to be operated on

It is possible to treat virtually all patients via the osseointegration technique, as long as the patients fulfill general requirements for surgery. Moreover, age does not appear to influence patient selection, nor does a large number of chronic health conditions. Thus, patients with medical conditions such as diabetes, arthritis, and cardiac and vascular diseases have been operated on, as well as patients on long-standing steroid medication, without any adverse long-term effects. Such patients will of course require conventional precautions throughout the entire surgical interventions.

The overall preoperative requirement regarding the local health state is that no pathological conditions are present in any of the hard or soft tissues of either jaw. Any such condition may adversely affect the establishment of a tissue integration response

Table 12-1   Indications for treatment

Clinical findings that singly or collectively preclude the predictable and comfortable wear of a removable prosthesis:

1. Severe morphologic compromise of denture supporting areas that significantly undermine denture retention.
2. Poor oral muscular coordination.
3. Low tolerance of mucosal tissues.
4. Parafunctional habits leading to recurrent soreness and instability of prosthesis.
5. Unrealistic prosthodontic expectations.
6. Active or hyperactive gag reflexes, elicited by a removable prosthesis.
7. Psychological inability to wear a removable prosthesis, even if adequate denture retention or stability is present.
8. Unfavorable number and location of potential abutments in a residual dentition. Adjunctive location of optimally placed osseointegrated root analogues would allow for provision of a fixed prosthesis.
9. Single tooth loss to avoid involving neighboring teeth as abutments.

of the fixtures. All oral lesions must therefore be treated in advance so that the tissues will have time to heal prior to fixture installation. The time factor usually observed is three to four weeks for mucosal lesions and three to four months for bone lesions.

Some of the oral conditions that must be treated include:

1. *Mucosal lesions,* such as cheilosis, herpetic stomatitis, candidiasis, denture induced stomatitis, and hyperplastic ridge replacement
2. *Bony lesions,* such as tooth root remnants, impacted teeth, cysts, and residual bone infections
3. Various types of *benign mucosal and bone tumors*

Furthermore, it must be emphasized that patients should be capable of carrying out

and maintaining optimal oral hygiene so that no gingivitis is present. Preferably, simultaneous treatment of the opposite jaw should also be done. This step can, however, be performed during the healing period following fixture installation as well, but must be completed before the second operation, i.e., the abutment connection. By restoring both jaws at the same time it is possible to ensure a complete rehabilitation of the masticatory functions.

The status of the attached mucosa overlying the potential fixture sites is of interest for the surgical planning, and may be either attached or unattached, and either thin or thick and mobile. Clinical experience suggests that a transepithelial fixture component that penetrates unattached mucosa is not a potential hazard, particularly if the protruding oral component is aligned so as not to interfere with active circumoral or circumlingual tissues. Wennström's conclusions on the relative importance of unattached gingival tissues around a natural tooth offer interesting information in this regard[3] (see chapters 3 and 7). Unattached circumfixtural epithelium can increase the risk of entrapment of food debris and foreign particles with obvious risks. This can be avoided by resorting to one of the grafting procedures to ensure an overlying area of attached grafted tissue at the proposed surgerized site. Such a procedure is preferably performed after the bridge has been attached, as it then can be used as a stent for the graft during healing. Usually extra vigilance on the patient's part vis-à-vis home care is adequate, and extra surgical interventions are avoided. If the mucosa is too thick it may have to be trimmed to avoid resorting to an ultralong oral abutment connection, which would be necessary for optimal hygiene maintenance. The extra length, however, could lead to a cosmetic or a mechanical (unfavorable crown/root ratio) compromise, or both.

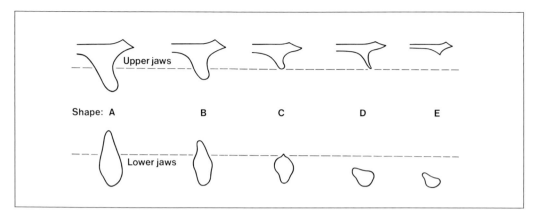

Fig. 12-1   A proposed classification of residual jaw shape and different rates of bone resorption following tooth extraction. The interrupted lines indicate the approximate demarcation between alveolar and basal bone: *(A)* most of the alveolar ridge is present; *(B)* moderate residual ridge resorption has occurred; *(C)* advanced residual ridge resorption has occurred and only basal bone remains; *(D)* some resorption of the basal bone has started; *(E)* extreme resorption of the basal bone has taken place.

Jaw anatomy

The feasibility of *fixture installation*[2] can be determined after studying the morphological structural features that are present. In general, all jaws irrespective of shape and bone quality can be treated according to the same standard procedures. The only exceptions to this general rule are those maxillary jaws with advanced residual ridge resorption, which is so excessive that a preliminary grafting procedure becomes necessary.

On the other hand, a great variety in jaw anatomy is encountered in so-called routine patients. It is therefore important to thoroughly analyze anatomical structures via clinical and radiographical examinations before any surgery is started. Clinical assessment consists of both palpation and probing through the mucosa to assess the thickness of the soft tissues at the proposed surgical sites. Radiographic analysis comprises a periapical series, an orthopantomogram, a lateral cephalostatic view, and, sometimes, tomogram and an occlusal view (see chapter 18). However, it must be remembered that even the most thorough preoperative analysis will fail to reveal subtle morphological details that only become evident when the bone site is surgically exposed.

It is convenient to consider the anatomical features of bone relevant to fixture preparation under the headings of *jaw shape* or *contour,* and *jawbone quality.* Experience suggests that five general groups of diverse jaw shapes are encountered (Fig. 12-1):

A. Most of the alveolar ridge is present.
B. Moderate residual ridge resorption has occurred.

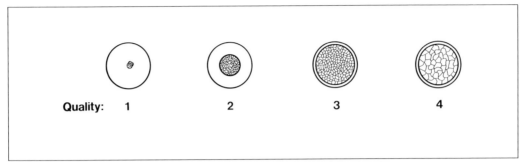

Fig. 12-2 A proposed classification of jawbone quality: *(1)* almost the entire jaw is comprised of homogenous compact bone; *(2)* a thick layer of compact bone surrounds a core of dense trabecular bone; *(3)* a thin layer of cortical bone surrounds a core of dense trabecular bone of favorable strength; *(4)* a thin layer of cortical bone surrounds a core of low density trabecular bone.

C. Advanced residual ridge resorption has occurred and only basal bone remains.
D. Some resorption of the basal bone has started.
E. Extreme resorption of the basal bone has taken place.

A classification of the jaws with regard to jawbone quality recognizes four groups (Fig. 12-2):

1. Almost the entire jaw is comprised of homogenous compact bone.
2. A thick layer of compact bone surrounds a core of dense trabecular bone.
3. A thin layer of cortical bone surrounds a core of dense trabecular bone of favorable strength.
4. A thin layer of cortical bone surrounds a core of low density trabecular bone.

The features of bone quality are not always possible to elucidate from radiographic assessments only, as the cortical layer of the surface of the jaw may mask the bone quality of the internal parts of the jaw. It is during explorative drilling in fixture site preparation that the true bone quality present in the jaw can be determined.

Jaw shape and bone quality combinations

Naturally, a great variety of combinations between jaw shapes and bone qualities exists. This clinical observation tends to make each jaw rather unique from an anatomical point of view. Still, some guidelines can be provided concerning the surgical aspects of the fixture installation procedure in relation to jaw shape and bone quality when selecting patients.

Certain combinations of jaw shapes and bone qualities provide a relatively uncomplicated surgical endeavor. These are the sort of clinical situations that should be undertaken during the early skill acquisition stages of learning the prescribed technique.

Thus, upper and lower jaws of shape groups *B* and *C*, when combined with quality groups *2* or *3* (Fig. 12-3), are considered straightforward therapeutic situations. These types of jaws (Figs. 12-4 and 12-5) allow for good stabilization of the equipment during drilling and fixture installation because of the favorable bone qualities pres-

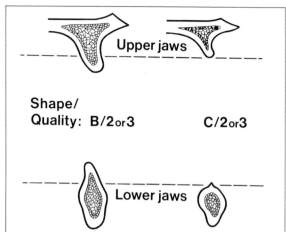

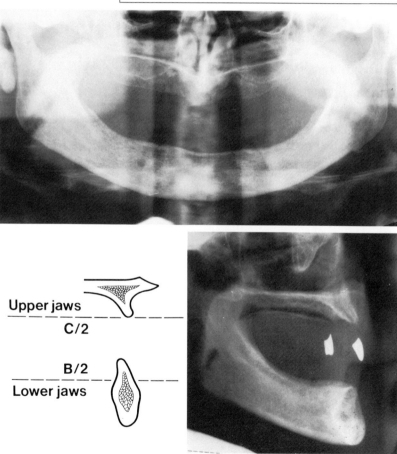

Fig. 12-3 Diagrams showing combinations of jaw shapes *(B, C)* and bone qualities *(2, 3)* of upper and lower jaws considered to be straightforward therapeutic situations.

Fig. 12-4 Radiographs and corresponding diagrams showing an upper jaw of shape *C*/quality *2 (C/ 2)*, and a lower jaw of shape *B*/quality *2 (B/2)*.

203

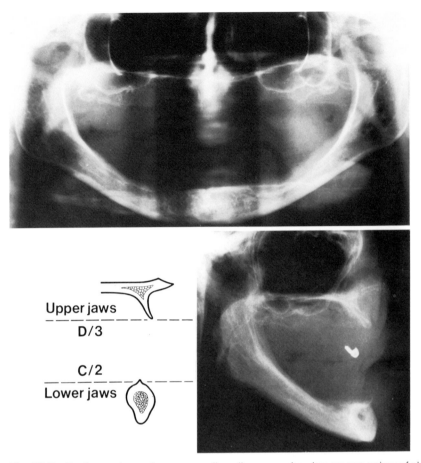

Fig. 12-5   Radiographs and corresponding diagrams showing an upper jaw of shape *D*/quality *3 (D/ 3)*, and a lower jaw of shape *C*/quality *2 (C/2)*.

ent. Furthermore, only standard instrumentation is needed in these situations.

In contrast to this, it can be difficult to install fixtures in upper and lower jaws of shape group *A*, especially when combined with quality group *4* (Fig. 12-6). In such situations (Fig. 12-7), the residual ridge, which mostly consists of a thin layer of cortical bone surrounding trabecular bone of unfavorable strength and low density, gives rise to instability during both the drilling and fixture in-

stallation procedures. Standard fixtures may therefore already become unsteady at installation time, which will preclude the establishment of tissue integration. In such situations, it is extremely important to use an accurate drilling technique in combination with long fixtures. The aim will be to reach the compact layer of the inferior border of the mandible or the basal bone of the maxillae in order to achieve fixture stabilization (see chapter 14).

204

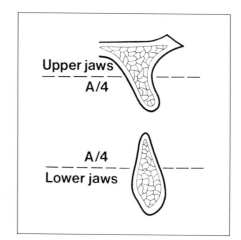

Fig. 12-6 Diagrams showing combinations of jaw shape *A* and bone quality *4* of upper and lower jaws considered to be difficult therapeutic situations.

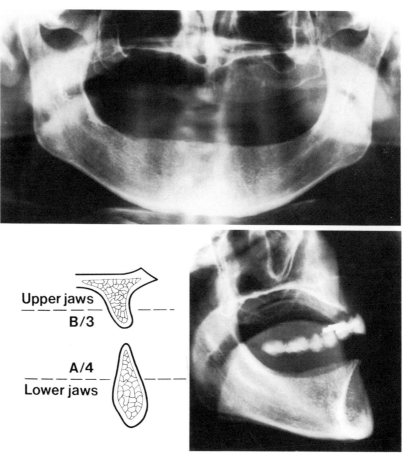

Fig. 12-7 Radiographs and corresponding diagrams showing an upper jaw of shape *B*/quality *3 (B/3)*, and a lower jaw of shape *A*/quality *4 (A/4)*.

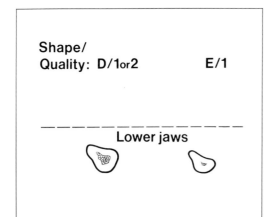

Shape/
Quality: D/1or2   E/1

Lower jaws

Fig. 12-8 Diagrams showing combinations of jaw shapes *(D, E)* and bone qualities *(1, 2)* of lower jaws considered to be very difficult therapeutic situations, but still possible to treat according to standardized procedures.

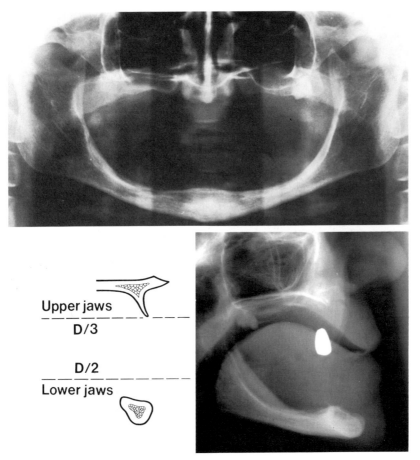

Upper jaws
D/3

D/2
Lower jaws

Fig. 12-9 Radiographs and corresponding diagrams showing an upper jaw of shape *D*/quality *3 (D/3)*, and a lower jaw of shape *D*/quality *2 (D/2)*.

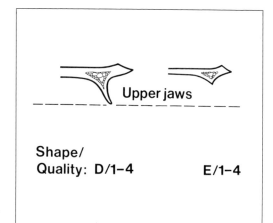

Fig. 12-10 Diagrams showing combinations of jaw shapes *(D, E)* and bone qualities *(1-4)* of upper jaws considered to be extremely difficult therapeutic situations, mostly necessitating a grafting procedure.

Shape/
Quality: D/1–4   **E/1–4**

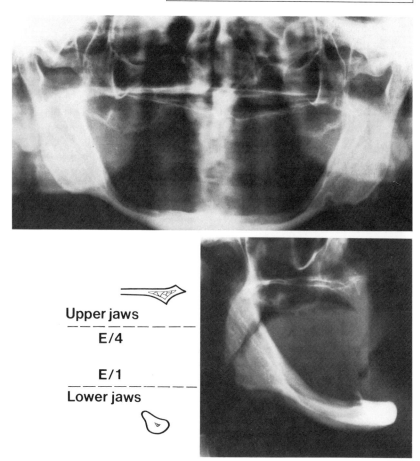

Fig. 12-11 Radiographs and corresponding diagrams showing an upper jaw of shape *E*/quality *4 (E/ 4),* and a lower jaw of shape *E*/quality *1 (E/1).*

207

Lower jaws of shape group *D*, mostly when combined with quality group *1* or *2* (Fig. 12-8), are considered to be rather difficult therapeutic situations. Still these jaws (Fig. 12-9) may be treated according to the standardized procedure. Mandibles of shape group *E*, especially when combined with quality group *1* (see Figs. 12-8 and 12-11), will make the surgical procedure even more difficult because of the obvious risks of overheating the bone site or fracturing the jawbone during the drilling procedure. An extremely gentle surgical technique should therefore be used in these situations.

Maxillae of shape groups *D* and *E*, irrespective of bone quality present (Fig. 12-10), are always found to be extremely difficult to work with. The bone volume in these cases (Fig. 12-11; see also Figs. 12-5 and 12-9) is mostly too small for fixture installation and may necessitate a grafting procedure.

Other anatomical features

In connection with the radiographic assessment of the anatomical feature of the jaw it should also be mentioned that, besides jaw shape and bone quality, it is important to identify the mental foramina, the anterior border of the maxillary sinuses, and the incisal canal, as these structures constitute limits for fixture installation. Furthermore, variations in the vertical height of the residual ridge within the same jaw do not require modification of the fixture installation procedure. Different resorption levels may be compensated for by using different abutment lengths, and via the design of the subsequent prosthetic work.

Patient preparation

The final step of patient selection and preparation consists of information about the nature of the treatment procedures and the possible results[2] that can be obtained in each single treatment situation. It is also important to thoroughly explain time schedules, surgical and prosthodontic treatment technique difficulties, and the protocol for the follow-up system. In this way the patient can be reassured and prepared for the procedure being offered.

If the patient during any phase of the preoperative assessment expresses unrealistic expectations of the proposed treatment, further consultation from other professionals, e.g., a psychiatrist, is sought.[4] Such a course of .action is also followed if early examination suggests the presence of mental health problems, or history of drug and/or alcohol addiction, as these conditions may contraindicate treatment (see chapter 9). In most cases, however, the patient may proceed to the first surgical stage after all preoperative examinations have been taken care of.

References

1. *Zarb, G. A.*
   The edentulous milieu. J. Prosthet. Dent. 49:825, 1983.

2. *Adell, R., et al.*
   A 15-year study of osseointegrated implants in the treatment of the edentulous jaw. Int. J. Oral Surg. 10:387, 1981.

3. *Wennström, J. L.*
   Keratinized and attached gingiva. Regenerative potential and significance for periodontal health. Thesis, University of Göteborg, Sweden, 1982.

4. *Blomberg, S., and Lindquist, L. W.*
   Psychological reactions to edentulousness and treatment with jawbone-anchored bridges. Acta Psychiatr. Scand. 68:251, 1983.

Chapter 13

Surgical Procedures

Ragnar Adell, Ulf Lekholm, and Per-Ingvar Brånemark

General requirements

The surgery for obtaining osseointegration of fixtures and adequately functioning barrier tissues around abutments requires:

1. Sterile conditions, as in a fully equipped operatory
2. Standardized recommended fixture installation and abutment connection equipment
3. Correctly manufactured fixtures and abutments with defined material properties, preoperatively prepared to remove any contaminants
4. An experienced oral surgeon, specifically trained in the osseointegration method, maintaining a nondamaging technique and respecting the individual characteristics of the tissues at hand
5. A thoroughly evaluated and prepared patient
6. A well-trained staff

Operation technique

The surgical procedures comprise *fixture installation* and *abutment connection*. Generally, these steps are undertaken under premedication and local anesthesia. In principle, almost all topographic variations in mandibles can be treated by the following technique without grafting. In about 5% to 10% of the maxillary cases the severely altered ridge morphology requires a grafting procedure.

Fixture installation

Preoperative care

The patient takes 10 mg diazepam orally the evening before the operation. About one hour preoperatively 20 to 25 mg diazepam and 2 g of phenoxymethylpenicillin are administered orally. The indicated diazepam dosage is for patients weighing 130 pounds and is adjusted individually. The patient changes to a disposable gown and receives a cap for the hair and socks for the feet. Local anesthesia is given according to the recommendations for mandibles and maxillae, respectively. After rinsing the mouth with 0.2% chlorhexidine solution the patient is taken into the operatory.

The patient's mouth is cleaned on the inside and outside with 0.1% chlorhexidine. The same attention should be paid to the jaw opposite the field of operation. At this point the operatory nurse changes gloves. A clinidrape is put under the patient's head and made into a turban. A sterile mask is placed over the patient's nose and eyes, and tied at the back and fastened to the upper lip with tape (steristrip). Ensure that a free air passage is maintained. A perforated

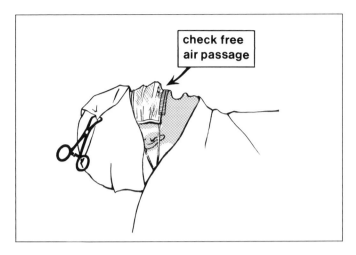

Fig. 13-1 Prepared patient with protective layers for eyes and nose.

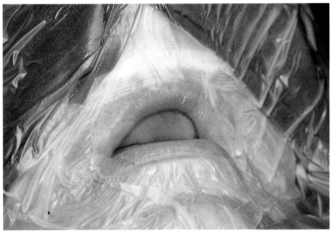

Fig. 13-2 Patient with steri-drape applied ready for operation.

wide tube introduced beneath the mask parallel with the upper lip may facilitate free air passage for the patient. The patient is covered with an operating sheet and the head with a clinidrape (Fig. 13-1). These are fastened to the turban with clips on both sides. A hole large enough for the patient's mouth is made in the steridrape. The protective sheet is removed and the steridrape applied around the operating field, with care taken to mold the sheet around the mouth and chin (Fig. 13-2). Two different suction devices are used, one for saliva and the other for the operation wound only.

Laying of instruments

The nurse puts on a cap, mask, and sterile operating gown. The nurse wipes all movables in the operatory with 70% alcohol on the morning of the operation, after which nobody is allowed into the operatory without sterile clothing. The operatory nurse scrubs

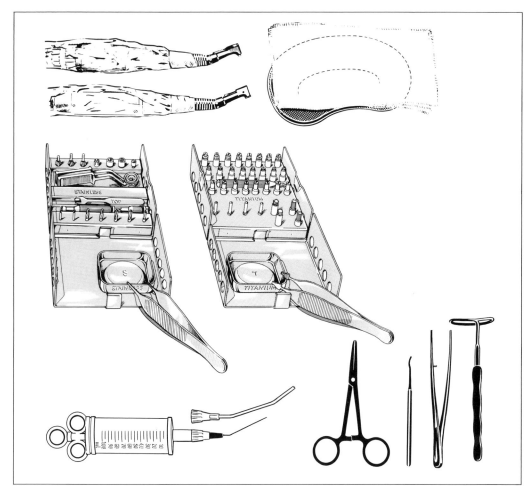

Fig. 13-3   Second set of instruments used for fixture site preparation.

and puts on a sterile gown and sterile gloves. All talcum is removed with gauze dressing, moistened in saline. Instruments and materials are unwrapped. The drill cord is covered with foil. Before the contra-angle handpieces are mounted, they are cleaned with gauze to remove any remaining oil. After the contra-angle handpiece is mounted on the engine, the foil is secured to the handpiece with tape. The motors are run a few minutes with the contra-angle handpiece held tipped down vertically in order to eliminate excess oil. Handpieces are then dried on the outside with a sterile gauze dressing.

All instruments, which will later be used for bone preparation except for the fixture box (second set of instruments) (Fig. 13-3), are placed farthest away on the assistant's table and covered with clinidrape. On top of these are placed those instruments that are to be used at the flap reflection stage (first set of instruments) (Fig. 13-4). All gauze dressings to be used are moistened with saline in order

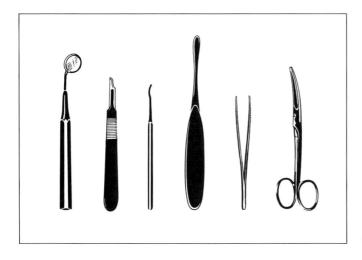

Fig. 13-4 First set of instruments used for reflection of flaps.

to enhance absorption quality, to bind loose fibers, and to keep tissue damage to a minimum.

The fixture box is prepared. The lid is taken off and fixture mounts attached to as many fixtures of presumed lengths that will be used preoperatively. One fixture mount at a time is taken up by the open-end wrench, put on the fixture, and rotated until the mount is locked around the hexagonal head of the fixture. The screw of the fixture mount is tightened, loosened, and retightened. This step is important, as a fixture mount too loose could rotate and damage the fixture hexagonal head during installation. A damaged head can cause problems at abutment connection. On the other hand, if the fixture mount is too tightly applied, considerable difficulties may arise when it is disconnected after the fixture has been installed into the bone, damaging the fixture site. The lid is replaced on the fixture box, and all instruments are covered until the operation starts.

Surgical technique in mandibles

Anesthesia

Inferior alveolar blocks are given bilaterally. When the anesthesia has taken full effect, the mental foramina are identified by palpation, and "scratches" are made in the overlying gingiva for later identification of these sites. Then the mental nerve is blocked on both sides and infiltration anesthesia is deposited into the lingual and buccal mucoperiosteum in the depths of the sulci. Altogether about 12 ml 2% lidocaine-adrenaline solution is given (1:80,000). It is important to infiltrate down to the base of the mandible, which is innervated by cervical nerves.

Soft-tissue reflection

The incision line is marked with a dissector in the depth of the buccal sulcus, inclining toward the crest in the region of the mental foramina. The mucous membrane is incised between the canine regions. Sharp dissection through the muscle fibers is performed under tight stretching of the lip. The muscle fibers are successively loosened in a hori-

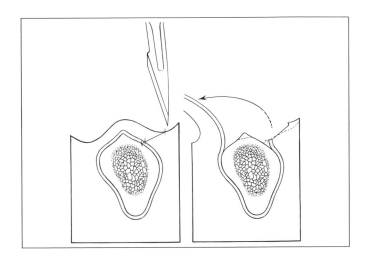

Fig. 13-5   Reflection of flap.

zontal direction and the periosteum is cut between the canine regions 5 to 6 mm below the ridge crest. With the help of a dissector, a very careful subperiosteal dissection is performed as close to the bone surface as possible in order to avoid damaging the periosteum.

The top of the crest is exposed with a dissector and by removing any fibrous adhesions. The lingual side of the alveolar ridge is exposed with a dissector so that a mucoperiosteal flap can be raised between the canine regions with a minimum of tissue damage (Fig. 13-5). The very thin periosteal layer on the lingual side of the jaw must be given special attention in order not to perforate it. The aim is to achieve an osteoperiosteal flap, i.e., the cambium layer of the periosteum should be included in the flap.

With a dissector, subperiosteal dissection is carried out in a lateral direction from the canine region to the mental foramen with its outcoming nerve and blood vessels. The incision is widened step by step until it encompasses the region just distal of the mental foramina. The direction of the anterior mental canal should be checked on each

side with a dissector. Where extreme absorption is present, perhaps with the mental nerve within fibrous tissue, great care must be taken at sharp dissection.

The objective is for a minimum of vertical dissection, as too much exposure of jawbone increases the risk of damage to periosteal circulation. Information concerning the topography of the operation site can generally be procured by careful vertical probing using a dissector. Special attention should be paid to possible concavities on the lingual side.

Sharp and thin parts of marginal crest top should be removed with bone forceps in order to create a surface for commencement of the drilling stage.

When the bone tissue within the operation field is completely exposed, the instruments belonging to the first set are taken away with the help of the clinidrape on which they rest. The second set of instruments is now ready for use. The instruments that lie in the fixture box are not to be touched with gloves. Instead, they are to be lifted from the box with a special titanium forceps. Used drills are put in cups containing saline solution and not directly on the assistant's table. Titanium

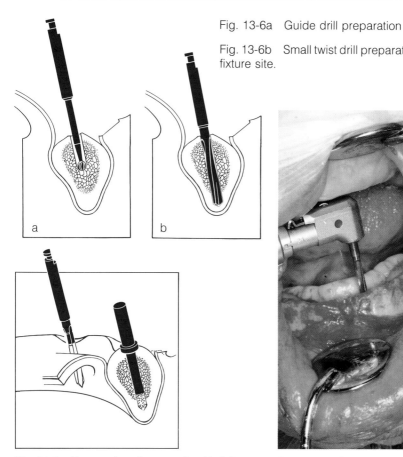

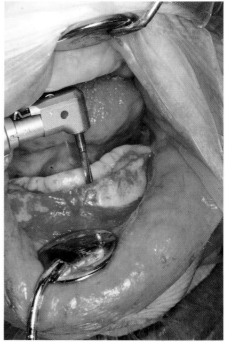

Fig. 13-6a   Guide drill preparation

Fig. 13-6b   Small twist drill preparation to final depth of fixture site.

Fig. 13-8   Preparation of a most distal left fixture site parallel with a direction indicator installed near the midline.

Fig. 13-7   Checking the direction of the fixture site with a small twist drill in relation to the opposite jaw.

drills should be placed in the titanium cup, and stainless steel drills in the stainless steel cup. With the change of instruments even the suction device for the wound is changed.

Drilling at high speed

Every time rotating instruments are used, profuse irrigation with saline solution must be applied. The jet is directed toward the point where the rotating instrument enters the marginal bone. Bone chips should be

removed frequently from the edge of the drill, and during drilling the bur should be moved up and down in the site so that saline can reach down to the cutting edge and cut bone can be removed. With regard to the anatomy of the bone and the topography of the opposite jaw, the preliminary direction of the fixture sites (usually six) is now chosen in between the mental foramina, and their entries are marked with a guide drill (Fig. 13-6a). This and the following steps are carried out at high speed, i.e., at the maximum of 2,000 rpm. The precision of bone preparation is facilitated if the surgeon uses magnifying glasses. The ideal distance between two fixture sites is about one fixture diameter, or 3.5 mm. If available space between the mental foramina does not allow the installation of six fixtures with sufficient interfixtural spaces, it is better to install five or even four fixtures, optimally situated. Using fewer than four fixtures is not recommended. The marginal compact layer plus some of the underlying spongy bone is penetrated by the guide drill. This enables the surgeon to form an idea about the character of the bone tissue at hand, especially the thickness of the marginal compact layer.

With the help of a small spiral drill (Fig. 13-6b) the fixture site closest to the midline is prepared first. The direction of this site is established by carefully checking the direction in relation to the opposite jaw (Fig. 13-7). The site should be vertical in the mesiodistal plane. If the topography of the mandible in extremely resorbed cases allows it, the direction of the fixture sites should be chosen so as to avoid the later abutments piercing the mucosa adjacent to the floor of the mouth. A direction indicator is placed into the prepared site. The most distal site on the left (for a right-handed surgeon) is prepared next with the aid of the small twist drill and with parallelism in all levels with respect to the direction indicator placed near the midline (Fig. 13-8). A new direction indicator is placed in the left most distal site with its direction corresponding to the direction indicator placed close to the midline. Should this not be the case, the direction of the most distal site on the left side is adjusted until mutual parallelism is achieved. The direction indicator at the midline is then removed. The remaining sites are gradually prepared from left to right, with a small twist drill, and with respect to reciprocal parallelism. The direction indicators are installed step by step in the prepared sites.

With the aid of a pilot drill (Fig. 13-9a) and with successive removal of the direction indicators, the marginal part of the future fixture sites are now prepared from right to left keeping the previously chosen directions in sight. The preparations are made as deep as indicated by the markings on the pilot drill, or just through the marginal compact layer, depending on its thickness.

Direction indicators are once more inserted in a site close to the midline, after which the most distal site of the left side is prepared by means of a large twist drill (Fig. 13-9b) observing parallelism as shown by the indicator. The latter is then transferred to the new site and fitted into its thickest part. The diameter for a standard twist drill is 3.0 mm for normal bone, but for very hard bone one with a diameter of 3.15 mm should be used. On both the small and the large twist drills there are markings indicating suitable preparation depths for long fixtures and short fixtures. With very low mandible height, the base cortical bone can be intentionally penetrated as the surgeon's left forefinger is pressed from below against the skin. This facilitates precision in the penetration of the compact basal bone. The aim is to create subperiosteal space to be filled with blood with the least possible injury to the periosteum. The dissector may be used to detach the periosteum through the prepared site.

In case of profuse bleeding from marrow vessels, the direction indicator can be used as a temporary hemostatic device. With mutual parallelism, the remaining sites are thereafter prepared with a large twist drill from left to right (Fig. 13-10), and with respect to the position of the direction indicator. New direction indicators are inserted successively.

Working from right to left, the direction indicators are gradually removed and the thickness of the marginal cortical bone is checked with a dissector. The entry to the fixture site is then prepared with a marginal countersink (Fig. 13-11). Observe that the

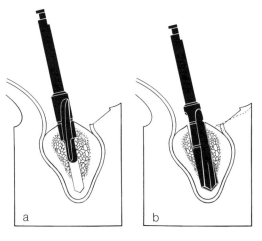

a

b

Fig. 13-9a   Pilot drill preparation.

Fig. 13-9b   Large twist drill preparation to final width of fixture site.

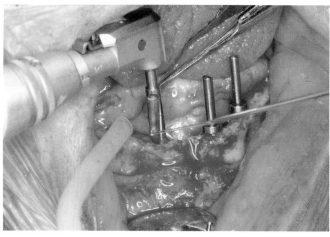

Fig. 13-10 Large twist drill preparation using direction indicators to achieve mutual parallelism.

shelf, created by the countersink, must remain within the marginal compact layer (Fig. 13-12). If possible, though, one should strive to achieve complete insertion of the cover screw. Corresponding height marking is given on the marginal countersink. If a short fixture is needed, a corresponding countersink must be used.

Drilling at low speed

The following steps, carried out at low speed (15-20 rpm), require a low-speed contra-angle handpiece. It is very important that those instruments used during low-speed preparation, i.e., tap, and fixture, are not touched with anything but titanium forceps. Profuse saline irrigation while using these instruments is imperative. The taps must be cleaned with a titanium needle before being used in the next fixture site so as to remove bone chips from the vertical outlets.

Starting on the left at the most distal site, the canal is threaded (Fig. 13-13) to a length corresponding with the length of the fixture.

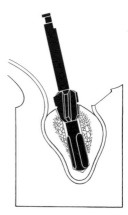

Fig. 13-11 Countersink preparation of the entrance of the fixture site.

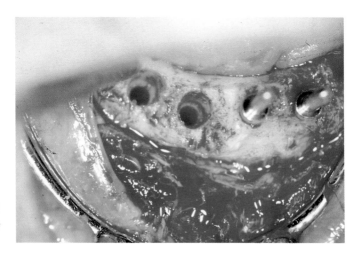

Fig. 13-12 Shelf in the marginal compact layer created by the countersink.

There is a mark for a short fixture on the standard tap. It is advantageous to check once again the direction and the relation to the inserted indicator close to the midline. The threaded profile in the bone should be checked visually (Fig. 13-14).

If the bone tissue in the prepared site does not bleed spontaneously, bleeding by carefully probing in the apical part of the site should be provoked with a titanium needle. The blood from the site must not be suctioned away, or flushed with saline. The first fixture is installed in the left distal site, paral-

leling the direction indicator at the midline. After negotiating the first threads, the fixture should be allowed to freely follow the pre-tapped preparation without undue force (Fig. 13-15). The fixture is primarily installed without irrigation until the horizontal canal of the fixture is well within the prepared site. This is done in order to avoid saline being pressed into the marrow compartments by the fixture. The remaining procedure of fixture installation is carried out under profuse irrigation. The fixture is mechanically driven into the bone until the engine of the hand-

219

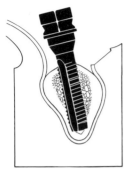

Fig. 13-13 Screw tap preparation.

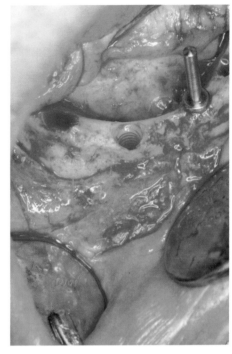

Fig. 13-14 Threaded site ready to receive a fixture.

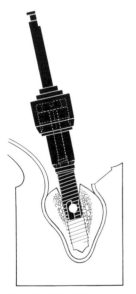

Fig. 13-15 Fixture under installation by a fixture mount and a handpiece connection.

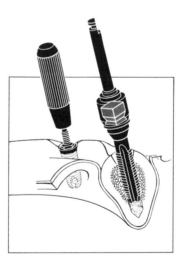

Fig. 13-16 Use of fixture direction indicator.

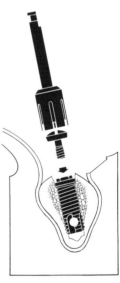

Fig. 13-17 Insertion of a cover screw.

piece stops, which often happens quite suddenly. If great resistance is encountered during fixture insertion, manual installation with a cylinder wrench may be performed after the fixture has become stable in the marginal threadings. The wrench is used under all circumstances to check the final tightening of the fixture in relation to the mechanical characteristics and the degree of vascularity of the specific fixture site. This is also done under profuse irrigation. It is important to maintain the previously achieved fixture installation direction by holding the thumb against the wrench and the forefinger around the jaw base. No cracking of the marginal compact bone should be allowed during use of the wrench. It is better to tighten too little than too much, since too hard a tightening may cause microfractures and destroy the entire thread profile.

The fixture mount is removed either mechanically with a screwdriver attached to the low-speed contra-angle handpiece, or manually with a screwdriver. In either situation, an open end wrench is used on the square part of the fixture mount to avoid torque force being transferred to the fixture itself.

When the screw of the fixture mount is unscrewed, it is extremely important to keep it stable with the open end wrench so that the fixture does not rotate in its site. Caution should also be observed in order not to loosen the fixture through a lever-arm effect. This is especially true if the fixture site consists of a thin layer of cortical bone, and of a loose marrow and cancellous bone tissue. The hexagonal fixture head is checked for possible damage from installation work.

The first inserted fixture is provided with a fixture direction indicator that can be screwed into its central canal (Fig. 13-16). Thereafter, the remaining sites are threaded and fixtures are successively installed respecting mutual parallelism.

The cover screws are applied to the fixtures with the help of the screw inserter (Fig. 13-17) in the handpiece. Final control tightening is performed manually with a screwdriver. The cover screw must be tight, but at the same time should be easily unscrewed.

Soft-tissue adaptation

The operation area is thoroughly irrigated and any sharp bone edges removed with forceps. Debris and cut bone, often found deeply beneath the lingual flap, should be eliminated.

The flap is replaced and sutured with 3/0 mattress sutures of polyamide, beginning at the midline (Fig. 13-18). Thereafter, suturing is performed from the distal border of the operation area towards the midline. It is important to catch the periosteum on the buccal side so that fixtures and cover screws are covered with periosteum (Fig. 13-19). The sutures are first inserted through the lingual flap, avoiding the cover screws so that the knots are placed on the remaining string of attached gingiva (Fig. 13-20). If the fixture is well embedded, the mucoperiosteum will rest on the jaw between the fixtures and not directly on the cover screws of the fixtures.

Postoperative measures

The patient rinses the mouth with sterile saline, is given 1 g of liquid paracetamol, and rinses the mouth again. The surgeon applies a roll of saline-moistened gauze over the operation area. Another gauze roll is applied, thick enough to just enter the maximally opened mouth of the patient (Fig. 13-21). If the roll is too thin the patient must actively compress the operation area, which could be strenuous. The postoperative compression is maintained for at least one hour, while the patient rests in the ward. The pa-

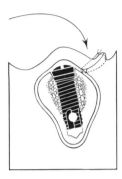

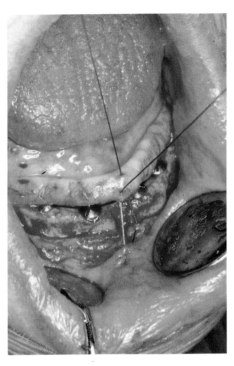

Fig. 13-18 Adaptation of the flap with vertical mattress sutures.

Fig. 13-19 Adaptation of the flap aiming at full periosteal covering of the cover screws.

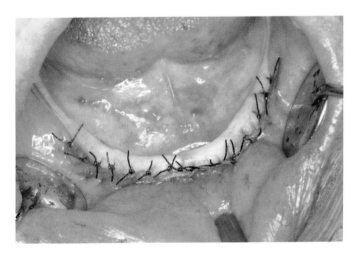

Fig. 13-20 Operation field after readaptation of the flap.

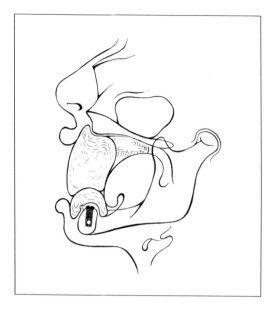

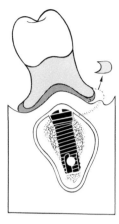

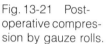

Fig. 13-21 Post-operative compression by gauze rolls.

Fig. 13-22 Adjusted and relined denture during healing of fixture sites.

tient is restricted from wearing the lower denture for the first two postoperative weeks. A prescription containing phenoxymethylpenicillin for 10 days (2 g × 2), analgesics (paracetamol 500 g and codeine 30 mg, 2 tablets × 3), and saline solution for mouth rinses are given to the patient.

Postoperative management

The day after the operation, the patient is checked for postoperative problems, as well as the extent of any edema or hematoma. Usually a glassy edema is found in the floor of the mouth with minor hematoma along the submandibular ducts. Sometimes the patient has a moderately swollen chin. Most of the time the patient only experiences minor postoperative pain for a few hours. The majority of patients sleep well on the night after the operation with no pain whatsoever. Minor paresthesia symptoms may temporarily occur in the lower lip. The operation site is checked for flap defects, cutting sutures, or other forms of wound dehiscences. The wound is cleaned only with saline, and where necessary resuturing is performed.

The sutures are removed on the seventh day after the operation, and the operation area is cleaned with 1.5% hydrogen-peroxide solution in saline. The operation area is again checked to ensure complete soft-tissue coverage of all fixtures. Should this not be the case a fresh flap must be raised and sutured completely to cover the fixture. It is

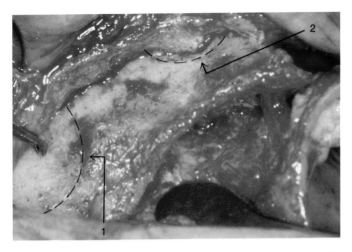

Fig. 13-23a Operation area showing anterior border of maxillary sinus *(1)* and lower border of piriform aperture *(2)*.

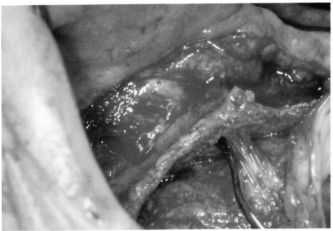

Fig. 13-23b Exploration of incisive canal with a dissector.

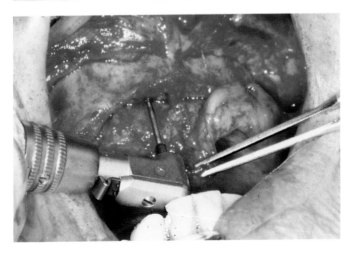

Fig. 13-23c Guide drill preparation starting palatally to the resected margin of the bone. The stretched neurovascular bundle from the incisive canal and the buccal concavity in the lateral incisor region are clearly visible.

extremely important that all suture material be removed, as suture remnants may have a deleterious effect on the prognosis of the fixture in question.

After the second postoperative week the denture is returned to the patient. It is first relieved excessively and relined with a tissue-conditioning material in the operation area (Fig. 13-22).

About four weeks after the operation either permanent relining may be performed with acrylic resin, or the temporary lining may be changed every three to four weeks.

Five weeks postoperatively the mucosa in the operation area is checked once more by the surgeon for possible minor perforations. Even a perforation the size of a pin can interfere with the desired osseointegration. Further checking of the mucosa may be appropriate at a later time.

Healing time after fixture installation in mandibles should never be less than three months, and it is strongly recommended that the surgeon—for all later references—draw a detailed operation chart from both transverse and profile aspects immediately after the operation. This will identify the positions of the fixtures in relation to neighboring anatomical structures.

Surgical technique in maxillae

Only deviations from the surgical technique as recommended for mandibles will be described.

Anatomical aspects

The maxilla differs from the mandible mainly with regard to the following anatomical factors:

1. Lack of a defined cortical shell
2. Inferior mechanical resistance
3. Often small vertical and horizontal dimensions

4. Sometimes wide nasal cavities
5. Not infrequently, anteriorly and inferiorly expanded maxillary sinuses

Taken together, the above factors make fixture installation in upper jaws more difficult and a greater challenge for the surgeon.

Anesthesia

Local infiltration anesthesia is given from the first molar on one side to the first molar on the other side. On the palatal side block anesthesia is given for the palatal nerves and for the nasopalatal nerve. It is advisable to make the infiltration anesthesia buccally up to the region of the infraorbital nerves. Altogether about 10 ml 2% lidocaine-adrenaline solution is given (1:80,000). It is also recommended to use tetracaine solution, applied topically on the anterior lower nasal mucosa.

Soft-tissue reflection

A horizontal incision is made in the depth of the buccal sulcus from the first molar on one side to the first molar on the other side. A palatally pedicled flap is raised, sufficiently detached from the incisive canal content and from the palatal osseous surface to get a full view from below of the residual alveolar process. After exposure of the bone, it is important to establish its topography properly. Special care should be taken to define the anterior borders of the maxillary sinuses and the lower borders of the piriform aperture (Fig. 13-23a). Possible lateral expansions of the incisive canal should be explored, preferably with a dissector (Fig. 13-23b). Possible buccal concavities in the lateral incisor regions should also be noted. By this exposure the width and topography of the canine strut can be established. The positions and number of fixtures are now chosen. Six fixtures is the recommended

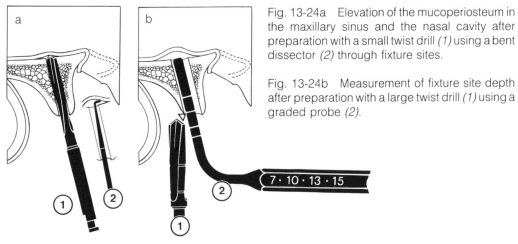

Fig. 13-24a   Elevation of the mucoperiosteum in the maxillary sinus and the nasal cavity after preparation with a small twist drill *(1)* using a bent dissector *(2)* through fixture sites.

Fig. 13-24b   Measurement of fixture site depth after preparation with a large twist drill *(1)* using a graded probe *(2)*.

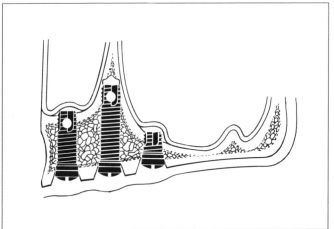

Fig. 13-25 Fixtures of various lengths adapted to different available bone topography.

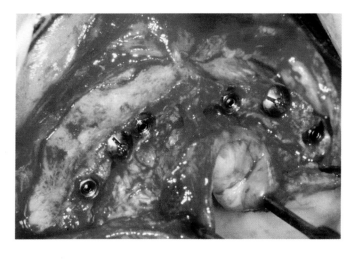

Fig. 13-26 Fixtures installed and supplied with either cover screws or pacemaker screws.

number. Due to the frequent lack of bone in upper jaws, however, it is better to install a smaller number, but never less than four fixtures. Fixture sites encroaching upon the incisive canal or the median suture should be avoided, as fixtures in such positions do not generally become osseointegrated.

Drilling at high speed

The preparation with the guide drill should generally start on the palatal aspect of the residual alveolar process (Fig. 13-23c). This is especially important in cases with a thin horizontal width in order to avoid later buccal perforations with wider drills.

When using the small and large twist drills, the compact layer toward the maxillary sinuses or the nasal cavities is deliberately perforated to avoid possible perforations of the mucoperiosteum in these cavities. The perforation of this compact layer is performed in order to have the fixture stabilized in a bone of sufficient mechanical strength. At the start of the preparation with the large twist drill, a change in direction can be made, if required, in order to avoid possible buccal perforations. Such a perforation, however, is not deleterious as long as full periosteal cover can be obtained.

The mucoperiosteum in the floor of the nasal cavity or in the maxillary sinuses is elevated through the preparations (Fig.13-24a) by use of a bent dissector to create a subperiosteal coagulum, which may later contribute to new bone formation. This new bone can support the apical end of the fixture. If sufficient bone volume is at hand the use of a longer large twist drill should be considered to create sites for later installation of long fixtures. Such long twist drills can generally be inserted into the canine struts. Fixtures of standard length (10 mm) are preferably used in other sites. Sometimes the bone volume in distal areas of the operation field, especially below the anterior recesses of the maxillary sinuses, allows only the installation of short fixtures (7.0 mm) (Fig. 13-25). The fixture lengths should be chosen according to measurements with the graded titanium explorer (Fig. 13-24b).

Any unnecessary countersinking should be avoided in order to save as much bone height as possible. The preparation of fixture sites should be made in such a manner as to avoid as much as possible any protrusion of fixtures or cover screws below the alveolar crest.

Drilling at low speed

In the case of soft maxillary bone only the coronal half of the fixture site should be threaded as the apical part of the fixture is self-tapping. It should be allowed to work its own way into the remaining part of the site. Generally, a lower torque force is required for the installation of maxillary fixtures both by engine and by manual tightening. When removing the fixture mounts care should be taken not to rotate the fixtures in the soft bone.

Depending on the depths of installation and to avoid unnecessary protrusion, the surgeon should choose between ordinary cover screws or pacemaker screws (Fig. 13-26).

Soft-tissue adaptation

Because the residual alveolar process in upper jaws is very thin in many cases, a rounded resection to a level just coronal to the cover screws is advisable before the flap is readapted.

Postoperative management

In cases where it has not been possible to fully embed the fixtures and/or the cover screws, it is of utmost importance that the surgeon informs the prosthodontist so that

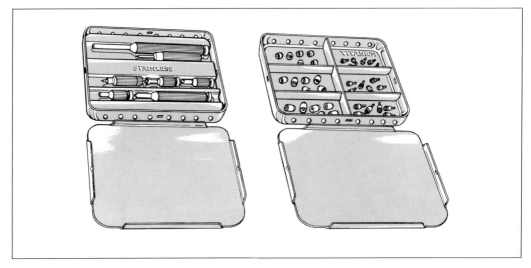

Fig. 13-27   Set of instruments for abutment preparation.

proper relief of the denture can be made over these fixture sites.

Healing time for upper jaws should never be less than six months so that the soft maxillary bone develops sufficient mechanical strength to cope with future occlusal load.

Abutment connection

In general, the surgical technique for abutment connection is the same for both jaws.

Preoperative care

The buccal and lingual mucosa in the operation area is infiltrated with about 5 ml 2% lidocaine-adrenaline solution (1:80,000).

The patient is cleaned extraorally and intraorally as for the fixture operation with 0.1% chlorhexidine solution and is dressed as for an ordinary oral surgical operation; the in-struments are laid out accordingly (Fig. 13-27).

Operation technique

The surgeon's diagram on the operation chart combined with palpation and probing (Fig. 13-28a) enable identification of the position of the cover screws. These will then appear as a number of bleeding points in the overlying gingival tissue.

Separate incisions, 0.5 cm long (Fig. 13-28b), or one continuous crestal incision, are made in the gingiva and slightly widened with dissectors (Fig. 13-28c). The incision is preferably made in the remaining attached gingiva, but within the cover screw's periphery. It is widened to half the diameter width of a fixture, after which the punch is inserted with its guide peg into the central hole of the cover screw (Fig. 13-28d). It is then pressed down to cut through the mucosa above the cover screw. Whenever pos-

228

Figs. 13-28a to f   Principal steps
at abutment connection.

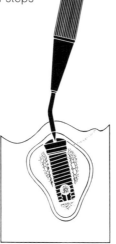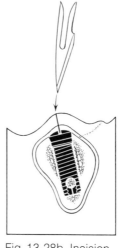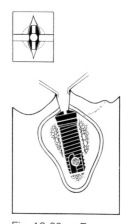

Fig. 13-28a
Relocation of cover
screw.

Fig. 13-28b Incision.

Fig. 13-28c   Expo-
sure of cover screw.

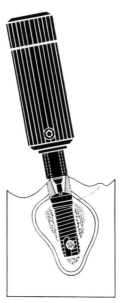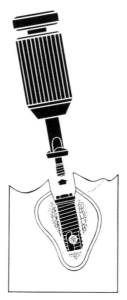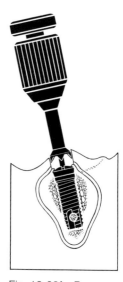

Fig. 13-28d
Punching.

Fig. 13-28e
Removal of cover
screw.

Fig. 13-28f   Remov-
al of osseous over-
growth with a cover-
screw mill.

229

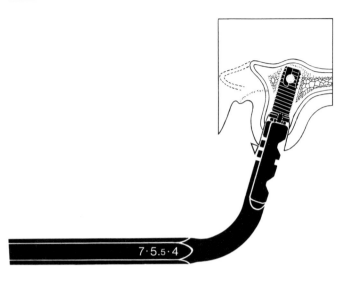

7·5.5·4

Fig. 13-29 Graded abutment probe.

sible, the openings for the abutments should be placed within attached mucosa in order to create a tight mucosal cuff around the abutments. The width of the residual attached gingiva is occasionally too narrow, or its localization is not compatible with the direction of the fixtures. In these cases the openings have to be placed in movable mucosa. This does not appear to impair the long-term prognosis of the mucoperiosteal barrier as long as oral hygiene is kept at a high level. In extremely resorbed jaws, the surgeon should avoid any incisions in the thin, fragile mucosa in the floor of the mouth. When this is unavoidable, attached gingiva should be transpositioned to protect this easily ulcerated mucosa, if this is surgically feasible.

The cover screws are removed with a screwdriver (Fig. 13-28e) and forceps. In some situations bone may have grown over the cover screws and can usually be removed by a hand instrument or by the punch. If bone overgrowth is more extensive a cover-screw mill (Fig. 13-28f) or, in extreme cases, a conventional round burr may be used.

Quite often a thin layer of connective tissue grows in between the cover screw and the fixture. This layer is again removed by punching against the upper part of the fixture. The guiding peg centers the punch in relation to the fixture. It is extremely important that all tissue found between cover screw and fixture be carefully removed so that the horizontal plate that surrounds the hexagonal upper part of the fixture is totally free from tissues. If not, tissue remnants may prevent a correct adaptation of the abutment to the fixture. Furthermore, the prepared gingival canal should be checked for any hard or soft tissue protuberances that could prevent correct placement of the abutment. If there is any doubt, the abutment entry should be cleaned manually with the punch or the cover-screw mill.

An abutment of suitable length is then chosen using the graded abutment probe (Fig. 13-29). Three different lengths of abutments are available. The top border of the abutment cylinder should be placed about 2 mm above the gingiva in lower jaws, and 1 mm coronal to it in upper jaws. Due to the usually mobile mucosa in the region of the mental

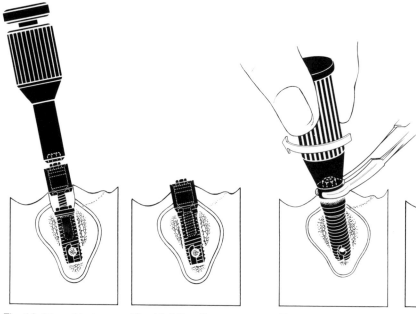

Fig. 13-30a Abutment assembly to be installed into the fixture.

Fig. 13-30b Correct position of the abutment cylinder grasping the head of the fixture.

Fig. 13-30c Final tightening of the abutment to the fixture. Possible torque of the fixture is prevented by use of the clamp instrument.

Fig. 13-30d Healing cap applied to the abutment as retention for surgical pack.

foramina use of longer abutments in these areas is recommended. In cases of considerable vertical height of the soft tissues at the fixture site, surgical reduction of the mucosa should be performed.

While the assisting nurse stretches the incision area and cleans out the abutment canal via the suction tube the abutment is installed by the surgeon. The complete abutment is preferably held with the hexagon screwdriver (Fig. 13-30a) and with a finger placed against the abutment cylinder. The abutment screw must never be forced into the fixture because of the softness of titanium. The surgeon should visually check the cor-

rect installation direction before the abutment screw is entered into the fixture.

The abutment screw is rotated until the abutment cylinder just reaches contact with the hexagonal fixture head. It is then unscrewed slightly and checked to ensure that the abutment cylinder can rotate freely. With the aid of an abutment clamp, the abutment cylinder is slightly rotated and, at the same time, pressed in an apical direction. This maneuver will enable the abutment cylinder to grasp the hexagonal head of the fixture. It then jumps onto the fixture and the abutment screw can be further tightened (Fig. 13-30b). Finally, the abutment screw is forceful-

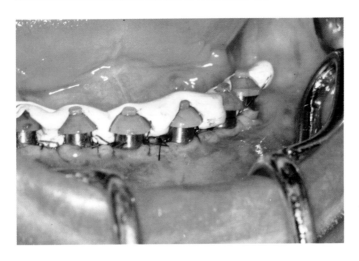

Fig. 13-31 All abutments provided with healing caps and the application of the surgical pack started lingually.

ly tightened with the hexagon screwdriver (Fig. 13-30c).

Holding the dissector lightly between two fingers, about 3 cm from its thinnest part, the abutment is tapped lightly. If the fixture is osseointegrated a high-pitched metallic sound will be heard. The remaining abutments are tapped in the same way. The abutment fixture assemblies should also be gently checked for stability, especially with regard to possible rotational movements.

The gingiva between the abutments is approximated with 3/0 or 4/0 polyamide sutures aiming at very close adaptation of the edges. Healing caps are screwed on to the abutments (Fig. 13-30d). If the abutments are placed very close together, the caps may have to be reduced with the bone forceps. Hard mixed surgical pack is applied between and over the healing caps and the gingiva (Fig. 13-31). The healing caps may even be used to directly compress the gingiva into place.

The patient is referred for a radiographic checkup of the abutment fixture connection through an orthopantomogram. No space should be accepted between the fixture and the abutment cylinder in the radiograph.

Postoperative checkups

Healing caps, pack, and sutures are removed after one week and the operation field is cleaned with 1% hydrogen-peroxide solution in saline. The healing caps and the surgical pack should be replaced and maintained during the early prosthodontic phase of treatment. After the first postoperative week, rinses with 0.1% chlorhexidine is prescribed (10 ml × 2 per day).

Patients with uncomplicated abutment connection through wide attached gingiva can have prosthodontic treatment started 10 days postoperatively. Other patients will require two weeks of gingival healing.

Chapter 14

Complications

Ulf Lekholm, Ragnar Adell, and Per-Ingvar Brånemark

The gentle surgical technique used in the osseointegration method will rarely induce complications.[1]

Adjacent structures

Complaints of persisting paresthesia or anesthesia in adjacent nerves have not occurred. Neither have penetrations of the maxillary sinus and nasal cavities provoked any adverse reactions. Allergic reactions related to the installation of titanium components have not been observed in either short- or long-term follow-up studies.

Complications related to fixture installation and primary healing period

Mobile fixtures

If the surgeon misjudges the jawbone anatomy or the mechanical properties of the local fixture site, or if the drilling procedure is not precise enough, the fixture site may turn out not to be congruent with the fixture. The fixture is then primarily unstable and this prevents osseointegration. Adequate treatment depends on installation of a long fixture, which reaches the basal compact layer of bone (Fig. 14-1). Provided favorable mechanical bone characteristics exist (shape/quality, C/2-3, according to jaw classification in chapter 12) and the threadings have been destroyed, fixtures of standard length but with increased diameter may also be used.

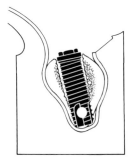

Fig. 14-1   When the standard fixture becomes mobile already at installation it should be replaced by a longer fixture. The site must be prepared deeper and retapped, reaching the basal compact layer of the jaw.

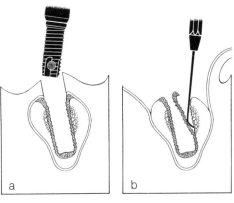

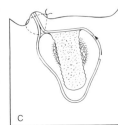

Figs. 14-2a to c   Treatment steps at a nonosseointegrated fixture.

Fig. 14-2a   Removal of the fixture.

Fig. 14-2b   Curettage of the fixture site to remove all nonmineralized connective tissue lining.

Fig. 14-2c   Closing of the site by a flap procedure.

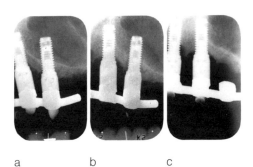

a   b   c

Figs. 14-3a to c   Series of radiograms.

Fig. 14-3a   Status at bridge connection.

Fig. 14-3b   Perifixtural radiolucent zone one year later.

Fig. 14-3c   Status one year after removal of the nonosseointegrated fixture. Observe the adjacent osseointegrated fixture.

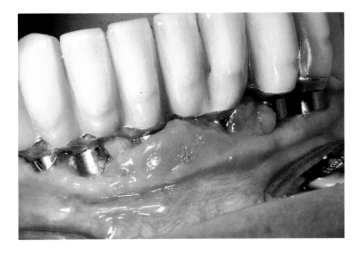

Fig. 14-4   Gingival hyperplasia due to too short abutments.

Mucosal perforation

Communication between the fixture and the oral cavity during the postfixture installation healing phase may be caused by defective flap adaptation, suture remnant granulomas, and/or decubital ulcer beneath the denture. Such perforations occurred in less than 5% of the treated patients.[1] Defective flap adaptation due to inadequate suturing should be treated during the follow-up visit the day after the fixture installation. Any communication with the oral cavity during the first six postoperative weeks should be treated by excision of the perforation site, flap mobilization, re-suturing, and proper adjustment of the denture. Later perforations are treated only by relief of the denture. If suture remnants are the cause of perforation they should be removed.

Complications related to abutment connection

Initial loss of anchorage function

At the abutment connection operations mobile fixtures are found infrequently. About half the number of recorded fixture losses occurred as initial loss of anchorage function.[1] The reasons for such a complication may be inadequate surgical technique or overloading during the healing stage by the denture. A nonosseointegrated fixture should be removed immediately (Fig. 14-2a). Usually, it cannot be extracted in an axial direction but must be rotated out with a pair of tongs. It is often advantageous if an abutment is mounted beforehand to provide better grip for the extraction instrument. All connective tissue of the fixture site must be removed (Fig. 14-2b), after which a mucoperiosteal flap is mobilized to close the site tightly (Fig. 14-2c). After a healing

period of about one year, the same site can be reused for another fixture installation.

Complications related to follow-up checks

Late loss of anchorage function

The remaining half of the fixture losses appeared as a late loss of anchorage function.[1] They are not usually associated with any subjective or clinical symptoms, but are revealed through the regular radiographic examinations as a thin perifixtural radiolucent area (Figs. 14-3a to c). The reason for this complication may be either a late symptom of surgical mishandling of the host tissues or an indication of subsequent traumatic stress concentration from an ill-fitting or improperly designed bridge. The treatment is the same as previously given (see Figs. 14-2a to c). Following loss of single fixtures, the patient generally can still wear the bridge on the remaining fixtures, possibly with shortened cantilevers.

Gingivitis

Marginal plaque-induced gingivitis should be treated by means of intensified oral hygiene. The access to the abutments, however, should also be checked and adjusted, if necessary. In a well-controlled material 80% of the abutments were found to be surrounded by clinically healthy gingiva.[2]

Hyperplasia formation

Gingival hyperplasia (Fig. 14-4) may be caused by the choice of too short abutments

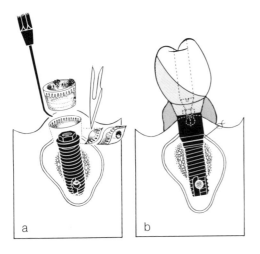

Figs. 14-5a and b Treatment steps at gingival hyperplasia and fistula.

Fig. 14-5a Excision of hyperplasia and fistula after removal of the abutment.

Fig. 14-5b Reduction of the gingival height and readaption of the abutment. The bridge is used as carrier for the surgical pack during the postoperative healing period.

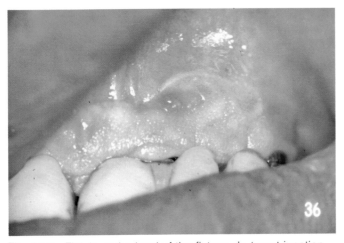

Fig. 14-6 Fistula at the level of the fixture-abutment junction.

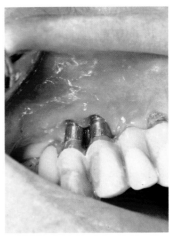

Fig. 14-7 Exposed buccal fixture threads causing traumatic ulceration and edema formation in the surrounding soft tissues.

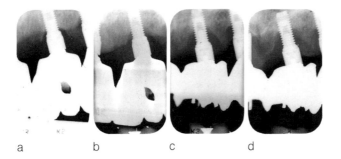

Figs. 14-8a to d Series of radiograms showing advancing marginal bone loss around a fixture, indicating stress concentrations in the bridge-abutment junction, which resulted in an abutment screw fracture.

or the omitting of healing caps and surgical pack during the first weeks after abutment connection. The mucosa then has a tendency to proliferate and cover the junction between abutment and bridge framework, which causes a traumatic ulceration. The frequency of this complication was about 7%.[1] Adequate treatment (Figs. 14-5a and b) is a gingivectomy or a flap procedure, and a change to a longer abutment should also be considered.

Fistulae

An untightened abutment screw with mobility of the abutment cylinder may cause the formation of granulation tissue at the abutment-fixture connection. Microorganisms may penetrate the capillary space around the mobile abutment screw with establishment of an infection in the granulation tissue at the level of the fixture-abutment junction. This may then propagate horizontally and appear as a fistula (Fig. 14-6) at the same level. The frequency of occurrence was less than 1%.[1] The treatment (see Figs. 14-5a and b) should, of course, include tightening of the abutment screw; however, the entire abutment should first be removed and sterilized and the granulation tissue excised. At the replacement of the abutment the proper sealing of the silicone ring should be checked.

Exposed threads

Exposed fixture threads (Fig. 14-7) due to marginal horizontal bone loss may cause traumatic ulceration of the soft tissues, especially if the unattached mucosa is susceptible to adjacent muscle pull. The associated presence of plaque in the depth of the threads may cause chronic inflammation, although the frequency encountered

was less than 1%.[1] This complication should not be overlooked and may be prevented by initially installing the fixtures deep enough, and by proper oral hygiene procedures. Treatment consists of conventional periodontal measures to create attached gingiva, i.e., free mucosal or skin grafts or a vestibuloplasty.

Fracture of abutment screw

Fractures of abutment screws that occur separately are usually asymptomatic and are seldom evident at roentgenographic examination (Figs. 14-8a to d). Consequently, they are only observed when a bridge is removed. This complication occurred in less than 3% of the screws used.[1]

If an abutment screw has fractured so that the remaining fragment is somewhat coronal to the fixture hexagonal head, the fragment can often be gripped with very narrow flat tongs and rotated out of the fixture. If the abutment screw has fractured level with the fixture head, or farther apically in the internal canal of the fixture (Fig. 14-9), a groove is cut in the abutment screw fragment using the smallest possible drill (2/0). A screwdriver, corresponding in size with the groove, is then used to rotate the abutment screw fragment out of the fixture.

After the abutment screw and the corresponding cylinder have been replaced, the reason for the fracture should be thoroughly investigated. One common cause is an incorrectly fitting bridge. Consequently, efforts should be taken to properly adjust the bridge or fabricate a new one.

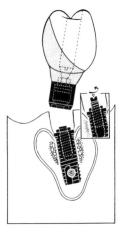

Fig. 14-9 Treatment steps at an abutment screw fracture. The apical fragment of the fractured screw is removed and a new abutment screw is applied. The fitting of the bridge must be adjusted.

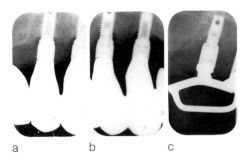

a   b   c

Figs. 14-10a to c   Series of radiograms.

Fig. 14-10a The condition two years after bridge connection.

Fig. 14-10b Status three years later, i.e., five years after bridge connection, with a fixture fracture and marginal bone loss.

Fig. 14-10c The repaired fixture supporting a new bridge.

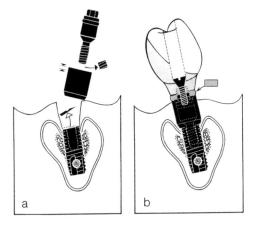

Figs. 14-11a and b   Treatment steps at fixture fracture.

Fig. 14-11a The abutment is removed. The coronal surface of the remaining part of the fixture is ground plain and a longer abutment cylinder is attached after its abutment screw has been shortened to fit the internal canal of the remaining apical fixture fragment.

Fig. 14-11b The abutment cylinder is connected to the fixture without being locked by any hexagonal head of the fixture. The fitting of the bridge is temporarily adjusted by self-curing acrylic resin.

Fracture of the fixture

Fixture fractures are mainly diagnosed at follow-up radiographic examinations (Figs. 14-10a to c) as a rapid marginal bone loss. Progressive marginal bone loss should always be considered an indication of undue stress concentration (see Figs. 14-8a to d), which eventually results in fixture fractures. Regular radiographic checkups during the first years after bridge connection and early treatment at the first sign(s) of marginal bone loss are recommended measures. A recent fracture of the fixture may be very difficult to determine radiographically, with the only sign being a rapid marginal bone loss. In all such cases it is advisable to unscrew the bridge and check the individual stability of each abutment fixture unit after the abutment screws have been tightened. Fixture fractures have been related to inadequately designed bridges and have occurred in about 3% of the patients studied.[1] With the recommended bridge techniques the frequency of these complications is expected to disappear.

Transverse horizontal fixture fractures, which occur apically to the internal threadings of the fixture, can only be treated by removal of both the coronal and the apical fixture fragment, the latter removed using a trephine bur. If necessary, the same site can be reused for another fixture installation at a later date following adequate healing. If the transverse fracture has occurred coronally to the apical end of the internal canal, the apical fixture fragment can still be used as a bridge support.

When such a problem is diagnosed, immediate treatment (Figs. 14-11a and b) is recommended by removal of the bridge, the abutment, and the coronal fixture fragment. With the aid of a small diamond cutter the coronal fracture surface of the apical fixture fragment is ground plain under profuse irrigation with saline. It is often necessary to expose the area by a flap or by punching out gingiva. Any perifixtural granulation tissue should be removed with a dissector, and a new longer abutment, which does not interfere with the bridge, should then be attached. It is, however, first necessary to shorten the abutment screw with a diamond cutter so that its length fits the remaining threads of the apical fixture fragment. The new abutment with its shortened screw is tightened without the use of a wrench against the fixture fragment, which now lacks an upper hexagonal head. After the abutment screw has been tightened, it should be checked carefully to ensure that the abutment cylinder cannot be rotated or moved in a vertical direction. A radiographic check (see Fig. 14-10c) of the junction between the abutment and the adjusted coronal fixture surface should be made. After adapting the mucosa to the new abutment, the bridge should then be reattached. The distance between the old bridge and the new abutment can be corrected temporarily with a layer of acrylic resin. Depending on the number of fractured fixtures and their locations a new bridge or a repair should always be considered.

The measures above must be taken immediately after the abutment has been removed or else gingival tissues will proliferate within a few days to almost completely cover the entrance to the fixture. Surgery is then needed to create access to the fixture; punching a canal through the covering gingiva or raising a flap are the recommended procedures.

References

1. *Adell, R., et al.*
   A 15-year study of osseointegrated implants in the treatment of the edentulous jaw. Int. J. Oral Surg. 10:387, 1981.

2. *Adell, R., et al.*
   Marginal tissue reactions at osseointegrated titanium fixtures. I. A three-year longitudinal prospective study. Int. J. Oral Surg. 1985 (in press).

Chapter 15

Prosthodontic Procedures

George A. Zarb and Tomas Jansson

Introduction

Over the years several diverse methods for the prosthodontic treatment of edentulous patients have evolved. These methods reflect a deep commitment to clinical excellence and optimal patient care. Collectively, these methods are an outgrowth of technical procedures as applied to a biologic appreciation of a compromised intraoral environment. The nature of the biomechanical compromise implied by edentulism is discussed in chapter 2.

Dentists, and prosthodontists in particular, have demonstrated considerable skill and versatility in their efforts to compensate for their patients' tooth losses. In other words, the dentist's challenge in prosthodontics has always been one of how best to cope with a depleted method of tooth attachment or a reduced area of periodontal ligament support. The search for a substitute attachment mechanism has led to the osseointegration method, which dramatically improves clinicians' clinical ability to *cure* patients rather than to merely *treat* them. This clearly offers a subtle but profound difference in the prognosis of prosthetic restorations, one which precludes the many adverse sequelae associated with edentulism. The challenge for the next several years is clearly going to be one of how to reconcile prosthodontics' enormous range of clinical and technical methodology with the advent and availability of techniques for achieving tissue-integrated tooth root analogues.

In this chapter the way in which time-proven standard clinical prosthodontic procedures have been adapted to the patient who now presents with several analogous tooth abutments protruding into the oral cavity (Figs. 15-1a to f) will be described.

Prosthodontic care for the patient is an integral part of the total treatment sequence as indicated in Table 15-1. Such care consists of early, or preliminary, and final treatment programs.

Table 15-1   Proposed flow chart outlining sequence of treatment

---

1. Patient examination by prosthodontist
   History, examination, radiographic evaluation
2. Patient examination by oral surgeon
3. Fixture operation(s)
   Healing period:
      3-month minimum for the mandible
      6-month minimum for the maxilla
   Prosthodontic maintenance
4. Abutment operation
   1 week later: change of surgical pack, preliminary impressions
   Weekly change of pack for 2 to 3 weeks
   Prosthodontic maintenance
5. Routine prosthodontic clinical/laboratory protocol
6. Patient recalls and maintenance program

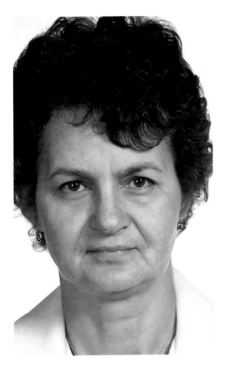

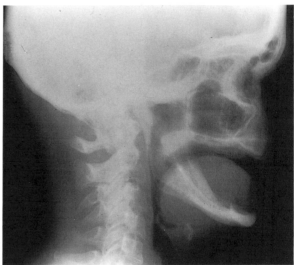

Figs. 15-1a and b   A middle-aged patient with advanced residual ridge resorption and a chronic inability to wear a complete lower denture typifies the prosthodontic aspects of osseointegration therapy.

Early, or preliminary, prosthodontic care

Experimental evidence and clinical experience indicate that a healing period of four to six months must be prescribed between the fixture and abutment operations. While a four-month healing period appears adequate for the mandible, a longer period is necessary for the maxilla. This period of waiting is usually uneventful, although tedious for the patient. However, it is essential if osseointegration is to take place, and every effort must be made to combine the objectives of undisturbed healing with clinical support for the patient. These objectives are achieved by (1) patient education regarding diet (quality and consistency), (2) care of oral tissues by means of good hygiene, gen-

tle massage, and frequent tissue rest, and (3) maintenance of function and cosmetic support. The latter is ensured by patient wear of a previous or an interim prosthesis. It is clear that a patient cannot simply give up wearing a denture while osseointegration is occurring. Some degree of function (even if the patient could not tolerate a removable prosthesis) and cosmetic support for the circumoral and facial tissues must be maintained. These short-term objectives are easily met by regular placement of a substantial thickness of tissue conditioner inside a liberally relieved prosthesis. The frequency of this procedure is important, not only because it ensures a soft and resilient stress reduction system overlying the operated sites, but also because it provides the prosthodontist with an opportunity to monitor the healing phase. The occurrence

Figs. 15-1c to e   The titanium tooth root analogues are fitted with a type of metallic framework (see Table 15-3) to which prosthetic teeth are added.

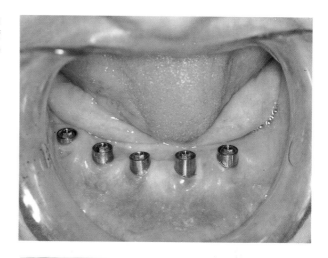

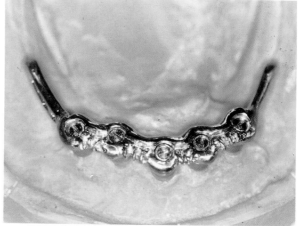

Fig. 15-1f *(below)*   Function and cosmetics are successfully restored.

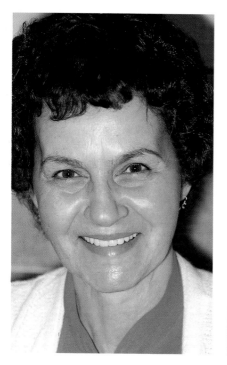

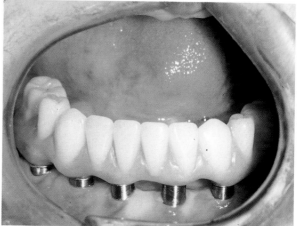

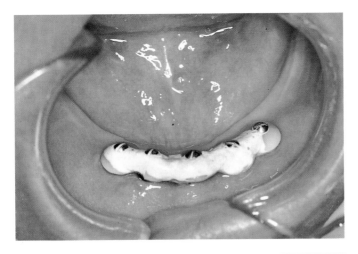

Fig. 15-2a Surgical pack is in place.

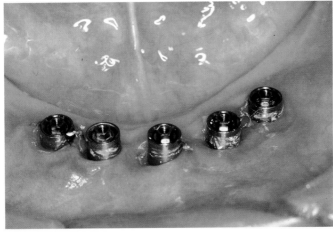

Fig. 15-2b Healing caps are removed to demonstrate progressive epithelial healing response at one week following the second surgical procedure.

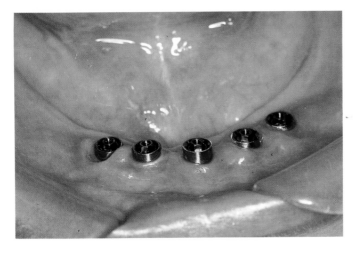

Fig. 15-2c At two weeks.

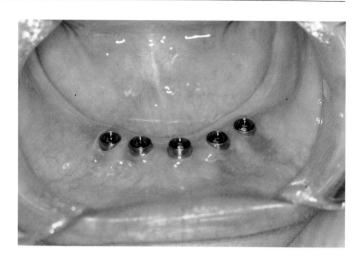

Fig. 15-2d At four weeks.

of complications during this stage is of course infrequent, and usually takes the form of a mucosal perforation which results from a defective flap adaptation, suture remnant granulomas, and/or a decubital ulceration (see chapter 14). The latter is the most frequent culprit and can be avoided by ensuring nonbrittle or rough-edge development from the lining resin; it is treated by correct denture adjustment. Any ulceration that occurs during the first six weeks after the fixture operation is treated by the oral surgeon by excision of the perforated site, and a minor soft-tissue flap procedure, along with the inevitable denture base relief. Following the abutment operation, the objective is to undertake and complete final prosthodontic treatment as quickly as possible. The only limitations to such an approach are the three- to four-week time period required for healing of the epithelial sites, patient comfort and availability, and the prosthodontist's office logistics. One week postoperatively, healing caps, surgical pack, and sutures are removed (Figs. 15-2a to d). This is a good time for preliminary impressions using a stock tray with a soft wax periphery and an irreversible hy-

drocolloid material. A fresh surgical pack is placed; care is taken to avoid hardened packs forming rough or sharp edges which might cause irritation. A routine procedure is followed at each subsequent appointment until the final prosthesis is inserted (Table 15-2). The healing caps are replaced and sometimes modified since fixture alignment and/or location may create a source of mucosal irritation when the standard healing cap is in place. Sometimes the location of a particular healing cap abuts onto the surrounding tissue quite adequately. A surgical pack will not be required in this location.

Although the healing gingival tissues are usually somewhat sore in the early postabutment exposure period, patients are encouraged to initiate a home care program which will become more aggressive as the tissues become firmer. The program (Fig. 15-3) consists of tissue massage (toothbrush and/or interproximal brush, rubber tip, frequent salt rinses) and impeccable cleanliness of the abutments (super floss, pipe cleaner, or gauze). At the second or third appointment (depending upon the progress of gingival healing) a final impression and preliminary jaw records are made. This can be used for

Table 15-2 Routine procedures for prosthodontic patient care

First postoperative (abutment) appointment	Removal of healing caps Pack removal Suture removal Tissue debridement with 0.1% H_2O_2 in saline Abutment cylinder tightening Preliminary impression Placement of a fresh pack ± adjustment of healing caps Prescription of rinses
Second appointment (5-10 days later)	Removal of healing caps and pack Abutment cylinder tightening Final impression
Third appointment, if needed (7-10 days later)	Preliminary centric relation record (elective) Patient instruction in home care procedures New surgical pack and final impression made if gingival response not optimal
Subsequent appointments	Routine final prosthodontic treatment program Abutment cylinder tightening Insertion of interim prosthesis (elective) Modification of old prosthesis Home care procedures

fabrication of a temporary all-resin prosthesis, or else it is sometimes possible to substantially relieve the patient's prior prosthesis and use it as an interim prosthesis. An infrequent occurrence during this phase of treatment is chronic epithelial irritation associated with one or more fixtures. This is due to *(1)* unfavorable fixture alignment—too far facially or lingually, or *(2)* failure to provide an abutment of adequate height. Both situations may encourage tongue, lip, or cheek rubbing against the abutment's edge. An abbreviated transfer

coping or a gold alloy cylinder may be used to avoid the irritation. Subsequent bridge design may avoid the problem, or else the fixture may not be used in the final design and simply "put to sleep" or ignored. In such a situation the coping or transepithelial sleeve is removed, the fixture is sealed via a screw cap, and the area is covered by a soft-tissue flap. This submerged fixture can always be employed should the need arise in the future.

Preprosthetic analysis

Before the final prosthodontic phase of care is undertaken, a careful reassessment of the patient's preoperative prosthetic status must be reconciled with a new postsurgical one. Some rather important points have to be kept in mind during this overall assessment. Osseointegrated fixtures can to a large extent be considered worthy substitutes for natural tooth abutments. But they differ in the nature of their attachment, in the number employed, and, very frequently, in their location, as well as in their cosmetic and mechanical considerations. Furthermore, if a fixture fails to integrate, or else loses its integration after a number of years, this can be remedied easily by removing it, waiting for healing to occur, and drilling a new host bone site. These clinical facts suggest a need for bridge design which must take all these factors into account.

Nature of attachment and number of fixtures

The interfacial response elicited by osseointegration is a reasonable substitute for the periodontal ligament. It also appears to be a very reliable one, although the relative resistance to diverse loads of both the natural

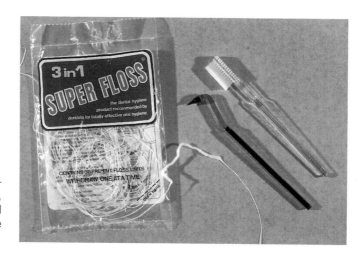

Fig. 15-3 A home care kit comprises a toothbrush, a rubber tip, and a material such as dental floss for wiping and polishing the titanium abutments.

tooth and an osseointegrated fixture are still being investigated. Clinical experience does suggest that four to six osseointegrated fixtures can easily and reliably function in a manner similar to the results obtained with a restored partial dentition, which depends on an intact or undermined state of the total area of periodontal ligament present. Previous chapters reviewed biomechanical aspects of this method as well as its longitudinal efficacy, leading to the conclusion that the ratio of functional occlusal contact surface area to the area of "contact osseointegration" can be large, indeed, without a compromise in the method's longevity. Doubts about the extent of loading that osseointegrated fixtures can sustain can be allayed by analyzing the rationality of arguments raised against the overloading of natural tooth abutments with extensive bridgework. A number of reports[1, 2] indicate that the limitations for fixed bridgework in patients with few abutment teeth and reduced periodontal tissues around these teeth are more related to technical and biomechanical prosthetic problems, rather than to the biological support

performance of the residual periodontium per se.

In fact, it has appeared justifiable to consider extensive bridges in patients with extremely reduced periodontal support as an alternative to removable prostheses. Such fixed prostheses, of a cross-arch design using mobile abutment teeth, provide a stable construction with very adequate functional capacity. Since the retention of a fixed prosthesis is superior to that of a removable one, both the function of the prosthesis, and the patient's psychological acceptance are improved. The prosthetic treatment phase in osseointegration is far easier to carry out and maintain than the one required for extensive fixed bridgework. This poses some rather provocative questions regarding the need for extensive, quasi-heroic, periodontal/prosthodontic interventions when treatment by osseointegration can be used adjunctively with, or even instead of, time-consuming and very expensive therapeutic undertakings. Clinical research in the next few years should provide some very interesting answers to these concerns.

247

Location of the osseointegrated fixtures

A major objective in prosthodontic reconstructions is a proper occlusal design that avoids undue stress concentrations in the remaining periodontal tissues supporting a prosthesis. Such a design is aided by optimal location of abutments that will preferably preclude cantilever extensions behind the most distal teeth. The extensive clinical experience and success with osseointegrated distal abutment fixtures placed in the bicuspid regions (for obvious morphologic reasons), and supporting cantilevered areas equal to two or three bicuspids in width, is a compelling argument for this design approach. Since patients with osseointegrated prostheses exert comparable loads to those exerted by individuals with natural dentitions (see chapter 9), high stress concentrations can occur, which in turn can induce ischemia by compression of the bone margins, or even microfractures along the fixture thread areas of bony contact. Furthermore, bone tissue is a nonuniform material, with cortical and cancellous bone responding differently to mechanical stresses. These points are reiterated so as to remind the prosthodontist that the interfacial response of osseointegration, while successful in its demonstrated ability to remodel into compact bone around the entire implant, does, on occasion, respond unfavorably to occlusal stresses. It is therefore mandatory that the prosthodontic effort include an absolutely passive fit of the prosthesis on the abutments, along with optimal occlusal design and contact relationship of the occlusion. If these criteria are combined with a plaque-free maintenance program, the objectives of routine excellent prosthodontic therapy are fulfilled.

Until the limits to functional and parafunctional loading on an individual osseointe-grated fixture can be determined, the prosthodontist will have to decide on the maximum number of abutment analogues with which to work. While six fixtures in each arch appear to be adequate, the relative orientation of the final number of fixtures may pose design and technical problems for the prosthodontist. Hence, professional teamwork is important in that the oral surgeon must perform in such a manner that will not only ensure osseointegration, but also avoid the problems that can sometimes occur.

Cosmetic and mechanical considerations

Surgical morphologic dictates frequently preclude the achieved objective of six parallel fixtures, adequately spaced interproximally, and oriented faciolingually so that they do not pose a risk of cosmetic or technical design compromise. Atraumatic surgery within the limits of residual ridge reduced morphology will lead to osseointegration, but occasionally with a regrettable, albeit unavoidable, failure on the part of the oral surgeon to comply with the prosthodontist's desires regarding fixture placement. The following problems may be encountered: *(1)* fixtures too close together; *(2)* imperfectly aligned fixtures, both mesiodistally and faciolingually; and *(3)* insufficient interarch distance, or considerable vertical and/or horizontal bone loss.

Fixtures too close together

When this occurs, the risk of interproximal plaque accumulation and home care maintenance problems increases (Fig. 15-4). The clinical problem is similar to the one encountered with overdentured anterior

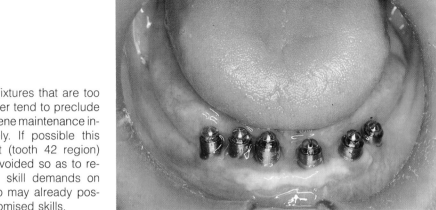

Fig. 15-4 Fixtures that are too close together tend to preclude optimal hygiene maintenance interproximately. If possible this arrangement (tooth 42 region) should be avoided so as to reduce digital skill demands on patients who may already possess compromised skills.

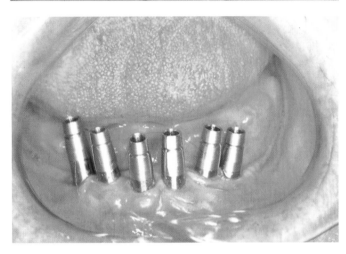

Fig. 15-5 Parallel fixture placement, a desired objective, is not always achieved. The "fanning out" result in this patient led to some technical prosthodontic problems that rendered treatment a little more complex.

mandibular teeth, where the risk of damaging interproximal gingival tissues appears to be higher. While it is tempting to want to take advantage of the stress-bearing services of each fixture, this may not be entirely desirable if crowding leads to a recurrent or untreatable localized problem. In such a case, the offending fixture (because of its location) is "put to sleep" (as described earlier).

Imperfectly aligned fixtures

A nonparallel, fan-shaped location of the fixtures is not conducive to optimal stress loading. Research identifying the range of nonparallelism that will lead to predictably good results is not available. However, clinical experience suggests a need for parallel, upright fixtures that are placed within the confines of the patient's neutral zone (Fig. 15-5). Buccally tipped fixtures can cause labial or buccal mucosal irritation to such an

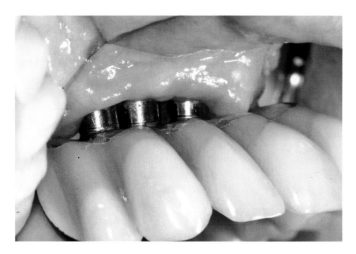

Fig. 15-6   The predictable patterns of residual ridge reduction frequently lead to a prosthesis design that places the teeth a long way from their attachment location.

extent that the fixture may have to be removed or not used. Here again, the risk of encroaching on tongue space or circumoral activity could prove to be a functional compromise. Above all, facially tipped fixtures will lead to cosmetic problems since access for the screw holes will occur in an esthetically compromised position.

Insufficient interarch distance

When such a clinical situation occurs, the short vertical distance between the arches can cause problems, especially in the maxilla. When severe bone loss has occurred, the prosthesis must compensate for tissue loss in both vertical and horizontal planes (Fig. 15-6). While this is technically feasible, it does lead to unfavorable cantilevering results with the risk of unpredictable responses from the tissue or materials. The maxilla appears to be particularly vulnerable, not only because of the relative prominence of the anterior teeth, but also because clinical experience has demonstrated a need for restricted cantilevers in the maxilla when compared to the mandible.

Finally, the morphology of circumoral activity must always be taken into account. Short active lips (especially upper ones) are more cosmetically demanding to work with, whereas thick, fleshy, relatively inactive lips lend themselves to easy optimal cosmetic tooth and gingival replacements.

Final prosthodontic care

The objective of this prosthodontic phase of treatment is the fabrication of a metallic framework to which prosthetic teeth and soft-tissue analogues can be added. The framework can be designed in one of two ways. It can comprise the bulk of the prosthesis, whereby the prosthetic teeth are virtually the only nonmetallic component (Fig. 15-7). This system borrows heavily from fixed prosthodontic technique protocol, and is therefore more appropriately prescribed for those patients where residual ridge reduction is mild to moderate. This will avoid a very large casting with its implied technical, economical, and cosmetic problems. The second method is an outgrowth of remov-

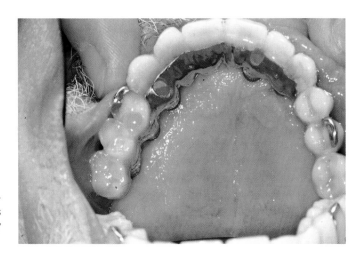

Fig. 15-7 A maxillary osseo-integrated prosthesis that uses fixed prosthodontic laboratory protocol in its construction.

able prosthodontic technique protocol (see Figs. 15-1a to f). It was developed because of the high cost of gold alloys and the frequent need to design a prosthetic framework that compensates for extensive ridge reduction. The bulk of such a prosthesis comprises the prosthetic teeth and acrylic resin replacing the missing soft tissues. The metal framework is abbreviated, and serves to reinforce the prosthesis as well as relate and attach it to the implants. In either case, the framework is made of a rigid and biomechanically compatible material which lends itself to casting accuracy, as well as design versatility.

The actual clinical protocol is virtually identical to the one employed in *Boucher's Prosthodontic Treatment for Edentulous Patients*.[3] Furthermore, the diverse techniques used in routine prosthodontics can easily be applied to the various stages entailed. The following procedures are used: *(1)* impression procedures, *(2)* jaw relations' registrations, *(3)* preliminary cosmetic assessment and try-in of framework, and *(4)* prosthesis insertion and patient instruction.

Impression procedures
(Figs. 15-8 to 15-20)

One week following the abutment operation the surgical pack is changed and the sutures are removed (see Table 15-1). Preliminary impressions are usually made at this stage in stock trays using one of the irreversible hydrocolloid impression materials. A custom tray is made on the preliminary stone cast which provides a good replica of the requisite landmarks for an impeccable final impression. These landmarks include critical detail of residual arch morphology, the location of surrounding unattached mucosa, and the retromolar pad. This detail is essential to enable the prosthodontist to accurately set up teeth in a manner that reconciles concepts of neutral zone, optimal cosmetic result, and correct location of occlusal plane height.[3] The custom tray is topless so that access to the screws inside the transfer copings is possible (Fig. 15-17). Final impressions can be made within three to four weeks depending on patient comfort, healing progress, and clinical judgment. Transfer copings are mounted on the implant abutments and retained by screws

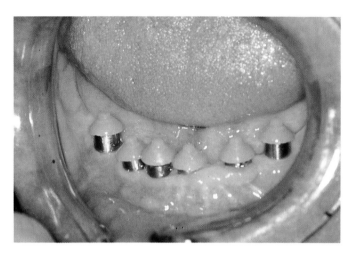

Figs. 15-8 to 15-21 The entire impression registration sequence.

Figs. 15-8 and 15-9 The healing caps are removed.

Fig. 15-9

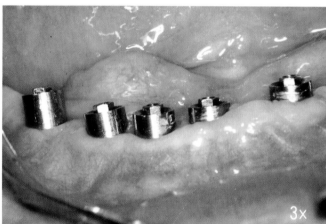

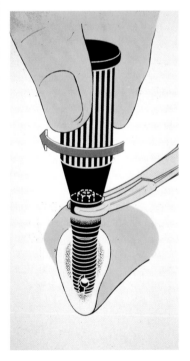

Fig. 15-10 Abutment cylinders are checked for tightness.

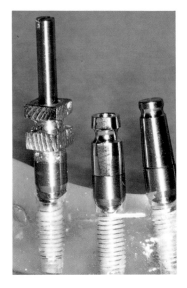

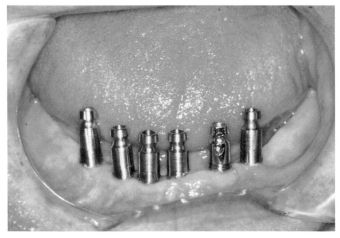

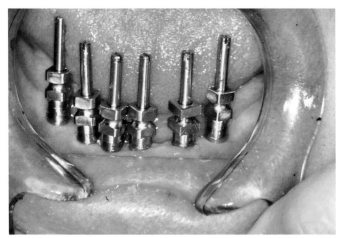

Figs. 15-11 to 15-13 The desired transfer coping is selected.

(Figs. 15-11 to 15-13). Abutment cylinders (the transepithelial components) are tightened; stability of each of these cylinders should be ascertained at each prosthodontic appointment (Fig. 15-10). Coping screw holes are blocked with wax or cotton pellets, and the custom tray with a softened wax lid is tried in the mouth so that the copings indent the wax cover (Fig. 15-18). Experience underscores the importance of linking the copings together intraorally before the impression is registered. This will ensure maximum accuracy and can be easily achieved by applying Duralay* to a scaffolding of dental tape or a closely adapted dental wire (Figs. 15-14 to 15-16). The tray, which may need minor additons to or deletions from its peripheries, is loaded with an impression material. A polyether variety has been used with great success but the choice is the clinician's (Fig. 15-19). The indentations in the wax lid or cover are used

* Reliance Dental Mfg. Co., Worth, Ill.

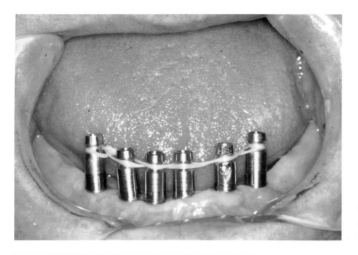

Figs. 15-14 to 15-16 The copings may be "splinted" together with Duralay.

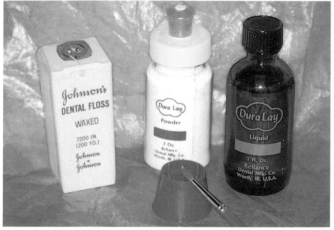

Fig. 15-15

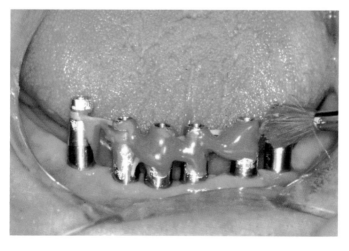

Fig. 15-16

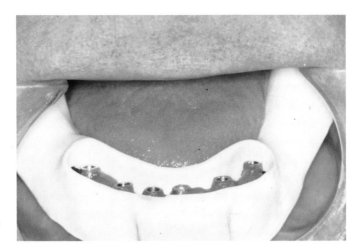

Fig. 15-17 The custom tray is tried in the mouth.

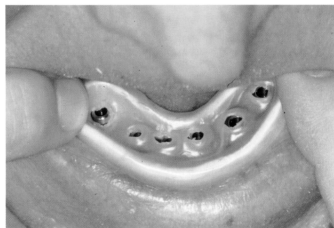

Fig. 15-18 The softened wax lid on the topless tray is indented for orientation purposes.

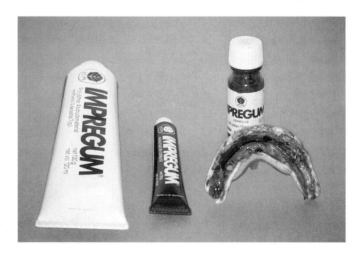

Fig. 15-19 One of several impression materials may be used.

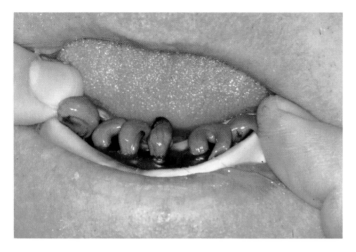

Fig. 15-20 When the impression material has set, the wax lid is removed along with the obturating cotton pellets, and the copings are unscrewed.

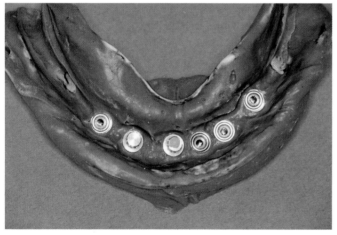

Fig. 15-21 Brass abutment analogues are mounted into the copings.

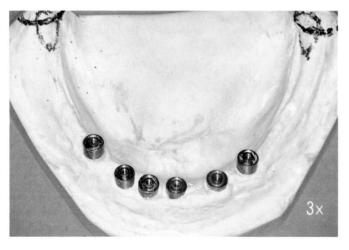

Fig. 15-22 The working cast is ready for fabrication of the prosthesis.

to locate the impression-filled tray in the mouth. After the material sets, the wax lid is removed, as are the wax or cotton pellets from the openings in the copings (Fig. 15-20). Each coping is unscrewed, and the tray is removed and inspected. Impression material must not cover the fit surface of any coping. Maximum coverage of the desired soft-tissue areas is essential, while "pressure spots" in the tray (resin material showing through the impression material) are not significant as the final prosthesis will *not* be mucosa borne. Brass abutment analogues are mounted on the copings and screwed into place (Fig. 15-21). The working cast is poured, and a replica of the arch to be restored is now available for framework and tooth replacement fabrication (Fig. 15-22). Occasionally an interim prosthesis can be made for a patient at this stage. Stock teeth are set up (after the casts are related on an articulator) and joined together by a matrix of acrylic resin which is reinforced by a thick stainless steel wire or bar. This interim prosthesis is processed

with guide pins in place. Once a final working cast (or casts) is produced, the speed of treatment completion becomes a matter of the prosthodontist's office logistics and patient convenience. The authors have used interim prostheses infrequently; instead they have been quite successful at hollowing out patients' previous prostheses and temporarily "refitting" them to accommodate the titanium abutment. Sometimes neither strategy is feasible and the patient accepts a few days of nonprosthesis wear until the final one is completed.

Jaw relations' registration (Figs. 15-23 to 15-32)

Wax occlusion rims on stabilized acrylic resin trial bases are used for recording centric relation. The occlusion rims can be employed either *(1)* with holes for three guide pins to enable the trial base to be screwed to the abutments, or *(2)* in an overdenture con-

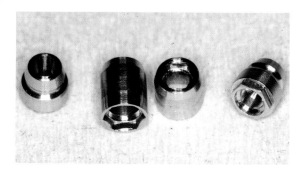
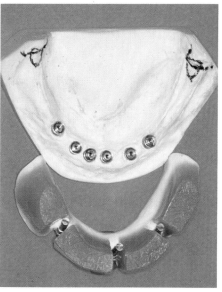

Fig. 15-23 Gold alloy cylinders will be used on the abutment analogues for the purposes of stabilizing the resin trial bases intraorally.

Figs. 15-24 to 15-32 Gold alloy cylinders will also be used on the working casts, during both recording of and in maintaining relations' registrations.

257

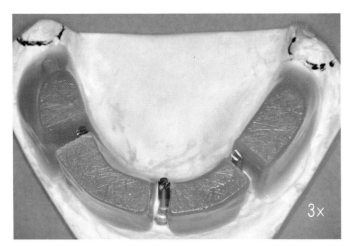

Fig. 15-25

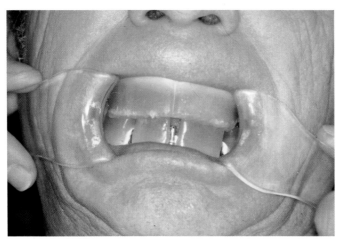

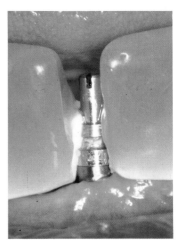

Figs. 15-26 and 15-27

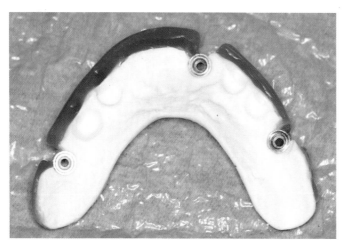

Fig. 15-28

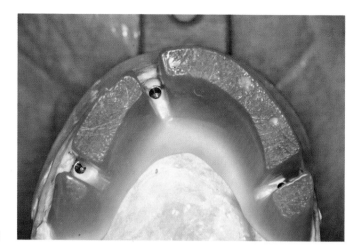

Fig. 15-29

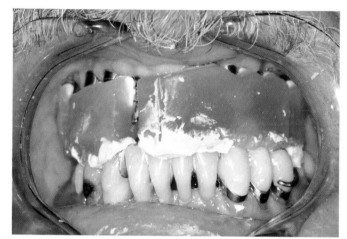

Fig. 15-30

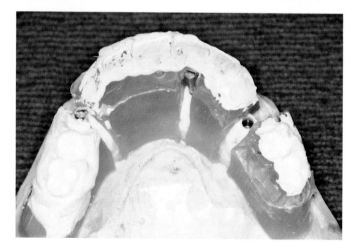

Fig. 15-31

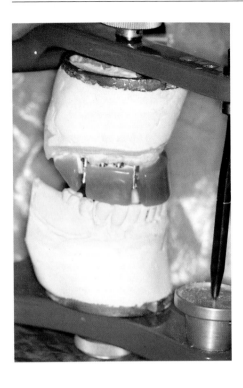

Fig. 15-32

text with or without gold alloy cylinders incorporated in the wax rim. The gold alloy cylinders will become an integral part of the framework, with the metal cast directly to the cylinders. An immobile occlusion rim dramatically facilitates the accurate and verifiable registration of jaw records. Accepted principles based on function, esthetics, patient comfort, and clinical judgment are used for establishing arch form, height of occlusal plane, freeway space, vertical dimension of occlusion, and preliminary centric relation record.[3, 4]

Preliminary cosmetic assessment and try-in of framework

The choice of which one of the two recommended framework design techniques will be employed will determine the next labora-

tory/clinical steps. If the fixed prosthodontic protocol technique is used (Table 15-3), a routine try-in of the tooth set-up is carried out before the framework is made. Acrylic resin artificial teeth (for rationale see chapter 5) are set up in wax on the trial denture base and tried in the mouth (Figs. 15-33 to 15-35). When both patient and dentist are satisfied with the result, a stone or silicone index is made. The wax and acrylic resin base are removed by "boiling out," gold alloy cylinders are screwed onto the abutment analogues, and waxing up of the framework is started. This wax-up is carried out in the context of the following objectives: *(1)* bulk of metal for strength, particularly in the region of distal abutments; *(2)* creation of adequate access location for hygiene purposes; *(3)* minimal display of gold on occlusal or facial surfaces for esthetic reasons; and *(4)* final strategic thinning out of the wax

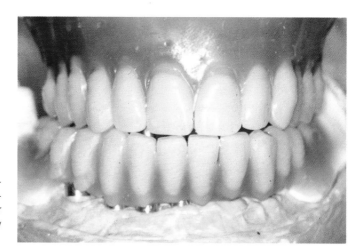

Figs. 15-33 to 15-35 Mandibular and maxillary setups are retained via guide pin screws or brass screws and the gold alloy cylinders.

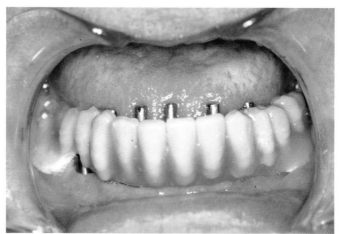

Fig. 15-34

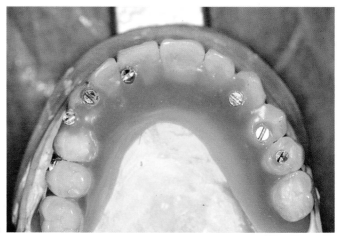

Fig. 15-35

Table 15-3   Choice of framework design fabrication

	Technique I	Technique II
Method	Fixed prosthodontic protocol	Removable prosthodontic protocol
Indication	Slight-to-moderate residual ridge reduction	Moderate-to-advanced residual ridge reduction
Material(s)	Gold alloy (type III) (substitute alloy)	Silver palladium (gold alloy—type III or IV—stelite alloy, substitute alloy)
Considerations	Accurate Proven load-bearing capacity (long-term) Can be expensive	Accurate Proven load-bearing capacity (short-term) Reduced cost

Table 15-4   Principles of optimal occlusion (Aimed at rehabilitating one or both dental arches with osseointegrated prostheses*)

1. Acceptable interocclusal distance.
2. Stable jaw relationship with bilateral contact in retruded closure.
3. Stable quadrant relationships providing axially directed forces.
4. Freedom in retrusive range of contact.
5. Multidirectional freedom of contact movement. This may be a unilateral or bilateral cuspid protected or group function (partial or complete), or a balanced occlusion may be present.

* From Beyron.[6]

to allow for retention of the acrylic resin teeth (see chapter 17 for laboratory procedures). Next, sprues are waxed onto the frame, which can be cast in one piece or as two or more separate units. The casting is next tried in the mouth to ensure a passive and impeccable fit. If this is not achieved, the framework has to be severed and an intra-oral index made. The same procedure is followed if the casting is made in more than one unit. Soldering can be done in the oven or with a pencil flame, and the soldered

prosthesis tried again in the mouth. When the prosthodontist is satisfied that an absolutely passive fit has been obtained, the prosthetic teeth are waxed onto the gold frame using the index. A final try-in can now be made to ensure esthetic and simulated functional satisfaction (Table 15-4). The prosthetic teeth are finally attached to the framework with heat-cured acrylic resin (Figs. 15-36 to 15-38). Figures 15-39 to 15-59 review similar clinical and alternative laboratory procedures.

If technique II is selected (see Table 15-3), inlay wax, wax partial denture forms, and/or Duralay are used to join the gold alloy cylinders together and extend posteriorly to the distal abutments on each side (Fig. 15-51). This trial prosthetic structure can be tried in the mouth to confirm the impression's accuracy, and then augmented with loops and beads for retentive purposes. Here again the objectives of wax-up design are similar to those described in technique I. Silver palladium has been used successfully in this technique because this alloy possesses physical properties that parallel those of type III gold alloys.[5] The cast frame is tried-in and if judged not a passive fit, it is accordingly cut and indexed in the mouth. In this

Figs. 15-36 to 15-38 Both completed mandibular and maxillary prostheses used in the previous illustrations have been processed and are ready for insertion. Cosmetic results in both patients are excellent.

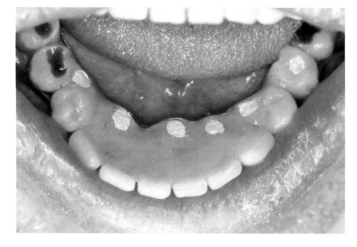

Fig. 15-36 The access holes to the fixture abutments through the framework casting are temporarily obturated.

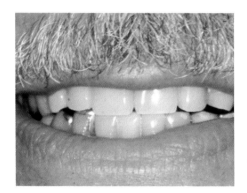

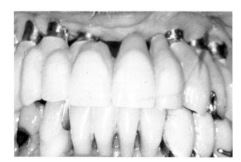

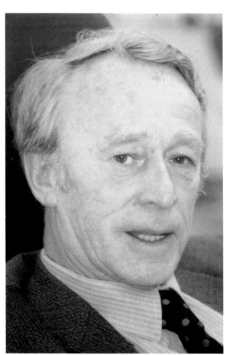

Fig. 15-37 Maxillary prosthesis.

Fig. 15-38 Mandibular prosthesis.

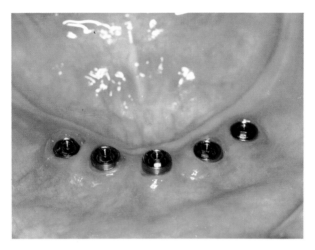

Figs. 15-39 to 15-59 Treatment for a young patient using technique II of the prosthodontic protocol.

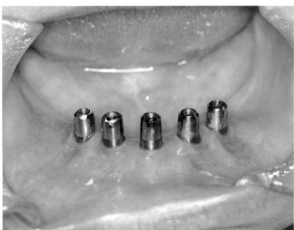

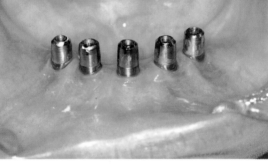

Fig. 15-39 A healthy gingival response may be compromised during the waiting period for prosthesis completion as a result of abutments' edges rubbing against adjacent detached mucosa.

Fig. 15-40 Shortened transfer copings will avoid such an occurrence. This may be a useful adjunct in such situations.

Figs. 15-41 to 15-44 A custom tray fits over splinted and obturated copings.

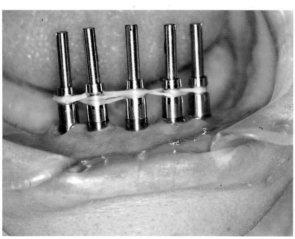

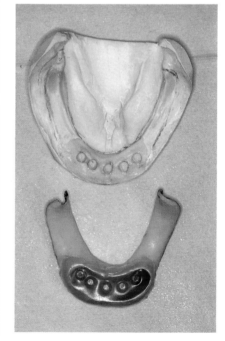

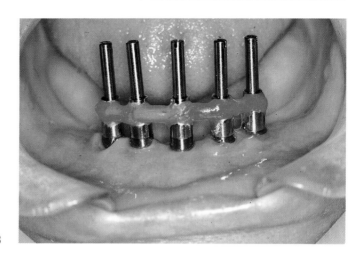

Fig. 15-43

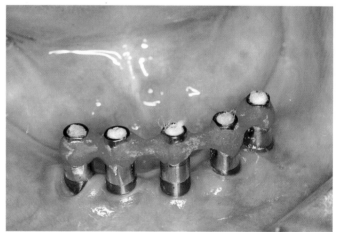

Fig. 15-44

Fig. 15-45　The final impression
is poured with brass analogues
in place.

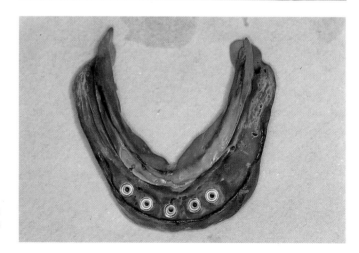

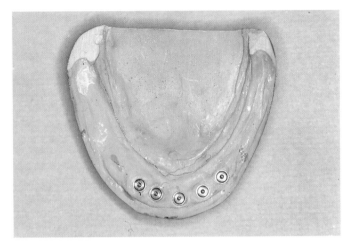

Fig. 15-46 The hard stone working cast.

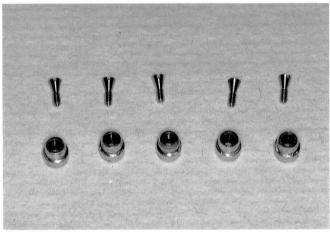

Fig. 15-47 Gold alloy cylinders and their screws.

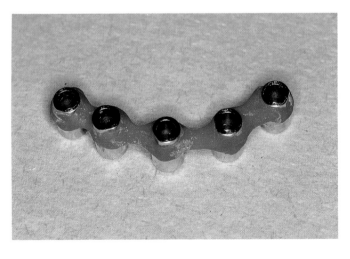

Fig. 15-48 These can be "splinted" on the working cast and returned to the mouth to confirm the accuracy of the working cast.

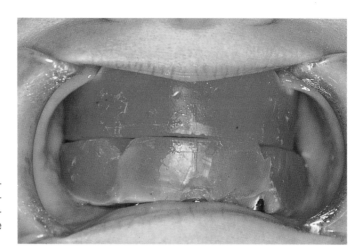

Figs. 15-49 and 15-50 An occlusion rim and a face-bow record are used to register jaw relation records and to relate the casts on an articulator.

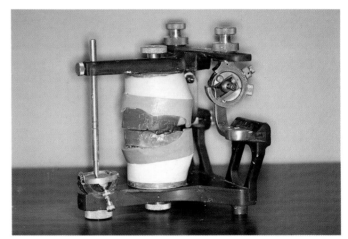

Fig. 15-50

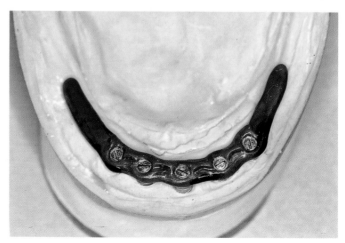

Fig. 15-51 A framework is waxed up.

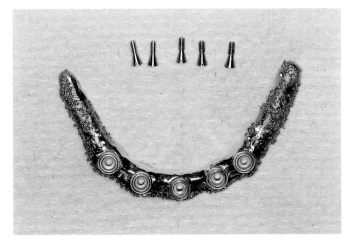

Fig. 15-52   Cast framework.

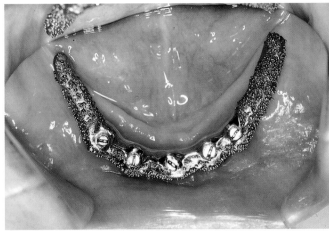

Figs. 15-53 and 15-54 Frame-work tried in the mouth.

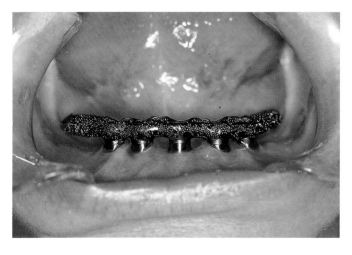

Fig. 15-54

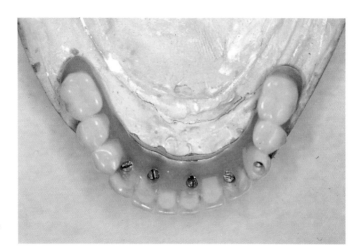

Figs. 15-55 and 15-56 The tooth set-up is completed.

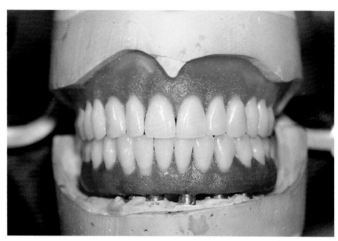

Fig. 15-56

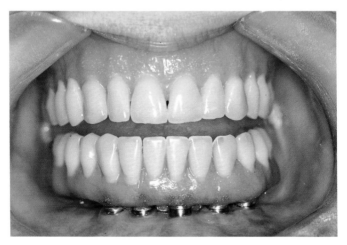

Fig. 15-57 The processed prosthesis is ready for insertion.

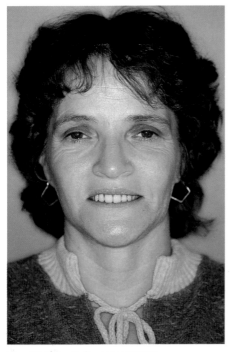

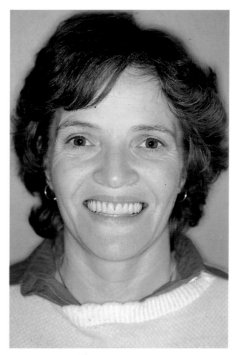

Fig. 15-58   Before treatment.   Fig. 15-59   After treatment.

technique the tooth setup is similar to conventional complete denture technique protocol, except that a metal frame occurs lingually (at least in the intercuspid areas) to the
tooth arch form (Fig. 15-55). Occasionally
the access location for an abutment's screw
is through a prosthetic tooth. This is unavoidable if either technique is used, and
the hole can be blocked with tooth-colored
resin or a composite material following final
seating of the prosthesis. The try-in appointment will ascertain the esthetic and simulated functional merits of the prosthesis. The
major advantage of this technique is that it
allows for a particularly cosmetic application of standard complete denture principles for those patients who have advanced
residual ridge resorption. The laboratory

steps involved in the processing of this
technique are described in the next chapter.

Prosthesis insertion

The completed prosthesis is checked on the
articulator and carefully inspected. Gross
premature (interceptive occlusal) contacts
in centric relation, detected by the use of
articulating paper between the teeth substitutes, are removed by grinding. The same
procedures are used to locate and remove
all occlusal interferences in lateral and pro-
trusive occlusions. The ground acrylic resin

tooth surfaces are polished, and the prosthesis is inserted in the mouth and tested for passivity of fit and screwed onto the abutments with gold screws. The occlusion is again checked with articulating paper and modified when necessary to ensure fulfillment of the objectives of an optimal occlusion[6] as listed in Table 15-4. Clearly basal surface errors do not apply in this technique, since the undersurface of the prosthesis will not contact the mucosa. However, attention must be paid to the possible presence of imperceptible discrepancies in the surface of the material(s). A magnifying glass is useful for this purpose. Such an occurrence would require careful polishing to ensure that scope for plaque accummulation is eliminated.

Careful attention must also be paid to the relationship of the gingival surface of the prosthesis and the mucosal tissues. In theory we aim at a "hygienic pontic" type of design, so as to ensure optimal scope for hygiene maintenance on the patient's part (Figs. 15-54 and 15-57; see also Fig. 15-1e). This is almost invariably feasible with mandibular prostheses unless a short, everted lower lip is present. This may not be the case with a maxillary prosthesis, especially when a short active upper lip combines with substantial presence of anterior residual ridge tissue. This problem is discussed later on in this chapter.

Patient education

Appearance

Patients must understand that their appearance with new bridges will become more natural with time.[3] Initially the bridges will feel strange and bulky in the mouth and will cause a feeling of fullness of the lips and cheeks. The lips will not adapt immediately to the fullness of the prosthesis borders and may initially present a distorted appearance. Muscle tension may cause an awkward appearance that will improve after the patient becomes relaxed and more self-confident.

Patients should therefore be instructed to refrain from exhibiting their bridges to curious friends until they are confident and competent to exhibit them at their best. When patients are not careful in following these instructions, they may likely become unfairly critical of the prostheses and develop an attitude that will be difficult for the dentist to overcome. During the edentulous or partially edentulous period, gradual reduction of the interarch distance and collapsing of the lips will have occurred. These changes have usually been so gradual that the family and friends were not aware that they have occurred. Therefore, a repositioning of the orbicularis oris muscle and a restoration of the former facial dimension and contour by the new bridges may cause too great a change in the patient's appearance. This can be overcome only with the passing of time, and patients are advised to persevere during this period of readjustment.

It should be emphasized that patients who are candidates for osseointegration treatment have frequently undergone years of developing parafunctional jaw and oral musculature activities to stabilize their dentures. These movements may carry over into the early weeks of wearing the new osseointegrated prosthesis, with resultant complaints of lip and cheek biting and unusual complaints about uncoordinated activity. Reassurance, patience, and prudence, particularly in relationship to mastication, should be stressed.

Mastication

Learning to chew with an osseointegrated prosthesis takes place fairly rapidly, but patients should be informed that a learning period is expected. New memory patterns often must be established for both the facial muscles and the muscles of mastication. Once the habit patterns become automatic in nature, chewing takes place without conscious effort. Mastication is additionally impaired because of the preliminary, interim period of excess salivary flow. The patient should be informed that in a few days normal salivary flow will resume.

The sudden ability to bite and chew hard foods might mislead patients occasionally to literally "bite off more than they can chew," causing possible damage to the prosthesis or a supporting fixture. Although a rare occurrence, patients should be aware of bolus size and consistency and hardness of the food being eaten, and adopt a careful strategy for biting large and/or hard amounts of food. Front-teeth biting should be avoided, particularly when the sagittal cantilevering effects of the anterior tooth/tissue replacement segments are pronounced.

Speech and oral hygiene

Fortunately, the problem of speaking with new prostheses is not as difficult as might be expected. The adaptability of the tongue to compensate for changes is so great that most patients master speech with new dentures within a few weeks. If correct speech required exact replacement of tissues and teeth in relation to tongue movement, no patient could ever learn to talk with artificial teeth. Even a 0.5-mm change at the linguogingival border of the anterior teeth would cause a speech defect, especially in the production of /S/ sounds, if it were not for

the extreme adaptability of the tongue to these changes. For that reason, tooth positions that restore appearance and masticatory function usually do not produce phonetic changes that are too great to be readily compensated. However, a study of tongue positions is valuable and gives an appreciation of the value of designing an arch form in the relation formerly occupied by the natural teeth.

Speaking normally with dentures or any large prosthesis requires practice. Patients should be advised to read aloud and repeat words or phrases that are difficult to pronounce. Patients usually are much more conscious of small irregularities in their speech sounds than those to whom they are speaking.

Some patients encounter difficulties with maxillary prostheses. These problems are usually related to the presence of a variable space between the maxillary prosthesis and the gingival tissues. Salivary spraying and some degree of lisping are the most common complaints. Obturation or "filling-in" of this critical area must be determined in the context of the patient's motivation and ability to maintain optimal oral hygiene, circumoral morphology and activity, and anteroposterior location of this segment carrying the prosthetic teeth. Sometimes a detachable labial flange or even an overdenture has been resorted to so as to solve this problem. Hygiene strategies are similar to those prescribed for patients treated for periodontal disease, and include the use of aids similar to those shown in Fig. 15-3. The objective is a plaque-free environment around each transepithelial titanium abutment. Clinically the surface characteristics of unalloyed titanium appear to discourage extensive plaque accumulation. But plaque accumulation does occur, and its presence may lead to compromise in gingival health, particularly if the abutment was placed in detached mucosa. Therefore a sustained, conscientious program of home care is mandatory. The openings in the prosthesis are blocked with gutta-percha during the first three to six months. This will allow for easy access to the screws should this be necessary (e.g., for screw tightening), or at a recall visit for inspection of tissues, optimal hygiene measures, etc.

When both prosthodontist and patient are satisfied with clinical functional progress, and that a good hygiene status can be maintained, the sealing of the screw holes is carried out.

The screw holes are filled with white gutta-percha or a cotton pellet, and then sealed with a thin layer of autopolymerizing acrylic resin. Patients are then recalled annually so that the mouth and the prosthesis can be inspected for any possible changes that require attention. At this time the therapeutic result is monitored (see Table 15-1).

Difficulties and special problems[7]

Mandibular prostheses

Very few problems have been encountered with mandibular prostheses. Osseointegration in the mandible appears to be easier to achieve and maintain than in the maxilla. This is probably because of differences in bone quality, density, and structure. While the minimal number of mandibular abutments required has not been scientifically ascertained, experience suggests that four abutments are essential. There have been occasions where only two or three abutments were osseointegrated, and while waiting for healing at the failed sites, prior to placing new fixtures, these patients have been successfully treated in the short term (18 to 24 months) with fixed or removable prostheses. The major technical problems relate to framework fit and design. Accuracy of fit is essential; a nonpassive fit will lead to stress concentration in one or more abutments with serious risks of abutment or screw fracture and loss of osseointegration. In the early stages of development of technique II (see Table 15-3) fractured prostheses were encountered, usually in the region of the distal abutment. Correct wax-up at this potentially vulnerable junctional site (see Figs. 15-52 to 15-54) is essential to preclude such a problem, and a rationale for correct design was developed (see chapter 16).

Other technical problems encountered are minor ones, and relate to the need for placing screw holes through a prosthetic tooth (Figs. 15-60 to 15-63) or a less than ideal pontic-abutment relationship with consequent cosmetic compromise (Figs. 15-64 and 15-65). Both problems are easily compensated for by clever use of tooth-colored acrylic resin and careful tooth placement and contouring.

Maxillary prostheses

Maxillary prostheses are prepared in the same manner as mandibular prostheses (Fig. 15-66 to 15-80). The same protocol applies if both upper and lower jaws are being treated at the same time. Longitudinal maxillary results have not been as good as mandibular ones, although the observed high success rate[8] remains quite impressive.

Bone quality and density in the maxilla seem to provide less than optimal local conditions for fixture anchorage. Bone volume is frequently unfavorable as well because of expanded location of maxillary sinuses, wide nasal cavities, and residual ridge reduction that results in compromised faciopalatal morphologic dimensions. These features frequently combine to limit the number of fixtures placed, resulting in restricted can-

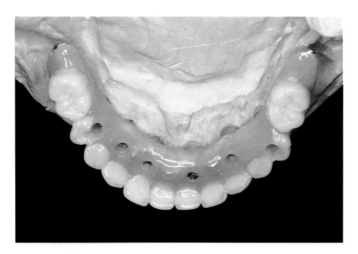

Figs. 15-60 to 15-63 Access holes for screws may occur through one or more prosthetic teeth.

Fig. 15-60

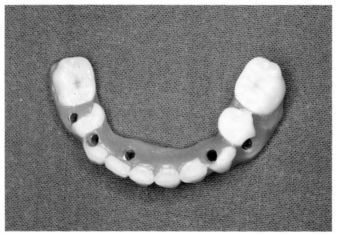

Fig. 15-61

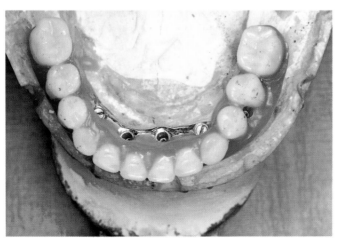

Fig. 15-62

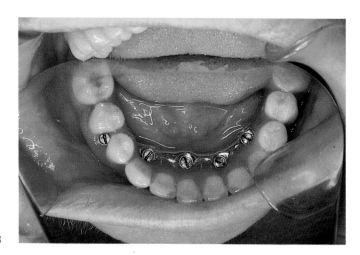

Fig. 15-63

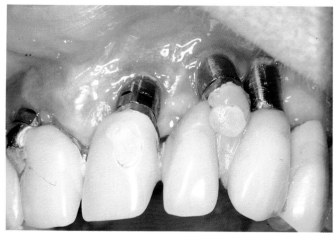

Figs. 15-64 and 15-65 Access to the abutment coincides with an interproximal area or the facial surface of a tooth. A favorable lip line frequently camouflages such an occurrence. Otherwise technical ingenuity has to be relied on.

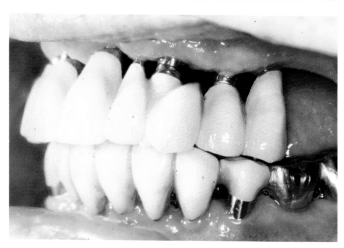

Fig. 15-65

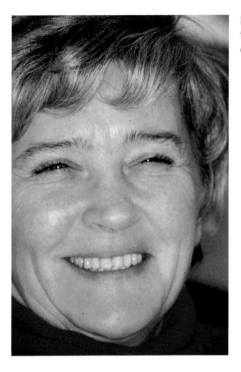

Figs. 15-66 to 15-80   Clinical examples of long-term treatment with maxillary prostheses demonstrating excellent tissue response and maintenance.

tilever extensions and an abbreviated size of the maxillary prosthesis (see Fig. 15-65). Patients for whom this unavoidable approach caused functional or cosmetic concerns are very rare. The authors feel that there is no need to provide these patients with extensive posterior tooth replacement, and have accepted limited bilateral occlusal contact areas.

Sometimes the oral surgeon cannot avoid fixture placement that is tipped labially or buccally. This usually leads to some construction problems, as well as a risk of clinical cosmetic compromise, since the screw holes will occur on the facial side of the tooth surfaces. These problems can be solved (see Fig. 15-64), but they are a nuisance and demand greater technical and esthetic attention to detail.

Phonetics is another problem. A complete denture usually easily restores original soft tissue and tooth arch contour relationships. This provides for easy tongue and simulated tissue landmark relationships which facilitate correct speech. An osseointegrated maxillary prosthesis rarely achieves this sort of relationship. Nonetheless, most treated patients adapt to the altered morphology, a clear tribute to lingual adaption and versatility. Patients who do not adapt run into prolonged problems with salivary sprays forced out of the space between the prosthesis and overlying tissues. Lisping is also a lingual failure to cope with the "hygienic" space present. Attempts to solve either problem have consisted of ridge-lapping the pontics on the prosthesis and filling in the interproximal areas, detachable labial or palatal veneers, or, in two or three unusual situations, conversion of the electively fixed prosthesis into an overdenture. This problem is rather difficult when a severely resorbed maxilla is treated, especially if a short active upper lip is present.

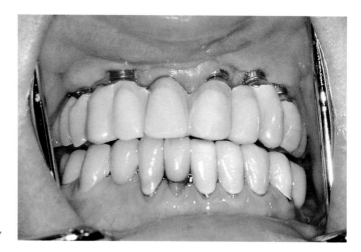

Fig. 15-67

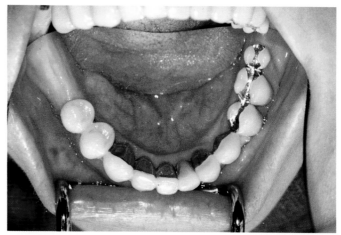

Fig. 15-68

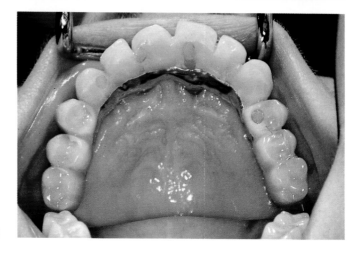

Fig. 15-69

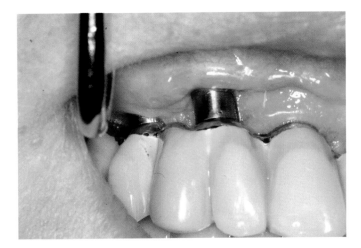

Fig. 15-70

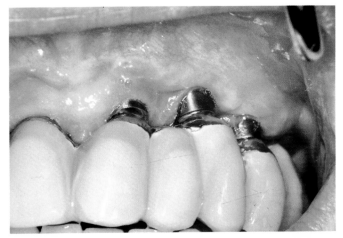

Fig. 15-71

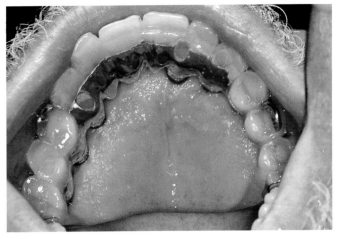

Fig. 15-72

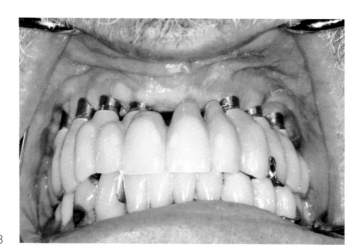

Fig. 15-73

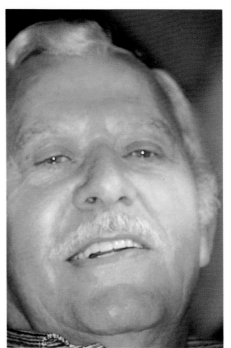

Fig. 15-74

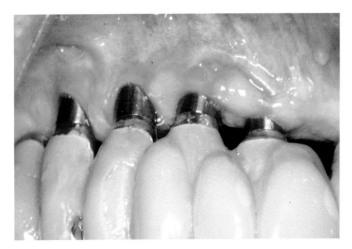

Fig. 15-75

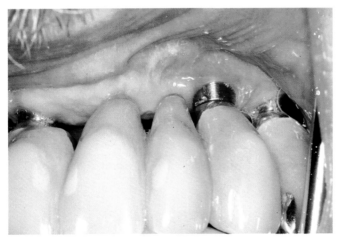

Fig. 15-76

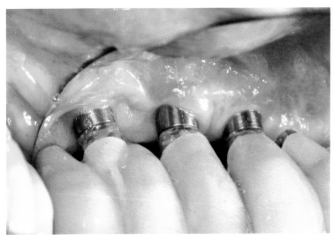

Fig. 15-77

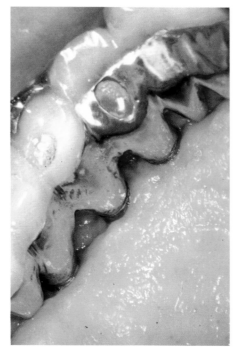

Fig. 15-78

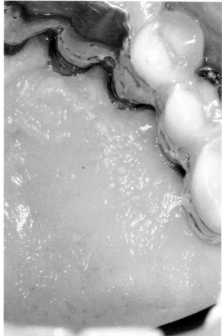

Fig. 15-79

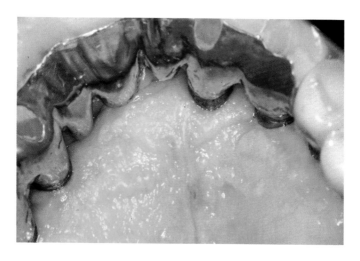

Fig. 15-80

References

1. *Nyman, S., and Ericsson, I.*
The capacity of reduced periodontal tissues to support fixed bridgework. J. Clin. Periodontol. 9(5):409-414, 1982.

2. *Lundgren, D., et al.*
Functional analysis of fixed bridges on abutment teeth with reduced periodontal support. J. Oral Rehabil. 2(2):105-116, 1975.

3. *Hickey, J. C., and Zarb, G. A.*
Boucher's Prosthodontic Treatment for Edentulous Patients, 8th ed. St. Louis: The C. V. Mosby Co., 1980.

4. *Zarb, G. A., et al.*
Prosthodontic Treatment for Partially Edentulous Patients. St. Louis: The C. V. Mosby Co., 1978.

5. *Meyers, G. W., and Cruickshanks-Boyd, D. W.*
Mechanical properties and casting characteristics of a silver-palladium bonding alloy. Br. Dent. J. 153:323, 1982.

6. *Beyron, H.*
Occlusion: Point of significance in planning restorative procedures. J. Prosthet. Dent. 30:641, 1973.

7. *Lundqvist, S., and Carlsson, G. E.*
Maxillary fixed prostheses on osseointegrated dental implants. J. Prosthet. Dent. 50:262, 1983.

8. *Adell, R., et al.*
A 15-year study of osseointegrated implants in the treatment of the edentulous jaw. Int. J. Oral Surg. 6:387, 1981.

Chapter 16

Other Prosthodontic Applications

George A. Zarb, Tomas Jansson, and Torsten Jemt

Introduction

The success of the osseointegration technique is predicated on "atraumatic surgery, followed by atraumatic prosthodontic treatment."[1] Its efficacy to date has been largely restricted to edentulous patients whose problems and complaints included severe morphologic compromise of the mandibular or maxillary denture-supporting areas, combined with one or more of the following features: poor oral coordination, low-tolerance mucosa, parafunctional habit(s), unrealistic prosthetic expectations, and the presence of a hyperactive gag reflex. The reported replicable clinical successes[2, 3] underscore the merits of this technique for patients who either cannot wear dentures or wear them with varying degrees of difficulty. These patients are clearly candidates for implant prescription. Furthermore, clinical experience indicates that several removable prosthesis-wearing patients frequently regret (and maybe even resent) their dependence on a removable prosthesis with all the implied consequences.

The introduction of the technique of osseointegration suggests a therapeutic breakthrough for the prosthodontic patient and the development of treatment plans that could significantly reduce the conventional role of removable prostheses.

The techniques and clinical applications described in chapter 15 are clearly a series of routine prosthodontic procedures which the authors moved "laterally" into this clinical endeavour. The challenge for prosthodontists now is to reconcile the established, applied biologic efficacy of osseointegration with the established range of time-proven prosthodontic treatment methods. Together with colleagues in several centers around the world, the authors are now investigating the longitudinal application of osseointegrated dental implants in the areas of overdenture application, treatment of partially edentulous patients, and single tooth replacement.

Overdentures

In the past few years a great deal has been written about the functional benefits obtained by a patient who wears a denture over retained teeth and/or roots. These benefits include improved denture stability, preservation of ridge height, and enhanced patient confidence and comfort. Experienced prosthodontists have long recognized that some patients' denture difficulties can be rectified easily if denture stability is improved. These patients do not necessarily need a conversion of their unstable complete denture into a rigid, fixed osseointegrated one. All they really need is the presence of a couple of overdentured abutments, which would be enough to restore good function and comfort to their masticatory system. It is therefore tempting for the prosthodontist to include such an "abbreviated" use of osseointegration in certain edentulous patients. Such an application offers both practical clinical as well as financial advantages. The surgical operation becomes reduced both time-wise and money-wise, and this approach may be kinder to the patient, particularly when considering the state of health and/or age. The dramatic impact of the option of shifting from an unsatisfactory complete denture to an eminently satisfactory fixed prosthesis should not lead to overlooking simpler, less dramatic, but, in the context of an individual patient's real needs, equally good prosthodontic treatment. Figures 16-1a to h show an intraoral view of a patient who had worn very well made and serviced complete dentures with varying success. Clinical judgment suggested that the patient would benefit

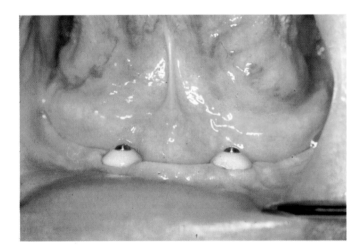

Figs. 16-1a to h   The sequence of clinical steps used in the application of osseointegration in overdenture treatment is illustrated.

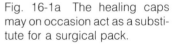

Fig. 16-1a   The healing caps may on occasion act as a substitute for a surgical pack.

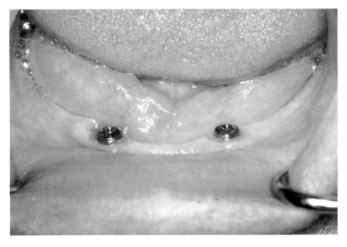

Fig. 16-1b   This allows for undisturbed epithelial healing to occur.

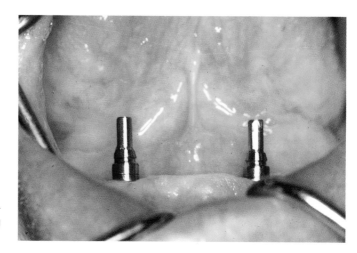

Fig. 16-1c   The gold alloy cylinders are stabilized with long guide pins (or screws).

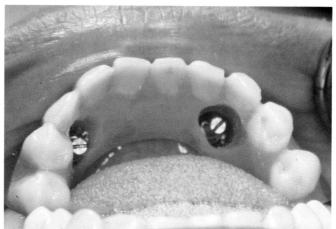

Fig. 16-1d   The original denture is "perforated" overlying the fixture sites.

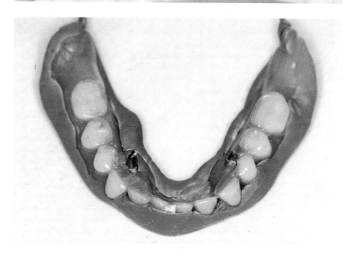

Fig. 16-1e   A conventional reline impression is made.

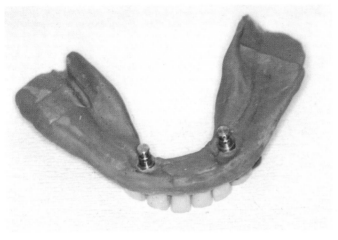

Fig. 16-1f   Brass analogues are related to the cylinders (note transfer copings could also be used).

Figs. 16-1g and h   A bar is cast to tie the cylinders together, and the denture is hollowed out to engage this bar with one or two clip retainers.

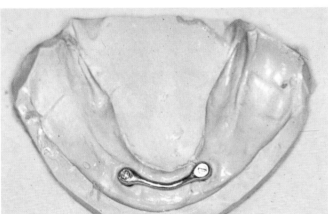

Fig. 16-1g

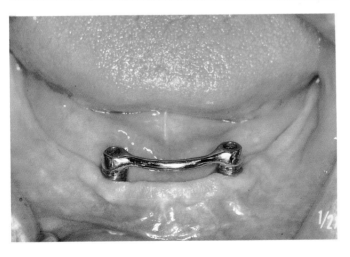

Fig. 16-1h

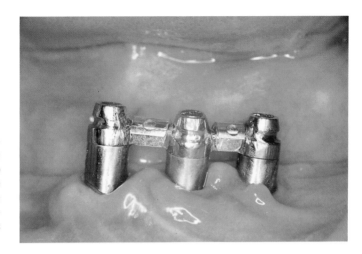

Fig. 16-2 Three out of five fixtures were used to support an interim overdenture until the two nonintegrated fixtures could be replaced. Patient experience in the long term indicated a preference for the overdentured status quo.

considerably from a little extra stability. Since this was easily achieved with a couple of osseointegrated fixtures, this treatment plan was the one prescribed for this patient. The fixtures either can be used separately or they can be joined together by a cast bar. The previous, technically adequate denture can then be hollowed out on the tissue surface side and relined so as to accommodate the overdenture abutments.

Whereas the enhanced risk of dental caries does not apply in such cases, the risk of plaque accumulation remains. Proper home care and plaque control must be emphasized. Above all, research in the quality and quantity of plaque accumulation around the titanium, and its relationship to the continuing health of the oral soft-tissue environment, must be undertaken.

In Fig. 16-2 the patient's mandible had been prepared for five fixtures. Two did not osseointegrate, and the remaining three were temporarily converted into overdenture abutments, while the original surgerized sites healed prior to a second surgical procedure. The patient was so delighted with her stable prosthesis that she declined having two new fixtures placed, and a subsequent fixed prosthesis. The authors have encountered similar experiences in the maxilla, and, here too, the overdenture technique can be combined with osseointegration to preclude some of the problems referred to in treating maxillary jaws.

Partially edentulous patients

The authors feel that the area of treatment of the partially edentulous state will evolve into a major area of application for the osseointegration technique. An understanding of the significance and implications of partial edentulism is an exciting challenge which repeatedly confronts the prosthodontist.[4] Equally exciting is the prescription for coping with the encountered problems—be it a fixed or a removable resolution or both. The introduction of tissue-integrated prostheses adds a new dimension to the notion of treating the partially edentulous milieu. However, it should be emphasized that several factors are still being studied. It is tempting to argue that "if four to six fixtures can be used as a foundation for restoring an entire dental

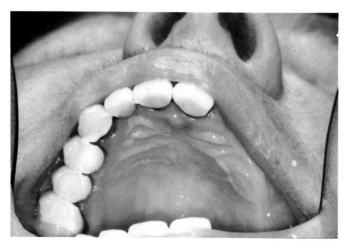

Figs. 16-3a to f In this extensive Class II type of partial edentulism, prosthesis design reconciled soft-tissue support with adequate access for optimal hygiene maintenance (reflected view).

Figs. 16-3a and b The loss of teeth in the maxillary quadrant was accompanied by excessive residual ridge resorption.

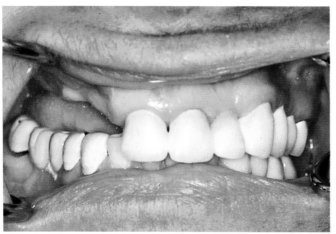

Fig. 16-3b

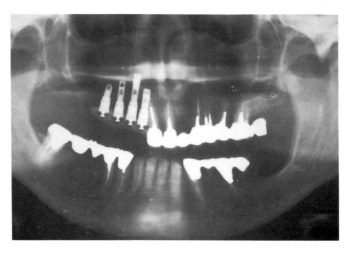

Fig. 16-3c   Four osseointegrated fixtures were placed.

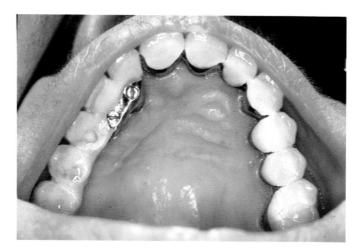

Figs. 16-3d to f A fixed prosthesis provided both functional and cosmetic rehabilitation.

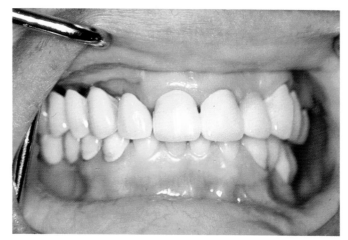

Fig. 16-3e

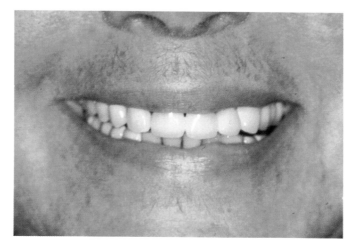

Fig. 16-3f

arch, then two or three can cope with just about any partially edentulous quadrant or segment in most mouths." This has certainly been our short-term experience (see Figs. 16-3a to f and 16-4a to e). Some compelling questions may arise, but clinical experience and research is bound to provide new solutions, techniques, and treatment rationales over time. The questions relate to items such as:

1. The limits to loading behavior of individual fixtures and a comparison of this behavior with that of other teeth (in similar or adja-

cent locations, in different stages of periodontal support) (see chapter 5).

2. The relationship between natural tooth abutment resiliency and the rigid anchorage of osseointegrated fixtures. A prosthesis that utilizes both types of abutments will demand that the prosthodontist have a keen understanding of the need for flexible connections (see chapter 5).

3. The implications of different materials used.

4. The development of new or modified instrumentation in the context of demands

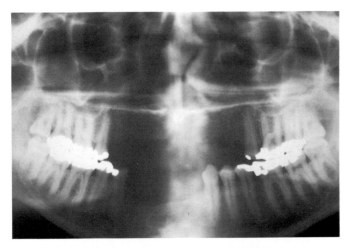

Fig. 16-4a   An automobile accident resulted in Class IV partially edentulous situations in both jaws of this young male patient.

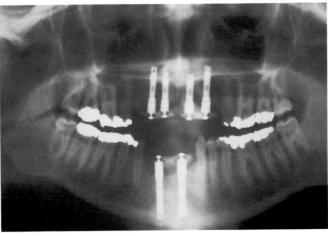

Figs. 16-4b and c   Long fixtures were placed to provide attachment for fixed prostheses.

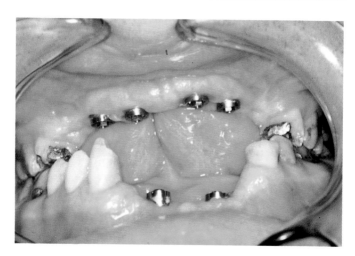

Fig. 16-4c

Figs. 16-4d and e Favorable circumoral activity in both patients allowed for excellent cosmetic results. (Note that in the authors' judgment all three prostheses [including Fig. 16-3] did not need natural tooth support. Clinical experience and theoretical considerations endorse such a clinical decision.)

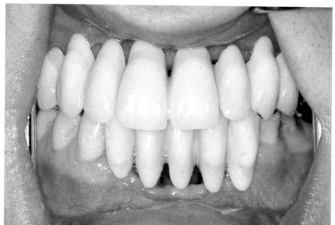

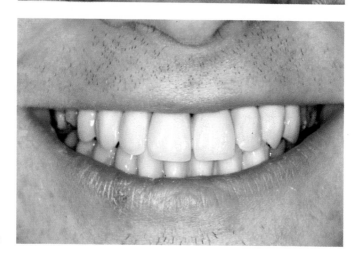

Fig. 16-4e

related to fixture location, access, interarch space, etc.

Single tooth replacement

Advances in bonding materials have been succesfully applied to "cemented" prostheses with good short-term results. The search for minimally invasive and reversible techniques for individual tooth replacement will of course go on. However, consideration should also be given to replacing a tooth root with an osseointegrated fixture as a foundation for an individually designed crown. Such application demands design considerations related to inter-tooth root space, extent and direction of interdental bone reduction, esthetic location of space, etc. Clinical research in this applied osseointegration is currently under way.

References

1. *Adell, R., et al.*
   A 15-year study of osseointegrated implants in the treatment of the edentulous jaw. Int. J. Oral Surg. 6:387, 1981.

2. *Adell, R.*
   Clinical results of osseointegrated implants supporting fixed prostheses in edentulous jaws. *In* Proc. of Toronto Conf. on Osseointegration in Clinical Dentistry. St. Louis: The C. V. Mosby Co., 1983.

3. *Zarb, G. A., and Symington, J. M.*
   Osseointegrated dental implants: Preliminary report on a replication study. *In* Proc. of Toronto Conf. on Osseointegration in Clinical Dentistry. St. Louis: The C. V. Mosby Co., 1983.

4. *Zarb, G. A., et al.*
   Prosthodontic Treatment for Partially Edentulous Patients. St. Louis: The C. V. Mosby Co., 1978.

Chapter 17

Laboratory Procedures and Protocol

George A. Zarb and Tomas Jansson

In chapter 15 the different clinical prosthodontic procedures employed were discussed: impression procedures, jaw relations' registrations, preliminary cosmetic assessment and try-in of framework, and completion of the prosthesis. The adjunctive
laboratory procedures that make the clinical
procedures possible follow a parallel pattern. Table 17-1 sums up the sequence of
steps that are carried out in the prosthodontic laboratory. For reasons of convenience
these steps are considered in two general
stages.

Stage 1

Preliminary cast and custom tray

An edentulous stock metal tray approximately 6 mm larger than the outside surface
of the residual ridges is selected. The tray is
refined by bending the peripheries as required and lining them with a soft boxing
wax to help confine the irreversible hydrocolloid impression material. The objective is to register the available basal seat
area for complete denture fabrication. The
cast is poured into artificial stone, and soft-
tissue undercut areas are blocked out with
wax. The tray outline is pencilled on the cast
to ensure the inclusion of important
anatomic landmarks (e.g., the retromolar
pads). An abbreviated wax occlusion rim

that liberally replicates the area to be occupied by the transfer copings is placed
over the transepithelial fixture component
sites. This rim is approximately 12 mm high
and 10 mm wide. A self-curing acrylic resin
tray material is mixed and uniformly adapted

Table 17-1   Sequence of prosthodontic
laboratory stages necessary to provide a prosthesis

Stage 1
1. Preliminary cast
2. Custom tray
3. Impression preparation
4. Final working cast
5. Fabrication of recording and transfer bases and occlusion rims
6. Transfer of jaw relation record(s) to articulator

Stage 2 will depend on selection of prosthesis
fabrication technique (see chapter 15, Table
15-3).

Stage 2	
Fixed prosthodontic protocol technique	Removable pros-thodontic protocol technique
1. Trial tooth set-up	1. Framework fabrica-tion
2. Indexing	
3. Framework fabrica-tion	2. Confirmation of or correction of framework fit
4. Confirmation of or correction of framework fit	3. Try-in with tooth set-up
5. Final processing	4. Final processing

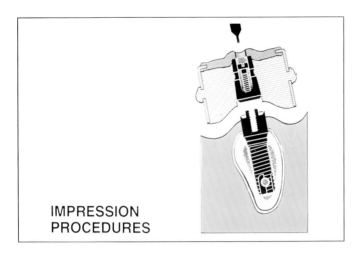

Fig. 17-3 Three different coping designs that satisfy diverse clinical needs.

IMPRESSION PROCEDURES

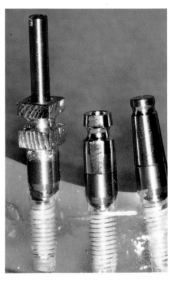

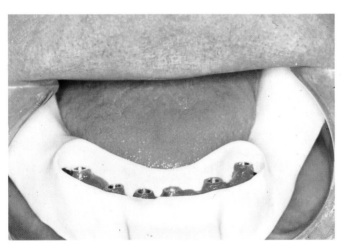

Fig. 17-2

over the cast and along the height of the wax rim so that the tray will be approximately 2 to 3 mm thick (Figs. 17-1 and 17-2). Note that the tray is open over the fixture sites. While it is possible to use a modified disposable edentulous tray, a custom tray is more likely to ensure the recording of those landmarks that enable the prosthodontist to best prescribe correct arch form and height of the occlusal table.

Several designs of transfer copings are available, and their selection is based on location of the fixtures and their angulation, access convenience, and clinical preference (Fig. 17-3). The objective is to accurately key the copings in the impression material, and to make sure that enough space is available around the copings in the tray. The copings' accurate relationship in the final impression is enhanced by the actual coping design (presence of grooves) and/or the use of a floss and resin splint (Figs. 17-4 and 17-5). After the impression has set, the copings are unscrewed, the tray

Figs. 17-4 and 17-5 A simulated clinical exercise of the "splinting" procedure which ensures an unchanged coping relationship to the fixture analogue.

Fig. 17-6 A transfer coping *(top left)*, a brass analogue *(bottom left)*, and a guide pin screw that can have its length modified.

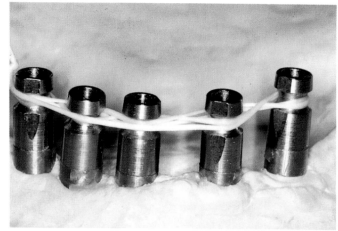

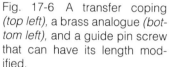

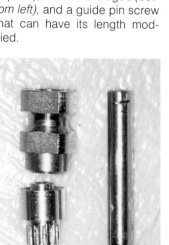

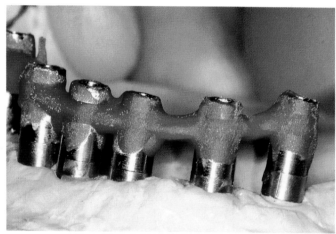

Fig. 17-5

is removed and inspected, and if the impression is acceptable, a final working cast is poured.

Impression preparation and final working cast fabrication

Brass fixture analogues are screwed into the transfer copings (Figs. 17-6 to 17-8). The objective is to replicate the intraoral coping/ fixture relationship in the laboratory for pros-

thesis fabrication (Fig. 17-9). The impression is poured in a hard stone. The final working cast is now ready for the preparation of the next prosthodontic step.

Recording and transfer bases and occlusion rims

Occlusion rims are employed as provisional substitutes for the planned prosthesis and used to record both the neutral zone and

295

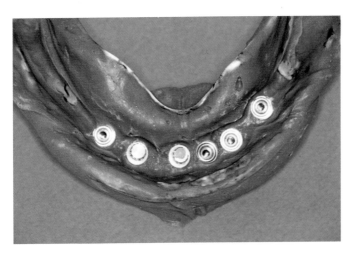

Figs. 17-7 to 17-9 Brass analogues are carefully attached via screws to the copings, and the impression is poured in a hard stone to form the working cast.

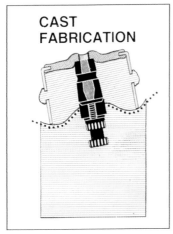

CAST FABRICATION

Fig. 17-8

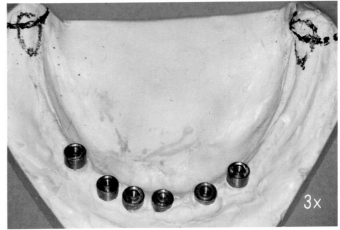

Fig. 17-9

maxillomandibular relations. They are made on the stone working cast and consist of a standard type acrylic resin denture base and a wax rim (Fig. 17-10). Two types of techniques for making registration records have been employed. In one type gold alloy cylinders (to be used as an integral part of the framework later) are incorporated into the wax rim (Figs. 17-11 and 17-12). Two or more screws can then be used to retain the rims firmly in place, or else the rim can be used in an overdenture context. The other

design uses three cylinders which are placed between four sections of occlusion rim and retained via guide pins (Fig. 17-13). The occlusion rims are used to establish *(1)* the level of the occlusal plane in the lower arch; *(2)* the arch form, which is related to the activity of the lips, cheeks, and tongue; *(3)* jaw relation records, which are preliminary at this stage; and *(4)* an estimate of the interocclusal distance.

While none of these determinations can be made in a precise, scientific manner, clinical

RECORDING OF JAW RELATIONS

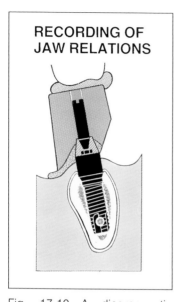

Fig. 17-10 A diagrammatic representation of an occlusion rim in the mouth showing the relationship of wax block, resin trial base, gold alloy cylinder, and guide pin that has been shortened.

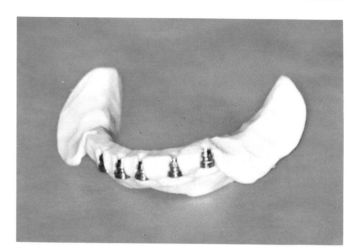

Fig. 17-12

Fig. 17-13

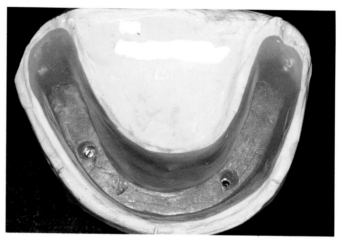

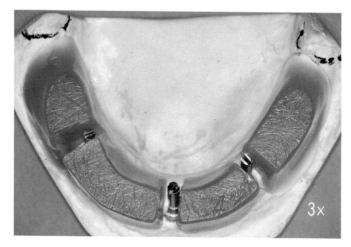

Figs. 17-11 *(top right)* to 17-13 A trial base attached to two or more cylinders can be used in two different types of occlusion rims.

SETTING TEETH IN WAX

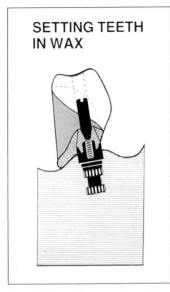

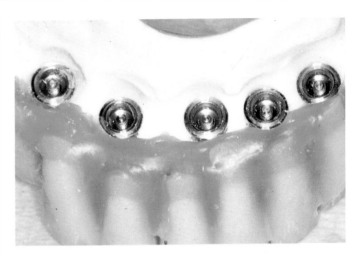

Fig. 17-14   The wax rim of Fig. 17-11 is replaced by prosthetic teeth and retaining/supporting wax as a soft-tissue analogue.

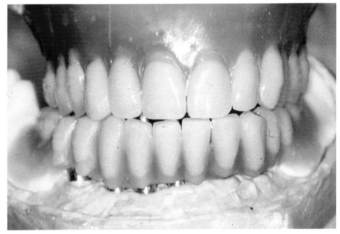

Fig. 17-16

Fig. 17-17

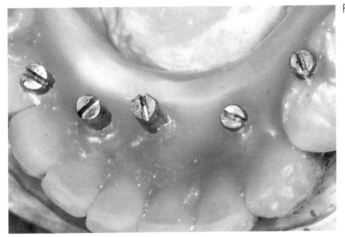

Figs. 17-15 *(top right)* to 17-17   The trial set-up is stabilized on the analogues in the laboratory, and in the mouth by alignment of the cylinders, and retention via guide pin screws.

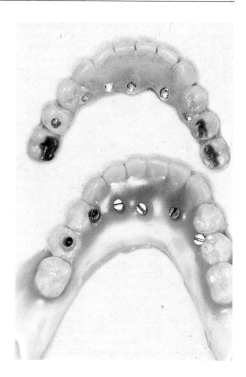

Fig. 17-18   The difference in bulk between the trial set-up and the completed prosthesis is readily seen.

experience has provided several basic principles that have become standard techniques.[1] The preliminary centric relation record is made after the occlusion rims have been contoured and designed to simulate the approximate position of the artificial teeth and tissues of the completed prostheses. A face-bow may be used to transfer the occlusion rims to a semiadjustable articulator of choice. Other records may be made, for example, of the jaw relation when the teeth are in an edge-to-edge incisal position. This record enables the dentist to accurately adjust the condylar guidances of the articulator. An articulator is used to simulate opening and closing and multidirectional tooth contact movements (simulated parafunctional movements).

Stage 2

Stage 2 of the laboratory protocol depends on which of the two techniques of framework design fabrication will be employed. If a fixed prosthodontic design protocol is selected, the sequence of events will be as follows (see Table 17-1).

Fixed prosthodontic design protocol

Trial setup

The selected teeth are set up on a trial base, which could be the same one used for the registrations (Figs. 17-14 to 17-17; see also Fig. 17-11). The trial prosthesis is retained via the guide pins, which may have to be shortened if their occlusal height leads to

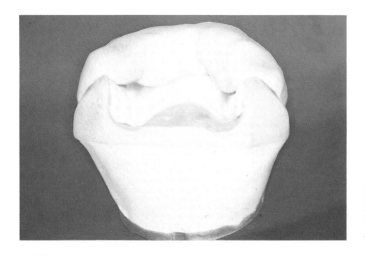

Figs. 17-19 to 17-22 The sequential steps of indexing, wax boil-out, and prosthetic teeth orientation in the index.

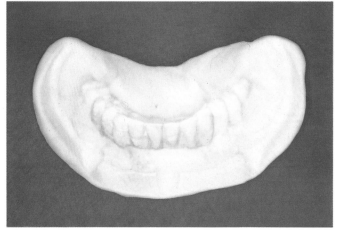

Fig. 17-20

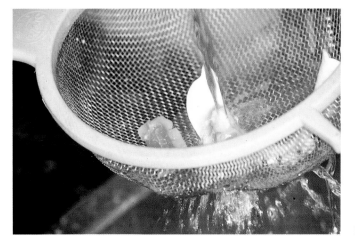

Fig. 17-21

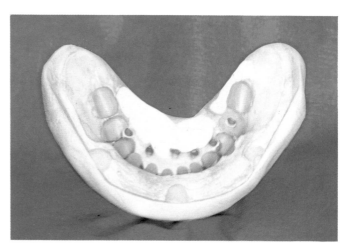

Fig. 17-22

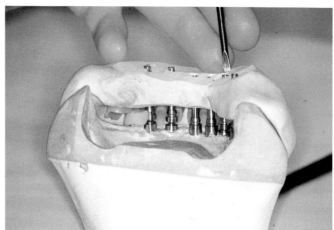

Fig. 17-23 The sequential steps on the working cast with guide pins in place.

occlusal interference. This stage is quite different in bulk from the final completed prosthesis (Fig. 17-18).

Indexing

A plaster, or preferably a silicone putty, index is made, the boil-out procedure is completed, and the prosthetic teeth are glued into the index, which is reoriented to the master cast (Figs. 17-19 to 17-23).

Framework fabrication

The frame is waxed up with the gold alloy cylinders screwed in place by means of guide pins in each fixture analogue. The objective is to join the prosthetic teeth together via a strong and rigid metallic unit that fulfills objectives of strength, support, nontissue impingement, and noninterference with the desired cosmetic result (Figs. 17-24 to 17-27). The wax-up is completed by adding retentive loops and beads, or by relieving the wax at the back of the pros-

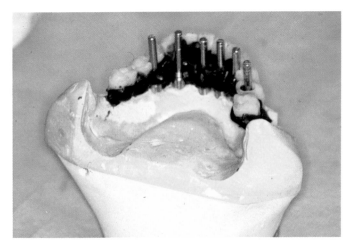

Figs. 17-24 to 17-28 The wax-up of the framework. The index is trimmed lingually to provide easy access for waxing up around the prosthetic teeth.

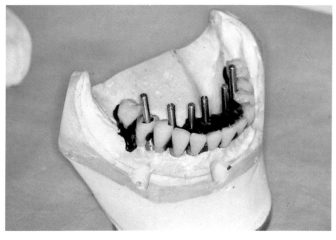

Fig. 17-25

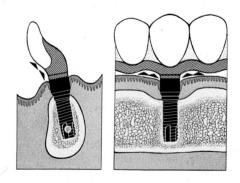

Fig. 17-26 The hygienic pontic design.

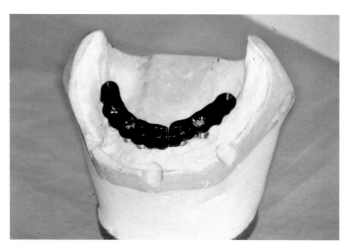

Fig. 17-27

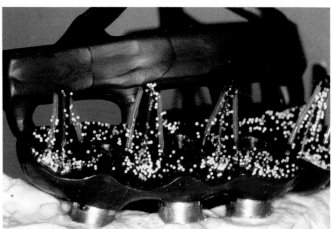

Fig. 17-28 The completed wax-up is made retentive via loops and beads.

thetic teeth. The wax-up is sprued, invested, and cast in the conventional manner, either as one piece or in sections (Figs. 17-28 to 17-32).

The casting is cleaned, the sprues are removed, and standard finishing procedures are carried out (Figs. 17-33 and 17-34). The casting is tried first on the working cast and next in the mouth (Figs. 17-35 to 17-37). A passive and impeccable fit is essential to avoid the buildup of adverse stress concentrations in one or more of the osseointe-

grated fixtures. If the casting fails to fit the cast it probably will not fit the mouth. It should be sectioned and assembled in the mouth with Duralay* (Figs. 17-38 to 17-40). In recent years the authors have routinely cast the frame in one piece, and then sectioned it in those few situations where an intraoral try-in revealed an imperfect fit.

Sectional assembly is followed by soldering and a new framework try-in (Figs. 17-41 and

* Reliance Dental Mfg. Co., Worth, Ill.

303

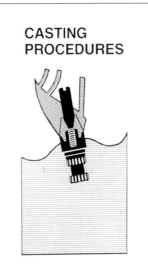

CASTING PROCEDURES

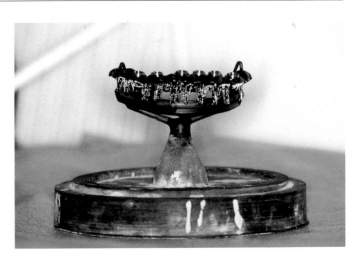

Figs. 17-29 to 17-34 Spruing, investing, casting, and polishing of the framework. The procedures follow standard fixed prosthodontic laboratory protocol.

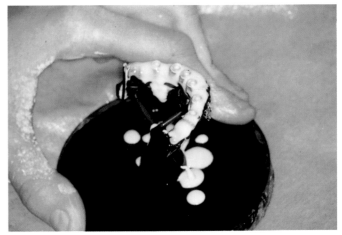

Fig. 17-31

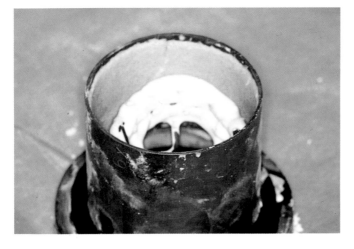

Fig. 17-32

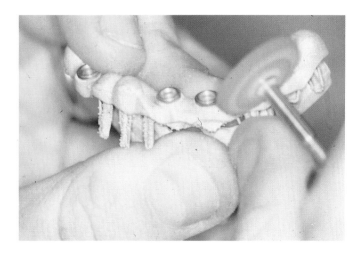

Fig. 17-33

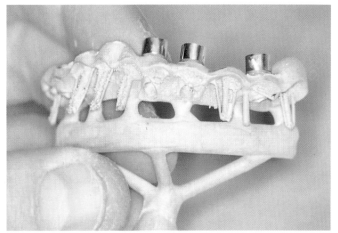

Fig. 17-34

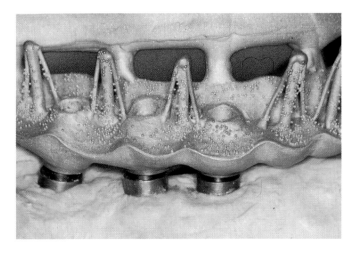

Fig. 17-35   The casting is tried on the working cast.

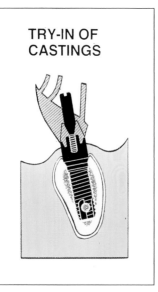

TRY-IN OF CASTINGS

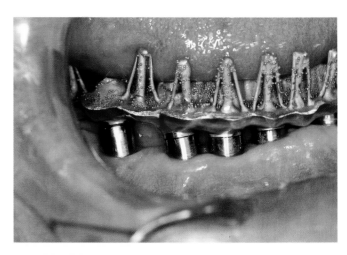

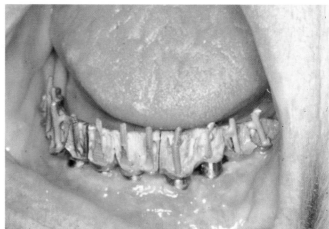

Figs. 17-36 to 17-38   The casting is tried on the mouth.

Fig. 17-37 *(top right)*   The one-piece casting shows an imperfect fit on the terminal abutment fixture.

Fig. 17-38   The sectional castings.

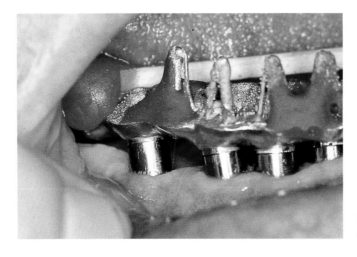

Fig. 17-39   It is sectioned, reassembled, and retried.

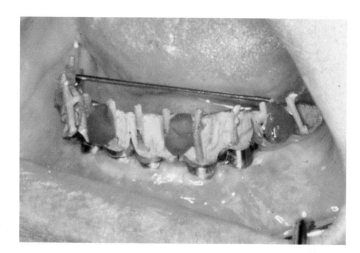

Fig. 17-40 The sectional castings are assembled intraorally.

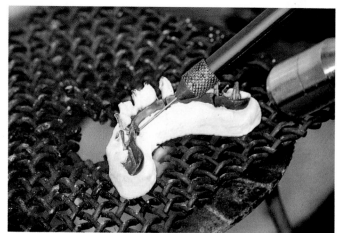

Figs. 17-41 and 17-42 The sectional castings are soldered and polished.

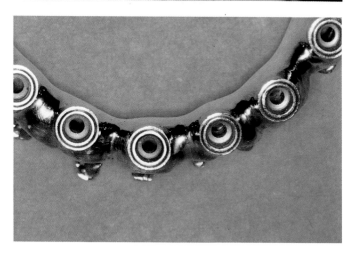

Fig. 17-42

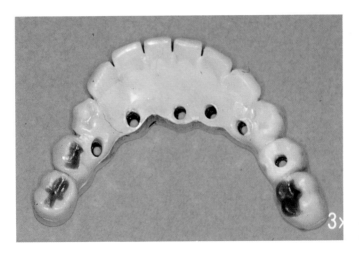

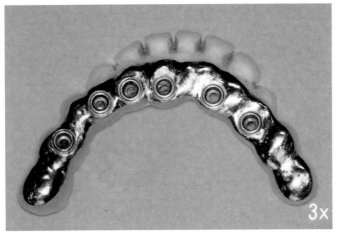

Figs. 17-43 and 17-44   The processed prosthesis.

Fig. 17-44

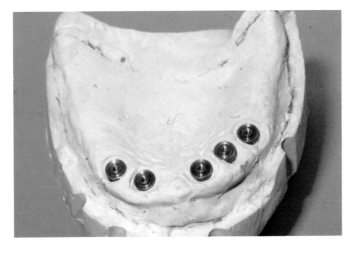

Figs. 17-45 to 17-50   The laboratory steps needed to fabricate a maxillary prosthesis are quite similar.

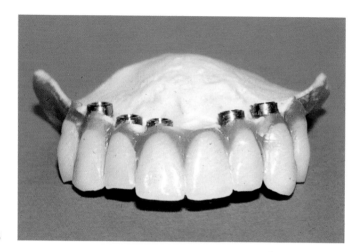

Fig. 17-46

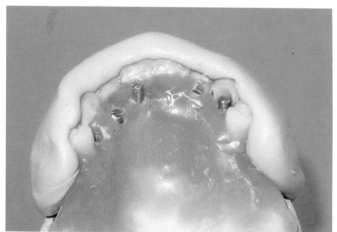

Fig. 17-47

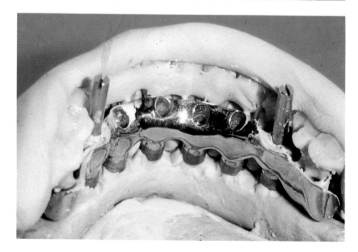

Fig. 17-48

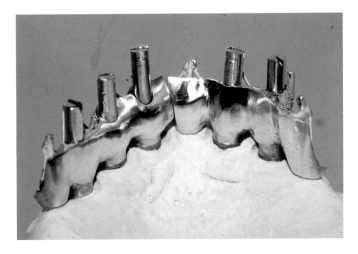

Fig. 17-49

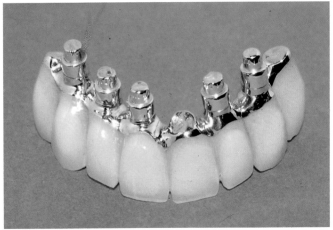

Fig. 17-50   The completed prosthesis is shown attached to polished brass analogues.

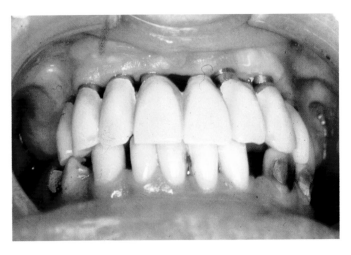

Fig. 17-51   The completed prosthesis shown intraorally.

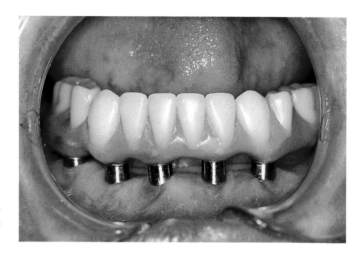

Fig. 17-52 The result when using removable prosthodontic protocol.

17-42). When the prosthodontist is satisfied with the frame's fit, it is returned to the laboratory for processing of the acrylic resin. The final acrylic resin processing technique is similar in both framework techniques if acrylic resin is used for both prosthetic tooth retention and soft-tissue replacement and/or augmentation (Figs. 17-43 and 17-44). Sometimes the final processing involves attaching the prosthetic teeth to the framework exclusively. In this case, the index will be used again while polymerization occurs. Identical procedures are used in fabricating maxillary prostheses. Figures 17-45 to 17-51 illustrate the laboratory steps undertaken.

Removable prosthodontic design protocol

The use of a removable prosthodontic design protocol (see Table 17-1) seeks to join standard complete denture technology with a quasi-partial denture type of casting which can be regarded as a reinforcement for the transverse strength of the prosthesis. The end result is a nontissue-borne complete denture substitute for missing teeth and soft tissues, which rests on transepithelial fixtures in a metallic bar embedded in the resin analogue (Fig. 17-52).

Framework fabrication

The high cost of gold alloys and the frequent need for versatility in design (e.g., a framework that compensates for extensive ridge reduction) suggested the need for different materials and design from the previously designed framework technique. The authors developed a more versatile and less expensive method that relies on a silver palladium framework. This metal (as is the gold in the other technique) is cast directly to the gold alloy cylinders. Laboratory and clinical evaluation of framework accuracy of fit, load-bearing capacities, and reduced cost underscored the advantages of using such a method.[2, 3] Silver palladium requires the use of phosphate-bonded investment materials and gas-oxygen torches. Careful consideration should be given to the regular use of this material. The frame is waxed up using standard laboratory wax forms and Duralay. It must be bulky enough to ensure

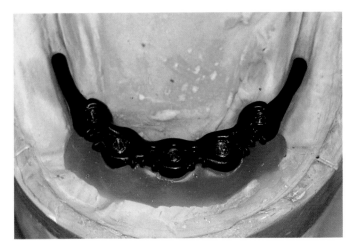

Fig. 17-53 The framework is waxed up to conform to design and strength objectives.

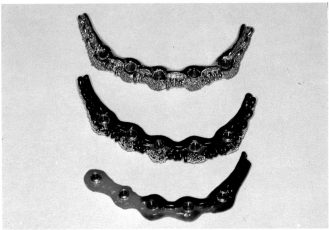

Fig. 17-54 A sequential development of the framework.

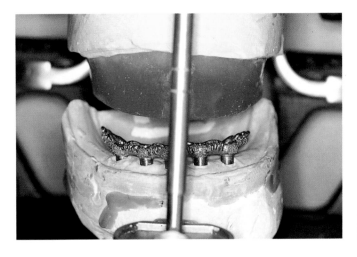

Fig. 17-55 The cast framework in place on the cast.

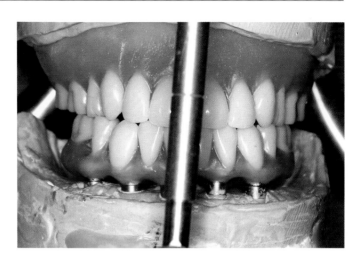

Fig. 17-56   The cast framework waxed up for try-in.

maximum strength, especially at the distal junction with the cantilever arms/beams. Consideration should be given to the structural advantages of using an I-shaped beam rather than an irregular-shaped beam. Theoretical considerations suggest that an I-shaped beam is more advantageous.

The wax and Duralay frame can be tried in the mouth to confirm the accuracy of the impression; it can also be corrected intraorally if this is deemed necessary (Figs. 17-53 and 17-54). The wax-up is refined to fulfill desired mechanical and cosmetic objectives. The frame is sprued, invested, cleaned, and polished.

Try-in of framework and tooth setup

The frame is tried in the mouth. Corrections are made where necessary, and the casting is screwed on the cast (Fig. 17-55). The prosthetic teeth are set up, and a cosmetic try-in carried out (Fig. 17-56). Relations are confirmed as are optimal cosmetic tooth arrangement and soft-tissue support. After patient approval, the prosthesis is returned to the laboratory for processing.

Final processing

The waxed-up prosthesis is screwed onto a new set of brass analogues and invested in a conventional denture flask for routine processing. In this way the "anchored" framework is in one half of the flask, and the prosthetic teeth in the other half. Deflasking, polishing, and finishing are routine (Figs. 17-57 to 17-60).

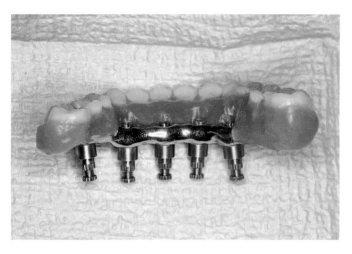

Fig. 17-57 The waxed-up prosthesis is connected to a new set of brass analogues.

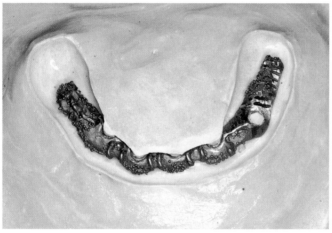

Figs. 17-58 and 17-59 It is flasked so that metal framework and prosthetic teeth are in opposite halves of the flask.

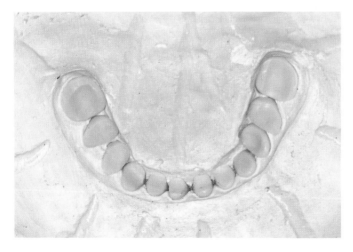

Fig. 17-59

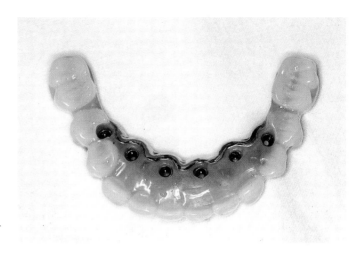

17-60 The completed prosthesis (see also Fig. 17-52).

References

1. *Hickey, J. C., and Zarb, G. A.*
   Boucher's Prosthodontic Treatment for Edentulous Patients. 8th ed. St. Louis: The C. V. Mosby Co., 1980.

2. *Leung, N., Zarb, G. A., and Watson, P. A.*
   Non-gold alloy systems for prosthetic frameworks. J. Dent. Res. (Abstr No. 1308) 60 (Special issue):324, 1982.

3. *Leung, N., Zarb, G. A., and Pilliar, R. M.*
   Casting of prosthetic superstructures in tissue-integrated dental prostheses. J. Dent. Res. (Abstr No. 1112) 62 (Special issue): 293, 1983.

Chapter 18

Radiographic Procedures

Karl-Gustav Strid

Radiological methods are an indispensable part of treatment with tissue-integrated prostheses, both at the preparatory stage and in the short-term or long-term assessment of the clinical result. For the preoperative examination, mapping of the prosthesis site is required so as to acquire detailed knowledge of dimensions and quality of bone, outlines of marrow spaces, locations of nerve and vascular passages, etc. In the postoperative follow-up, interest focuses on the development of bone anchorage and other tissue reactions as well as function of the prosthesis. It is particularly desirable to obtain information on the density and architecture of bone and on the appearance of the anchorage zone. An important objective is a long-term prognosis of prosthesis function. Specific radiographic procedures are recommended *(1)* preoperatively, *(2)* following abutment connection, and *(3)* at regular checkup appointments.

General principles

It is important that all roentgenograms be produced by a standardized procedure so that roentgenograms obtained on different occasions may be readily compared. Therefore, the radiographic examination of jaw-fixture patients should preferably be entrusted to a designated member of the therapeutic team. Radiographic routines

should be established and strictly adhered to.

Since the healing tissue may be expected to respond unfavorably to radiation exposure, and since information obtained from roentgenograms taken during the healing period will not serve any clinical purpose, radiography should probably not be performed from fixture installation to abutment connection. At present, little is known about the effects of low doses of ionizing radiation on the tissue-implant interface zone. It is therefore desirable that the radiation dose be kept low, and this may be achieved by careful application of the standardized technique. It is also essential that records be kept of any radiological procedures involving the interface zone. To this end, notes concerning all radiographic examinations of the jaw should be made in the patient's record, indicating the occurrence of unsuccessful roentgenograms as well.

The radiologist should be acquainted with the mechanical anatomy and functional relations of the implant and its associated components (Fig. 18-1) so that he or she may be able to disclose any mechanical failure expressed in the roentgenograms.

Equipment

In addition to the standard dental apparatus, the radiographic equipment re-

317

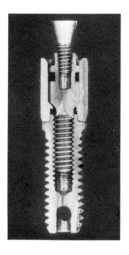 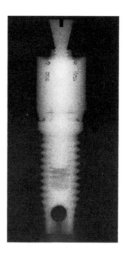

Fig. 18-1   Sectional view *(left)* of titanium fixture and its associated components and the roentgenographic appearance *(right)* of the assembled implant structure. Magnification × 3.

quired for the various examination procedures includes a stand for profile radiography (e.g., a cephalostat) and equipment for panoramic recording (e.g., an Orthopantomograph). For upper jaw cases, apparatus for tomography (laminagraphy) would also be required.

The standard dental apparatus should be provided with a collimator whose aperture is either circular, 40 mm (1-5/8 in.) in diameter, or rectangular, 22 × 35 mm (7/8 in. × 1-3/8 in.); the focus-to-aperture distance preferably should be 0.30 m (12 in.). The collimator is used as a direction finder in conjunction with a film holder, which is described in the next section.

Preoperative radiography

The preoperative radiographic examination comprises a panoramic survey, a profile view, and intraoral roentgenograms. In upper jaw cases, and in certain lower jaw cases, tomographic recordings are furnished at the surgeon's request.

The panoramic survey (Fig. 18-2) provides an overview of bone topography of the jaw and furnishes information on the location of important anatomical structures; in lower jaw cases these include the inferior border of the mandible, the mental foramina, and the mandibular canal; and in upper jaw cases, the nasal cavity, the maxillary sinuses, and the septa in the canine regions. A profile roentgenogram (Figs. 18-3 and 18-4) provides information on the height and width of the jawbone in the incisal region, as well as information on the relationship of the jaw to be treated to the bone or the remaining teeth in the opposite jaw. Moreover, the soft-tissue profile is displayed in the roentgenogram, the hard palate is demonstrated, and the position of the mental foramen in relation to the anterior part of the mandible (regions 33 through 43) is indicated as well. The diaphragm of the roentgen tube is used to outline a field containing the anterior part of the vertebral column, the hyoid bone, the nasion, and the tip of the nose. If the patient is already wearing a denture, a recording should be made with it in place, providing information on the

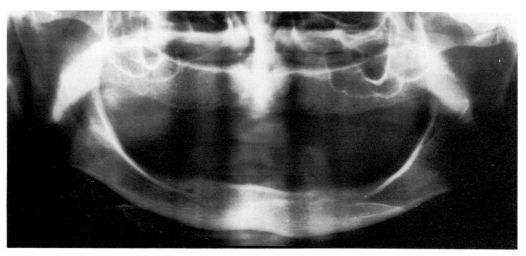

Fig. 18-2 Panoramic survey of completely edentulous jaws providing an overview of jawbone topography and furnishing information on the location of important anatomical structures.

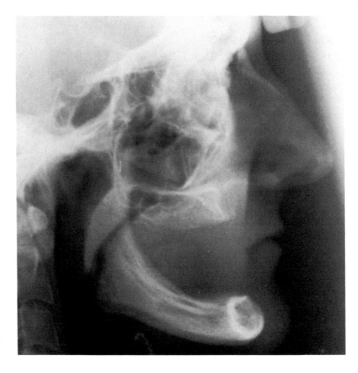

Fig. 18-3 Profile roentgenogram. In addition to providing information on bone structures, this roentgenogram displays the soft-tissue profile.

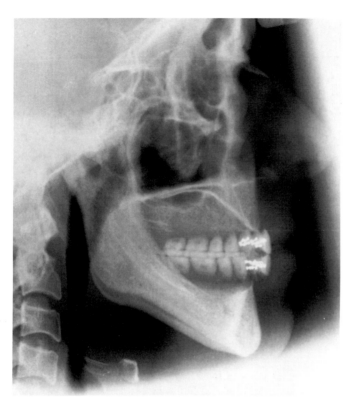

Fig. 18-4 Profile recording showing removable dentures in place, revealing the preoperative relationships between maxilla and mandible, and demonstrating the soft-tissue outline.

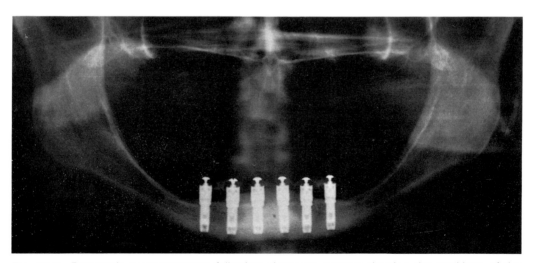

Fig. 18-5 Panoramic roentgenogram following abutment surgery showing the positions of the fixtures and their alignment in the jawbone. This roentgenogram should be carefully inspected with regard to the fit between fixtures and the respective abutments.

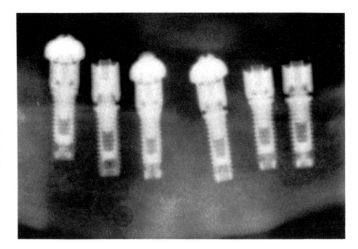

Fig. 18-6 Detail of panoramic roentgenogram demonstrating fixture-abutment misfit at the second, fourth, and sixth implants from the left. Note that the internal structure of the anchoring assemblies is clearly visible. Magnification × 1.5.

preoperative relationships between maxilla and mandible (see Fig. 18-4).

In upper jaw cases the panoramic and profile roentgenograms are supplemented by frontal tomograms in the canine regions, as indicated by the surgeon's findings at the clinical examination (see chapter 12). In lower jaw cases with a very thin crest, a tomogram in the sagittal plane will facilitate surgery.

The preoperative radiographic examination should also include an intraoral investigation of the operating site, using the standard apparatus and 35-mm films. The jawbone in the premolar, canine, and incisive regions is radiographed by the orthoradial technique.

Radiography after abutment connection

For reasons previously indicated, radiographic procedure preferably should not be carried out during the healing period, i.e., from fixture installation to abutment connection.

Radiography on removal of packing

The first radiographic check following surgery takes place when the packing is removed after abutment connection. A panoramic roentgenogram (Fig. 18-5) provides information on the positions of the fixtures and their alignment in the jawbone. Moreover, this roentgenogram should be carefully inspected with regard to the fit between fixture and abutment. It is important to ensure that the hexagonal socket of the abutment is correctly seated on the head of the fixture with no intervening gap. In the case of an incorrect fixture-abutment contact (Figs. 18-6 and 18-7a and b), this must be corrected before any prosthodontic measures are begun.

Radiography immediately after bridge connection

Perifixtural radiography immediately after bridge connection will demonstrate the condition of the perifixtural tissues and the functional relations between the fixture, abutment, and bridge components. The roent-

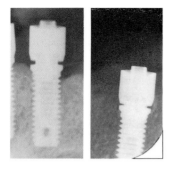

Figs. 18-7a and b   Two cases of improper fixture-abutment contact, which must be corrected before any prosthodontic measures are commenced. Magnification × 2.

Fig. 18-7a   *(left)* The hexagonal socket of the abutment rests with incorrect orientation on the head of the fixture.

Fig. 18-7b   *(right)* The abutment is correctly oriented but does not make contact with the bearing surface of the fixture head. Therefore, it is unable to transfer any loading forces from the bridge structure to the fixture.

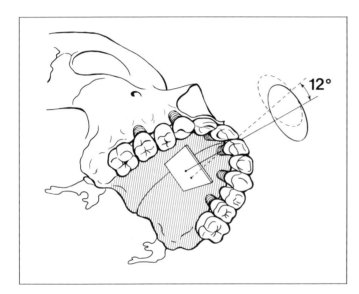

Fig. 18-8 Orientation of film and beam direction with respect to the fixture to be imaged. The film is applied orthoradially to the fixture with its longer edges parallel to the fixture's longitudinal axis. A stereoscopic pair of roentgenograms is produced at a 12° viewing angle.

genograms of this examination will serve as references for any future checkup radiography.

Radiography is performed as a periapical examination employing the right angle technique.

The x-ray tube should be operated at no less than 60 kV, preferably at 65 to 70 kV. If the roentgenograms are to be used for computer-aided image analysis (see chapter 11), it is desirable that the tube voltage remain the same for all exposures relating to the individual patient; the voltage used should be entered into the patient's record.

The fixtures should be individually imaged on intraorally placed films, preferably 22 × 35 mm (7/8 in. × 1-3/8 in.). The film is applied orthoradially to the respective fixture with its longer edges parallel to the fixture's longitudinal axis (Fig. 18-8). The beam direction must be perpendicular to this axis so that the threads are clearly depicted at both edges of the fixture (Figs. 18-9a to d). In the horizontal plane, the nominal beam direction should be perpendicular to the jaw arch in the region under examination. The image area should extend at least 5 mm (3/16 in.) into the bone at both sides of

Figs. 18-9a to d   To make a roentgenogram useful for assessment of the anchorage function, the threads must be clearly depicted at both edges of the fixture so that the bone tissue may be inspected at the bottom of the thread. Moreover, the image area should extend at least 5 mm into the bone at both sides of the implant or to the neighboring fixtures.

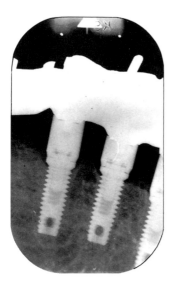

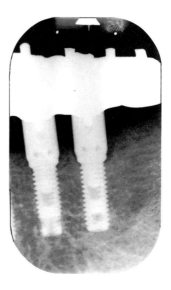

Fig. 18-9a *(top left)* Both implants are reproduced with a good projection and depicted ideally for computer-aided assessment.

Fig. 18-9b *(top right)* The fixtures are obliquely projected, as is visible especially at their right edges. The roentgenogram is marginally useful for assessment.

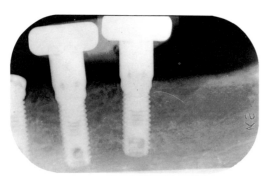

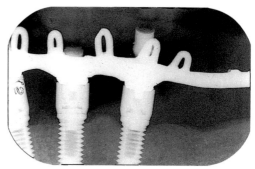

Fig. 18-9c   The fixtures are obliquely projected. This roentgenogram would not be useful for assessment of the fixtures.

Fig. 18-9d   If a satisfactory projection cannot be obtained otherwise, the apical part of the fixture may be excluded from the image area, provided the roentgenogram reproduces at least 3 mm of adhering marginal bone along the fixture. Although the apical parts of the fixtures are absent in this roentgenogram, the depicted area is sufficient for assessment.

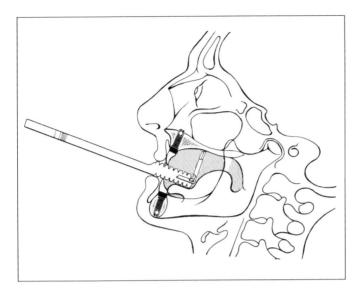

Fig. 18-10 Positioning the film with regard to the fixture in the upper jaw.

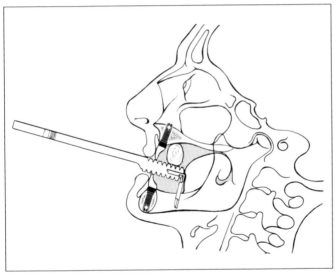

Fig. 18-11 Positioning the film with regard to the fixture in the lower jaw.

the implant or to the neighboring fixtures. A stereoscopic image pair is produced by taking two roentgenograms with the same film position, one with the nominal (orthoradial) beam direction, the other with the beam direction displaced horizontally some 12° off the nominal direction. A skilled radiographer may obtain a stereoscopic angle of this size without the use of a stereographic directional aid; otherwise a stereographic film holder may be used.

Especially in severely resorbed lower jaws, attempts at depicting the entire length of the fixture may cause discomfort and even severe pain to the patient. In most cases, however, the anchorage function can be

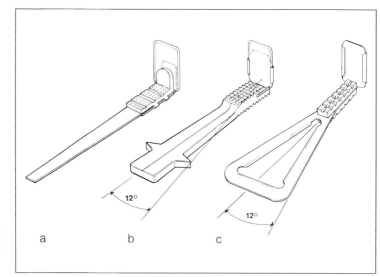

Figs. 18-12a to c An Eggen holder (Fig. 18-12a) or a stereographic film holder (Figs. 18-12b and c) will facilitate the positioning of the x-ray tube. It is essential that the film be kept flat in the holder.

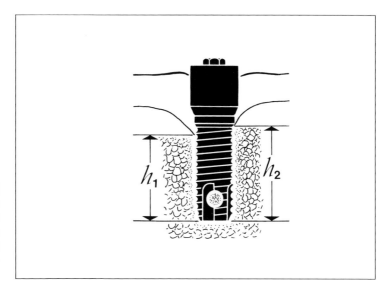

Fig. 18-13 The marginal bone height should be measured both mesially and distally. The values (h_1 and h_2) should be noted in the patient's record.

adequately assessed even if the apical part of the fixture is omitted in the roentgenogram (Fig. 18-9d).

In order to define the film position reproducibly, the use of a film holder (Figs. 18-10 and 18-11) is required. An Eggen holder[1] (Fig. 18-12a) or the stereographic film holder devised by Rockler[2] (Figs. 18-12b and c) will facilitate

positioning of the x-ray tube. It is essential that the film be kept flat in the holder.

The exposure time should be determined so that the internal mechanical structure of the fixture is clearly visible (see Fig. 18-9a). Otherwise mechanical failure such as fixture fractures or untightened screws may escape detection. Machine development of

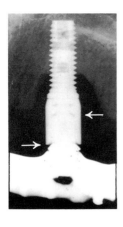

Fig. 18-14   A case of misfit between bridge and abutment. Note the space between bridge and abutment *(left arrow)* and the internal space between abutment and abutment screw *(right arrow)*. Magnification × 2.

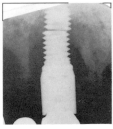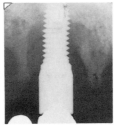

Fig. 18-15   Stereoscopic pair of roentgenograms of a fractured fixture, demonstrating the importance of stereoradiography. Although the roentgenograms differ only some 12° in projecting directions, the fracture will pass virtually unobserved at the first inspection of the right picture.

the films is recommended, and any pertinent parameters, such as developing time and developer temperature, should be standardized.

Once local radiographic routines have been established, it is important that they be strictly adhered to.

The perifixtural roentgenograms are used for assessing the condition of the perifixtural tissues. The marginal bone height (Fig. 18-13) is of special interest; it should be measured both mesially and distally and noted in the patient's record. In doubtful cases, where the marginal bone height cannot be readily determined from a single roentgenogram due to the superposition of anatomical structures, the stereoscopic pair is used to localize the bone margin. Furthermore, the stereoroentgenograms are helpful in the detection of infrabony pockets or the disclosure of a soft-tissue layer between

fixture and bone, indicative of failed osseointegration.[3]

The roentgenograms are also inspected for the functional relations of the mechanical parts (Fig. 18-14) and for a possible fixture fracture (Fig. 18-15).

Radiography at regular checkups

Regular radiographic examinations of the patients treated with jawbone-anchored bridges form part of the checkup program prescribed to such patients. The examinations are scheduled according to Table 18-1.

Checkup radiography is carried out as a perifixtural examination using the same routines as for radiography after bridge connection. The roentgenograms are

Table 18-1 Schedule for radiographic checkups of patients treated with jawbone-anchored bridges

Reference examination:
    immediately after bridge connection

Checkup examinations:
    6 months ⎫
    12 months ⎬ after bridge connection
    3 years ⎭
    subsequently at 3-year intervals

scrutinized with regard to the condition of perifixtural tissues and the state of the mechanical parts. The marginal bone height is measured and entered into the patient's record.

Computerized image analysis

Perifixtural roentgenograms are routinely assessed at The Institute for Applied Biotechnology, Göteborg, Sweden, by means of a computer-based image analysis system (see chapter 11). For each fixture, density profiles are measured through the anchorage zone.

Roentgenograms intended for computer-aided analysis should be mounted in suitable frames, marked with the patient's name and identity number, the reference number of the jaw, the date of examination, and the reference numbers of the respective fixtures. The x-ray tube voltage should be indicated on the frames.

References

1. *Eggen, S.*
   Standardiserad intraoral röntgenteknik. Sveriges Tandläkarförb. Tidn. 61:867-872, 1969.

2. *Rockler, B.*
   Personal communication, 1981.

3. *Hollender, L., and Rockler, B.*
   Radiographic evaluation of osseointegrated implants of the jaws. Dento-Maxillo-Fac. Radiol. 9:91-95, 1980.

Aspects of Prosthodontic Design

Per-Olof Glantz

The previous chapters emphasize the contention that, from a general prosthodontic point of view, there exist hardly any major fundamental differences between the clinical objectives and problems of treating patients with remaining natural teeth, and those of treating patients with osseointegrated implants. All principles common to patient treatment with fixed and/or removable partial dentures apply to the patient whose analogous tooth abutments are osseointegrated implants.[1]

Rigidity

The surgical anatomy of the edentulous oral cavity makes it difficult to achieve osseointegration distal to the mental foramina or in the distal parts of the maxilla. Consequently, fixed partial dentures are almost invariably extended distal to the most distal implant in order to create the optimal functional balance between the mandible and the maxilla. It is therefore essential to have a thorough knowledge of the detailed principles involved in the design of cantilever bridges.[2, 3] At present, there is no precise equation for describing the functional deformations, and deformation patterns, of fixed partial dentures with cantilevered pontics. However, sufficient knowledge exists to summarize certain mathematical relations between the relevant factors involved. In general this relationship is approximately represented by the following equation:

$$D = \frac{F \times L^3 \times \text{const}}{E \times W \times H^3}$$

where D is the amount of deformation exhibited by the prosthesis, F is the amount of loading of the prosthesis, E is the modulus of elasticity of the material used in the prosthesis, and L, W, and H (length, width, and height) are the dimensions of the cantilevered part of the prosthesis in the relevant loading direction.

An analysis of this equation shows that critical deformation levels may be approached, especially under circumstances when there are limited possibilities to establish compensational increases of the height of the prosthesis in its loading direction or in the range of loading directions. Obvious examples include unfavorable intermaxillary relationships, or when a compensatory increase in the height of the prosthesis undermines or reduces possibilities of maintaining an acceptable oral hygiene level. Whenever cantilevered pontics are used, a compensating increase in the height of the prosthesis in its loading directions must be made.[3] Clinically this means that patients with extensive vertical overbites should have their vertical intermaxillary relation problems successfully resolved before treatment with cantilevered bridges. The components in the equation also affect the design and morphology of the occlusal surfaces of both the osseointegrated prosthesis and its antagonist in the opposing arch. Lateral functional stresses transmitted to the cantilevered areas easily cause critical bending in a direction that is often difficult, or sometimes even impossible, to compensate for. Therefore, it becomes essential to keep cuspal inclinations to a minimum when bridges with cantilevered pontics are used.

It has sometimes been assumed that since mandibular osseointegrated fixed partial dentures are often functioning against complete maxillary dentures, lower functional loading levels are exhibited on these osseointegrated dentures rather than in cases with opposing natural teeth. Recent clinical studies of patients using strain-gauged dentures have demonstrated, however, that this assumption is not entirely correct.[4] It is true that individuals wearing complete maxillary and/or mandibular dentures demonstrate impaired ability to bite on solid objects. In centric occlusion, however, or in other contact relations where there is balanced support for the denture(s), complete-denture wearers can exhibit even higher local loading levels than dentate persons. This is probably based on the biomechanical phenomenon that loading of teeth is controlled by the action of the mechanoreceptors in the periodontal membranes, which are of course not present in edentulous subjects. Local or general overload may therefore be exerted on dentures during empty mouth chewing or during various types of parafunctional movements. Optimal design of the prostheses is therefore also essential in those cases where functional contacts are exhibited with removable dentures.

Hygiene

In chapter 4 the special surface chemical and surface physical characteristics of titanium and titanium dioxide were described. These characteristics further the possibilities for obtaining long-term osseointegration. Most of the hygienic aspects considered in prosthetic treatment with osseointegrated implants are similar to those in most types of routine prosthodontic treatment.

To prevent plaque retention, the initial and corrective phases of standard prosthodontic treatment are immediately followed by a maintenance phase that generally aims at preventing recurrence of caries and/or periodontal disease. There is no fundamental difference between the maintenance programs for patients wearing fixed partial dentures retained either by osseointegrated titanium implants or by teeth with reduced periodontal support.[5]

It appears, then, that the major differences between conventional prosthetic treatment and treatment for patients wearing osseointegrated titanium implants are as follows:

1. The natural tooth is mechanically connected with the supporting alveolar bone through resilient periodontal ligament while the osseointegrated implant is rigidly contained within the surrounding bone. This fundamental difference means that subjects with osseointegrated implants require increased precision and accuracy in every stage of their prosthodontic treatment procedures.

2. There is a considerable difference between the dimensions and geometry of prepared natural teeth and of the so-called abutment portions of osseointegrated titanium implants. The standardized geometry and dimensions of the latter make it possible to work with at least

partly prefabricated components for the prosthetic superstructure to these implants, and thus to reduce the high production cost traditionally associated with extensive restorative treatment.

3. From a strict materials point of view there exists a risk that titanium implants and the metallic components of the prosthodontic superstructure may produce an unusual type of oral corrosive process. The high inherited corrosion resistance of titanium, and of most dental alloys used for the production of fixed prostheses, make it unlikely that these corrosion processes will cause significant clinical or technical damage.[6]

References

1. *Zarb, G., et al.*
   Prosthodontic Treatment for Partially Edentulous Patients. St. Louis: The C. V. Mosby Co., 1978.

2. *Glantz, P.-O., and Nyman, S.*
   Technical and biophysical aspects of fixed partial dentures of patients with reduced periodontal support. J. Prosthet. Dent. 47:47, 1982.

3. *Glantz, P.-O., et al.*
   On functional strain in fixed mandibular reconstructions. Acta Odontol. Scand. 1985 (in press).

4. *Stafford, G. D., et al.*
   Influence of treatment with osseointegrated mandibular bridges on the clinical deformation of maxillary complete dentures. Swed. Dent. J. 1985 (in press).

5. *Lindhe, J. (ed.)*
   Textbook of Clinical Periodontology. Copenhagen: Munksgaard, 1983.

6. *Nilner, K., and Lekholm, U.*
   Electrical current creation in patients treated with osseointegrated dental bridges. (Suppl.) Swed. Dent. J. 1985 (in press).

Chapter 20

Other Applications of Osseointegrated Implants

Anders Tjellström

Introduction

The successful clinical application of osseointegration as an alternative to conventional prosthodontic treatment, or as a solution for difficult or untreatable prosthodontic patients, suggests exciting therapeutic possibilities in other health fields. At least three clinical applications have been investigated with early encouraging results: (1) applications in otolaryngology, (2) applications in maxillofacial prosthodontics, and (3) applications in orthopedics. The last of these, applications in the orthopedic field, is still in the experimental stage, although a clinical trial with osseointegrated metacarpophalangeal joint reconstruction has started at the University of Göteborg, Sweden. Various other joint arthroplasties based on the osseointegration principle are also being analyzed experimentally.

This chapter will present two clinically available applications of osseointegrated implants, one in otolaryngology and one in maxillofacial prosthodontics. Both of these treatment procedures are based on a permanent bone integration of titanium implants in combination with permanent skin penetration. Percutaneous passages have previously been possible to maintain only during follow-up periods of a few months, after which time the implants have been lost because of infection. The material presented here comprises the first ever with a positive outcome of percutaneous implants with a long-term follow-up patient series.

The prospect of establishing and maintaining permanent communication with inside the human body has fascinated medical science for years. Some medical disciplines demonstrate a routine need for such an objective, i.e., those dealing with patients treated with hemodialysis.[1] Others would like to be able to facilitate and improve an established technique, i.e., the recharging of cardiac pacemakers.[2] Direct electrical stimulation of nerves and muscles is a third field where permanent percutaneous connection would be of great value for both the scientist and the clinician.[3, 4] The attachment of artificial limbs to the skeleton is still another area that would be completely changed if stable skin penetration could be achieved.[3]

Patients who for some reason need a prolonged urinary diversion procedure would also benefit greatly from a percutaneous device.[5] In the otolaryngology discipline, many of the problems with electrical stimulation of the inner ear in totally deaf patients have been related to the difficulty of transferring the acoustic signal reaching the patient's hearing aid into electrical impulses in the cochlea. A direct coupling would ensure precisely controlled stimulation and tissue impedance measurements.[6]

The reported successful long-term results with dental implants[7] proved that it was pos-

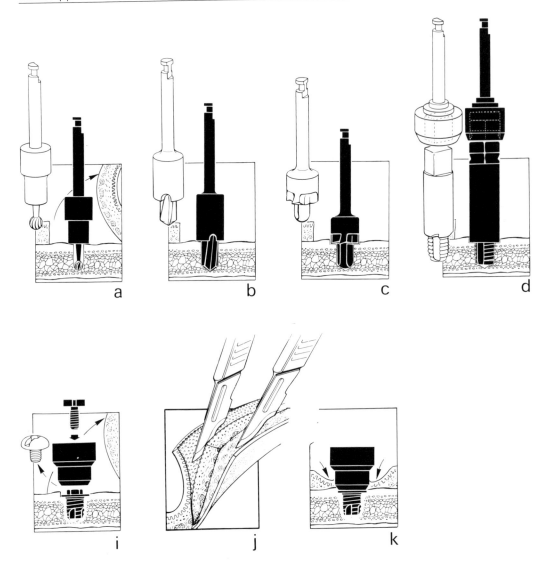

a   b   c   d

i   j   k

sible to clinically achieve prolonged transepithelial penetration without any adverse reaction. We speculated that if it was possible to maintain a reaction-free penetration of the mucosa in the oral cavity, it might be equally possible to achieve the same results with an implant in the mastoid process penetrating the covering skin, provided a similar technique was used.

Application in otolaryngology

At present, there is no surgical procedure available for sensorineural hearing losses, although great effort and considerable economic resources are devoted to experimental work on cochlear implants. These implants, not incorporated in clinical routine procedures, are only reserved for totally

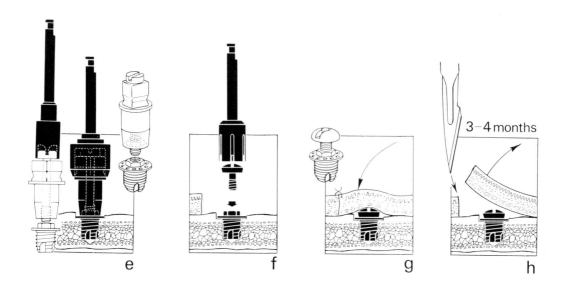

Figs. 20-1a to j   Schematic of the surgical technique to ensure osseointegration and permanent skin penetration. (Fig. 20-1a) After the skin has been elevated and the bone surface exposed a hole is prepared with a 1.8-mm bur supplied with a shield allowing penetration of 4 mm. (Fig. 20-1b) A spiral drill is then introduced perpendicular to the surface. (Fig. 20-1c) If the bone surface is uneven a countersink is used. Once again the spiral drill is utilized to ensure an exact depth of the hole. (Fig. 20-1d) The hole is gently threaded with a tap. (Fig. 20-1e) The titanium implant is inserted. (Fig. 20-1f) An internal cover screw is put in place. (Fig. 20-1g) The periosteum is sutured over the implant and the skin incision is closed. (Fig. 20-1h) The second surgical stage is initiated by removing the cover screw. (Fig. 20-1i) Subcutaneous soft-tissue reduction is performed. (Fig. 20-1j) The skin is permanently penetrated by a titanium abutment.

bilateral deaf patients. The majority of the patients with sensorineural hearing loss are older individuals, people who have been exposed to high levels of noise, and people whose hair cells in the basal turn of the cochlea have degenerated.

Chronic ear infection can be defined as perforation of the tympanic membrane that will not heal. Sometimes the disease is actively present, with drainage from the ear; at other times the ear is dry causing the patient fewer problems. Nevertheless, most of these patients have a hearing loss that varies, depending on the size and the location of the drum perforation, and on the status of the ossicles. The degree of secretion from the middle ear also influences the hearing level. The prevalence of this condition varies in different parts of the world, but is generally not very well known. In western Sweden, for example, the prevalence has been estimated to be 2%,[8] and the majority of these patients can be helped through surgery. In some patients this is not possible, and the patient has to be equipped with a hearing aid where the amplified sound is delivered through a plastic mold in the ear canal. However, a small number of patients cannot tolerate such a device, and have to wear a bone conduction hearing aid. Such an aid has its transducer placed on the skin over the bone, behind the external ear. The transducer is kept in place with a steel spring over the head or with heavy frames on glasses. This type of arrangement has several drawbacks. The position of the aid is insecure, and the pressure needed for its efficacy and retention is often very disturbing, possibly giving rise to ulcers in the skin. A most disturbing drawback is that the quality of the reinforced sound is generally very poor. The sound has to travel through a layer of soft tissue with great energy losses before it reaches the bone where the sound is transmitted with small losses. Therefore, an ordinary bone conduction hearing aid has to work with a relatively high output, which gives greater distortion and a poor sound quality.

A hearing aid attached directly to the bone would overcome the inherent poor qualities of conventional bone conduction systems. Since 1977 we have treated 57 patients with such a bone-anchored hearing aid.

Surgical procedure

The surgical procedure is very similar to the one used for dental implants, and the drill and the basic instruments are the same. A special flanged fixture has been developed, which is used with a special bur. The procedure is performed in two steps. At the first stage, generally performed under local anesthesia, a short incision is made behind the ear. The bone is exposed and a hole is prepared and threaded. A 3- or 4-mm-long titanium screw of special design is introduced with a gentle surgical technique described by Lindström et al.[9] A cover screw is inserted to protect the internal threadings and the periosteum and skin are sutured. The implant is left unloaded for three to four months, when the second stage procedure is performed. Once again under local anesthesia, the implant is identified, the covering screw is removed, and an abutment, constructed as a coupling for the hearing aid, is put on top of the fixture. At the same time a reduction of the subcutaneous tissue is performed to avoid inflammation and infection around the skin penetration. A detailed description of the surgical procedure was reported in 1983.[10] In Figs. 20-1a to j, a diagram of the procedure is presented. When primary healing has taken place after two to four weeks, the new hearing aid is fitted to the connector (Figs. 20-2 and 20-3a and b). The hearing aid has been developed in close cooperation with the Department of Applied Electronics, Chalmers University of Technology, Göteborg, Sweden.

All implants were observed to be integrated at the time of the second surgical stage, and percutaneous penetrating hearing aid couplings have been in place in all treated patients who wear the new hearing aid and prefer it over the old one. A five-year report on our experiences with this device was published,[10] the hearing thresholds analyzed,[11] and the point impedance has been measured also.[12]

Applications in maxillofacial prosthodontics

The loss of one or both ears is a significant cosmetic handicap. Three main reasons account for a patient's lack of an auri-

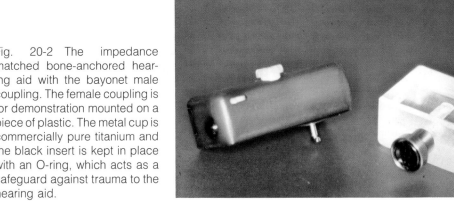

Fig. 20-2 The impedance matched bone-anchored hearing aid with the bayonet male coupling. The female coupling is for demonstration mounted on a piece of plastic. The metal cup is commercially pure titanium and the black insert is kept in place with an O-ring, which acts as a safeguard against trauma to the hearing aid.

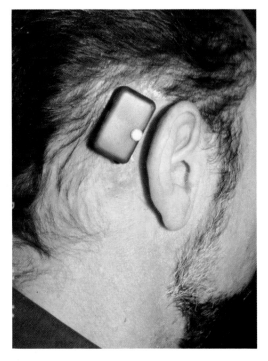

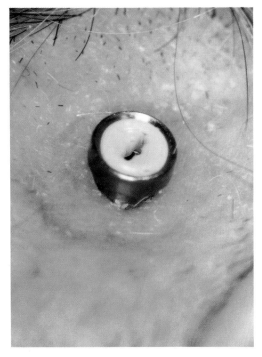

Fig. 20-3a A patient wearing his bone conduction hearing aid on a tissue-integrated implant.

Fig. 20-3b A close-up picture of the percutaneous coupling. Note the lack of inflammation or other adverse tissue reactions around the implant, which was installed six years ago. Due to subcutaneous tissue reduction the very thin skin is adherent to the bone tissue as well as to the implant surface.

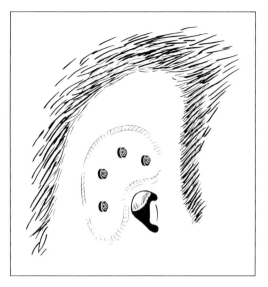

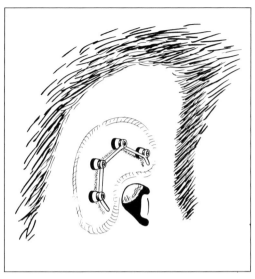

Fig. 20-4a   Situation with the titanium abutments penetrating the skin which is adherent to the periosteum because of the soft-tissue reduction surgery.

Fig. 20-4b   Gold tops have been attached to the abutments and the bar construction is soldered to the gold tops.

cle—congenital malformations, trauma, or tumor surgery. The exact number of patients with total auricular defects is not known, but the yearly incidence has been estimated to be six for every one million inhabitants.[13] Plastic surgical procedures are generally not very satisfactory if no part of the cartilage skeleton is available. Using autogenous rib cartilage has been attempted[14-16] as well as silicone rubber implants,[17] but to date no established successful routine procedure is available for total auricular reconstruction. For most patients with such defects the best solution is a prosthesis. With modern silicone and plastic materials, the prosthesis can be made to look very natural; however, the great problem of prosthesis retention has persisted. Attachment to glasses is the most common method employed, but then the patient will not be able to remove the glasses in public. Furthermore, the position of the prosthesis is often insecure, and it is

hard to obtain a snug fit. Gluing is another possibility, but even this type of retention has certain disadvantages. The dermal adhesive might not tolerate sweat and moisture, and negative skin reactions to the adhesive are common. Discoloring of the prosthesis is another problem, especially on its thinner parts.

Tissue-integrated titanium implants that penetrate the skin in the mastoid process have been used for the retention of auricular prostheses. The surgical technique is identical to that for achieving osseointegration (see chapter 13), except that with the auricular prosthesis shorter and slimmer abutments are used. After healing around the abutments, the casting of a bar between the abutments is undertaken, as well as the design of the prosthesis and its attachments.[18] The prostheses shown in Figs. 20-4a to e, 20-5a to c, and 20-6a to c were made by E. Yontchev, D.D.S., at the Clinic of

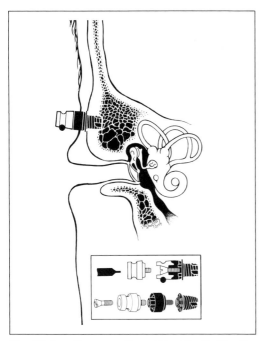

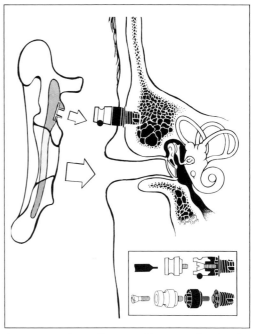

Fig. 20-4c Cross-section of Fig. 20-4b. The fixture is integrated with the bone tissue, and the abutment secured to the fixture and attached to the gold top with the bar in its small groove.

Fig. 20-4d The silicone rubber prosthesis with its acrylic plate and one of its snap fasteners ready to be attached to the bar.

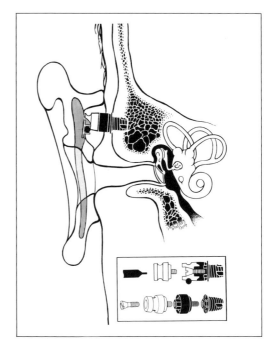

Fig. 20-4e The auricular prosthesis attached to the tissue-integrated implants.

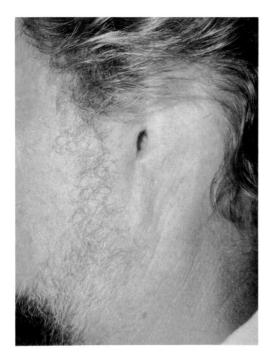

Figs. 20-5a to c   Fifty-eight-year-old male who lost his left external ear due to surgery for malignant melanoma.

Fig. 20-5a   Status post-tumor surgery.

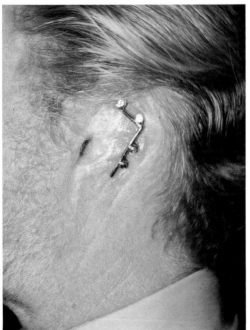

Fig. 20-5b   Implants, percutaneous abutments, and dental bar for retention of the prosthesis.

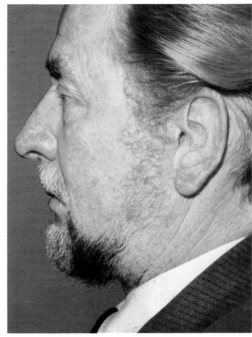

Fig. 20-5c   Appearance with silicone rubber prosthesis in place.

Figs. 20-6a to c Sixty-nine-year-old male who lost his left external ear due to surgery for a squamous cell carcinoma. The area received postoperative radiation 6,000 rads. When no signs of tumor recurrence was observed 18 months postoperatively, titanium implants were inserted for retention of an auricular prosthesis.

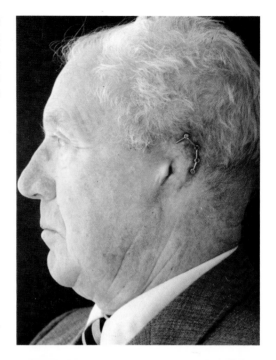

Fig. 20-6a Percutaneous implants and the dental bar attached to the abutments.

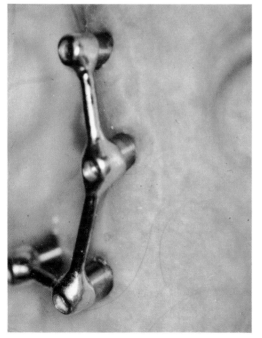

Fig. 20-6b Close-up view of the same area.

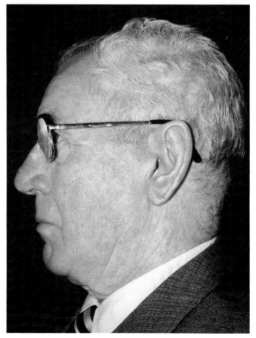

Fig. 20-6c The patient with his silicone rubber prosthesis in place.

Odontology, University of Göteborg, Sweden. Forty-one patients have been treated; 12 had lost their ears due to tumor surgery, two defects were due to accidents, and the remaining 27 were congenital defects. The youngest patient was 11 years old and the oldest 74. The longest follow-up time of this treatment group is five years. Only one of 102 implants was found to be not integrated. This was in a young girl with Treacher Collins' syndrome; her skull was just 1.5 mm thick at the implant site. However, the remaining three implants were all osseointegrated, and were used for her auricular prosthesis. In one of the patients there was some soft-tissue reaction between two of the four abutments. The reason for this reaction was probably that the space between the abutments was too narrow (1 to 2 mm); therefore, one implant was removed. This resolved the patient's problem.

Orbital and nasal prostheses

The same type of retention system has been used for orbital prostheses. Six patients are presently wearing their prostheses, and another seven have had their implants installed and are at different stages of rehabilitation. One person who lost his nose due to tumor surgery has been treated according to the same principle.

Future considerations

The possibility of a permanent reaction-free percutaneous connection has led to change in treatment strategies in the otolaryngology field, as well as in many other medical areas. A direct connector for the electrical impulses for cochlear stimulation in the deaf patient is one very obvious achievement. Direct stimulation of the inner ear for patients with severe tinnitus comprises a large therapeutic field where this technique could prove to be a dramatic treatment breakthrough.

References

1. *Striker, G. E., and Tenckhoff, H. A. M.*
   A transcutaneous prosthesis for prolonged access to the peritoneal cavity. Surgery 69:70-74, 1971.

2. *Rogers, A., and Morris, L. B.*
   Percutaneous leads for power control of artificial hearts. Trans. Amer. Soc. Artif. Int. Organs 13:146-150, 1967.

3. *Mooney, V., et al.*
   The use of pure carbon for permanent percutaneous electrical connector systems. Arch. Surg. 108:148-153, 1974.

4. *Mooney, V., et al.*
   Percutaneous implant devices. Ann. Biomed. Eng. 5:34-36, 1977.

5. *Kobashi, L. I., and Raible, D. A.*
   Biocarbon urinary conduit. Urology 16 (1), 1980.

6. *Balkany, T. J.*
   An overview of the electronic cochlear prosthesis: Clinical and research considerations. Otolaryngol. Clin. North Am. 16 (1), 1983.

7. *Adell, R., et al.*
   A 15-year study of osseointegrated implants in the treatment of the edentulous jaw. Int. J. Oral Surg. 10:387, 1981.

8. *Tjellström, A.*
   Tympanoplasty with preformed autologous ossicles. Medical Dissertion, University of Göteborg, Sweden, 1977.

9. *Lindström, J., Brånemark, P.-I., and Albrektsson, T.*
   Mandibular reconstruction using the preformed autologous bone graft. Scand. J. Plast. Reconstr. Surg. 15:29, 1981.

10. *Tjellström, A., et al.*
    Five-year experience with skin-penetrating bone-anchored implants in the temporal bone. Acta Otolaryngol. 95:568-575, 1983.

11. *Håkansson, B., Tjellström, A., and Rosenhall, U.*
    Hearing thresholds with direct bone conduction versus conventional bone conduction. Scand. Audiol. 1985 (in press).

12. *Håkansson, B., and Tjellström, A.*
    The bone-anchored hearing aid. A study of the mechanical point impedance of the human head with and without skin penetration. J. Acoust. Soc. Am. 73 (Suppl. 1), 1983.

13. *Tjellström, A., et al.*
    Directly bone-anchored implants for fixation of aural epistheses. Biomaterials 4 (Jan.), 1983.

14. *Tanzer, R. C., and Edgertson, M. T. (eds.)*
    Symposium on Reconstruction of the Auricle. St. Louis: The C. V. Mosby Co., 1974.

15. *Furnas, D. W. (ed.)*
    Clinics in Plastic Surgery: Symposium on Deformities of the External Ear. Philadelphia: W. B. Saunders Co., 1978.

16. *Brent, B.*
    A personal approach to total auricular construction. Plast. Surg. 8:211-221, 1981.

17. *Ohmori, S., Nakai, H., and Takada, H.*
    A refined approach to ear reconstruction with silastic frames in major degress of microtia. Br. J. Plast. Surg. 32:267, 1979.

18. *Tjellström, A., et al.*
    Five-years' experience with bone-anchored auricular prosthesis. 1985 (in press).

Index

Quinte$$ential to denti$try.....

Edited by Paul J. W. Stoelinga

Proceedings Consensus Conference

The Relative Roles of Vestibuloplasty and Ridge Augmentation in the Management of the Atrophic Mandible

The second of the two volumes published from the 8th International I.A.O.M.S. Conference is a compilation of guidelines for logical selection of preprosthetic therapy. Nine internationally recognized prosthodontists and oral and maxillofacial surgeons arrived at their consensus of recommendations after two days of intensive discussion.

The book examines selection criteria based on the research and clinical experience of the nine surgeons in chapters on various aspects of vestibuloplasty, skin and mucosal grafting, and bone grafting for ridge augmentation. The scientists address such questions as: How much alveolar atrophy is an indication for augmentation? What are the indications for soft tissue grafting? What should be weighed when deciding whether vestibuloplasty or ridge augmentation will be the best treatment? **Contents also include:** methods for deepening the floor of the mouth / mandibular visor osteotomy / prosthetic follow-up / reduction of prolapse in soft tissues of the chin / hydroxylapatite particles as bone substitute
Contributors: R. Brusati / R. J. Grisius / F. Härle / S. Hillerup / R. Hopkins / H. A. de Koomen / C. Martis / P. J. W. Stoelinga / B. C. Terry

ISBN 0-86715-155-2
157 pages, 194 illustrations

Order 2516/1552

Quintessence Publishing Co., Inc.
8 South Michigan Avenue, Suite 2301
Chicago, Illinois 60603

Quintessential to dentistry......

Krüger/Worthington

Oral Surgery in Dental Practice

A textbook of oral surgery for dentists must above all be directed to the special needs of general dental practice.

The practitioner needs a description of surgical techniques and a review of pain control methods, but equally important are the descriptions of aftercare and those complications which may arise in practice. To this end the dentist needs some background knowledge of general surgery if he wishes to successfully use his specialized dentoalveolar surgery.

This book contains the essential information for a course in oral surgery for dentists, including dental implantology and periodontal surgery – as well as those basic elements of general surgery which are particularly significant for the dentist. It results from years of accumulated experience in the practical teaching of dental students and in designing continuing education courses for dentists in practice. It is intended to help the student through the oral surgery course and to serve as a reference work for the dentist in his daily practice.

ISBN 0-931386-19-5   Order 1286/0195
392 pages, 330 illustrations

quintessence
books

Quintessence Publishing Co., Inc.
8 South Michigan Avenue, Suite 2301
Chicago, Illinois 60603